Experimental Organic and Medicinal Chemistry: Principles and Practice

Second Edition

Experimental Organic and Medicinal Chemistry: Principles and Practice

Second Edition

T. Durai Ananda Kumar
M. Pharm., Ph.D.
Associate Professor
Department of Pharmaceutical Chemistry,
JSS College of Pharmacy,
Udhagamandalam, Tamil Nadu.

N. Swathi
M. Pharm., Ph.D.
Professor
Department of Pharmaceutical Chemistry,
Gokaraju Rangaraju College of Pharmacy,
Hyderabad, Telangana.

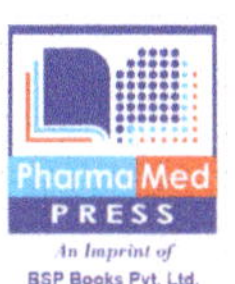

™ **PharmaMed Press**
An imprint of BSP Books Pvt. Ltd.,
4-4-309/316, Giriraj Lane,
Sultan Bazar, Hyderabad - 500 001.

Experimental Organic and Medicinal Chemistry: Principles and Practice, Second Edition
***by* T. Durai Ananda Kumar and N. Swathi**

Published by:

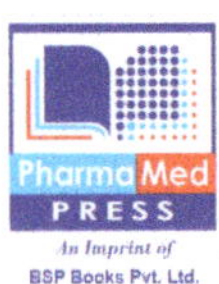

™ **PharmaMed Press**

An imprint of BSP Books Pvt. Ltd.,
4-4-309/316, Giriraj Lane, Sultan Bazar, Hyderabad - 500 001.
Phone: 040-23445688
E-mail: info@pharmamedpress.com
www.pharmamedpress.com/pharmamedpress.net

ISBN: 978-93-49562-30-1 (Hardback)

Foreword

Prof K. Chinnaswamy, B.Pharm,. M.Sc. (Pharmacy)

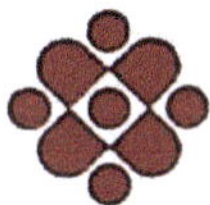

Professor & Head (Retd)
Department of Pharmaceutical Sciences
Madras Medical College, Chennai
President, Indian Association of Colleges of Pharmacy, Chennai

Organic and Medicinal Chemistry deals with facets of chemistry, biology, and pharmacology. The application of Organic and Medicinal Chemistry in the field of molecular discovery has no boundary. Therefore, acquiring knowledge on the synthesis of small organic molecules, explaining the reaction mechanism, employing reagents & catalysts in reactions, and study of natural products are essential parameters for the pharmacy graduates and others involved in the drug / medicinal chemistry research.

Dr. T. Durai Ananda Kumar and Dr. N. Swathi have come out with the enlarged-revised (second) edition of the book titled **Experimental Organic and Medicinal Chemistry:** ***Principles and Practice*** with the goal of improving chemistry instruction and practice in academia. This book will also be useful for chemists and biologists in industry. The book fulfills all the needs for a comprehensive resource on the topic, and it is an indispensable asset.

All the chapters are very well Introduced and cover the latest aspects. It is good to read the interesting perspective and presentation of experiments for simple adaptation in the laboratory by faculty and learners. The sixty-four chapters in this book cover a wide range of topics, including general laboratory practice, safety procedures, synthesis of pharmaceuticals & drug intermediates through name reactions, chemical & drug analysis, and isolation & degradation of natural products.

This book provides applications of the experiments in drug research alongside key points. Considering this, I recommend this book for undergraduate and postgraduate pharmacy students for their pharmaceutical chemistry and medicinal chemistry practicals. Also, I trust that this book would serve as a companion for postgraduate dissertation students and research scholars.

Best Wishes and Greetings
Chennai
13-03-2025

Prof K. Chinnaswamy

Preface

தொட்டனைத் தூறு மணற்கேணி மாந்தர்க்குக்
கற்றனைத் தூறும் அறிவு - குறள் 396

In sandy soil, when deep you delve, you reach the springs below;
The more you learn, the freer streams of wisdom flow

– Couplet 396

We authors submit our pranams to His Holiness Jagadguru Sri Shivarathri Deshikendra Mahaswamigalu, Jagadguru Sri Veerasimhasan Muth, Sutturu, Karnataka and Chancellor, JSSAHER, Mysuru, Karnataka.

Blessing of our parents enabled us to present this enlarged second edition of book entitled "***Experimental Organic and Medicinal Chemistry*****:** ***Principles and Practice***".

Organic-Medicinal chemistry research utilizes discovery of lead molecules and convert them into therapeutically potential molecules (lead optimization). Adequate knowledge in organic-medicinal chemistry (synthetic and analytical concepts) is essential for pharmacy graduates (B. Pharmacy and M. Pharmacy) and graduates of allied fields to cater academic and industrial sectors. The reference books and manuals available for practice is complex in nature or inadequate. This stimulated us to construct this book with literature information and experiments conducted in our laboratories guided us further. We author strongly believe that this book serves as a primer for the students of B. Pharmacy, M. Pharmacy (Pharmaceutical Chemistry, Medicinal Chemistry) and other organic-medicinal chemistry disciplines. This book also serves as a reference guide for the research scholars and research scientists in industry.

The synthetic and analytical concepts are described in five sections spreading through 64 chapters. General laboratory practices section imparts knowledge about various chemicals, their hazardous effects, and the relevant first-aid measures. Synthetic chemistry section emphasizes the experiments on named reactions emphasizing reaction mechanisms with the prototype examples. The next section, describes qualitative analysis of inorganic and organic compounds along with titrimetric estimations (quantitative analysis) of drugs and drug formulations. Natural products chemistry section deals with the isolation of active constituents along with their qualitative and quantitative determination.

Salient features

a) Synthetic approaches (synthesis of drugs and drug intermediates) are described with their pharmaceutical relevance and reaction mechanisms.

b) Green synthetic strategy is emphasized through highlighting the alternative reagents, synthetic strategies and hazards associated.

c) Limit tests, qualitative analysis of inorganic, natural and synthetic organic compounds are described in a lucid manner.

d) Estimations of natural and organic-medicinal compounds along with isolation of active principles are detailed in a reader-friendly manner.

e) Safety measurements and general laboratory practices is given in a comprehensive manner for the ready reference.

f) The experiments described are very simple to carry out and does not require any special equipment's.

The constant encouragement received from Dr. K. Satyanarayana, Former Vice President, Natco Research Centre, Hyderabad, is highly acknowledged. Our sincere gratitude to management and Principals of JSS College of Pharmacy, Udhagamandalam (Ooty), Tamil Nadu, JSS College of Pharmacy, Mysuru, Karnataka and Gokaraju Rangaraju College of Pharmacy, Hyderabad, Telangana. We extend our special thanks to Mr. Anil Shah, Director, BSP Books (P) Ltd, Hyderabad. We gratefully acknowledge the support and co-operation extended by team of BSP Books (P) Ltd, Hyderabad, specially Mr. Naresh Daveragave and Mrs. Rajitha/ B. Gayatri. The love and understanding of our family members enabled us to complete this book successfully, and we acknowledge them.

Adequate measures are taken to print error free material. However, if anything is found, kindly communicate your suggestions and critical points.

- Dr. T. Durai Ananda Kumar
- Dr. N. Swathi

Contents

Chapter - 16

Fischer-Speier Esterification

Chapter - 17

Haloform Reaction

Chapter - 18

Hantzsch 1,4-Dihydropyridine Synthesis

Chapter - 19

Hydrolysis

Chapter - 20

Knoevenagel Condensation

Chapter - 21

Mannich Reaction

Chapter - 22

Oxidation

Chapter - 23

Paal-Knorr Pyrazole Synthesis

Chapter - 24

Paal-Knorr Pyrrole Synthesis

Chapter - 62

Physicochemical Characterization of Natural Products

Chapter - 63

Quantitative Determination of Natural Products

Chapter - 64

Degradation of Natural Products

1 Laboratory Practices

The synthesis and analysis of compounds (inorganic and organic) is an important element of the pharmaceutical courses. The medicinal-organic chemistry laboratory provides a good platform for gaining knowledge about different chemical reactions. The representative reactions and analysis procedure provides adequate knowledge and practice. In general, chemical synthesis and analysis are conducted by dissolving the reactants and analytes in a suitable solvent. The temperature and pressure maintenance for the chemical reactions are important factors. The sequence of addition and speed in which the chemicals and reagents are added are major deciding factor. These factors decide the accuracy of the conclusions, both in synthesis and chemical analysis.

The organic reactions can be conveniently grouped into

1. Microscale reactions
2. Semi-microscale reactions
3. Macroscale reactions

It is very essential to know about the different components of synthesis and chemical analysis. Following are the important components.

1. Knowledge about chemicals
2. Solvents
3. Glassware and equipments
4. Glassware cleaning
5. Purification
6. Drying
7. Determination of melting point and boiling point
8. Yield calculation
9. First aid

1.1 Knowledge about Chemicals

***Class 1* Explosives:** The chemicals may explode under the stimulus of heat, impact or friction. The examples include peroxide, acetylide, azide, diazonium, nitroso, nitro, perchlorate and ozonide compounds. Autoxidation of ethers, tetrahydrofuran (THF) and related compounds forms explosive peroxides. Chromic acid and perchloric acid are known violent explosives.

Label	*Background colour*	*Symbol*
EXPLOSIVE 1.3F 1; 1.6 EXPLOSIVE 1; 1.4 EXPLOSIVE G 1	Orange	Exploding ball

***Class 2* Gases - inhalation:** Gases that are highly flammable, non-flammable and poisonous are included in this class.

Flammable: Hydrogen, butane, methane, ethylene and chlorine trifluoride

Non-flammable: Nitrogen, carbon dioxide, compressed air and helium.

Poisonous: Arsine, chlorine, phosphine, nitrogen dioxide, hydrogen cyanide and hydrogen azide.

Type	*Label*	*Background color*	*Symbol*
Flammable gases	FLAMMABLE GAS 2; OXYGEN 2	Red or Yellow	Flame
Non-flammable gases	NON-FLAMMABLE GAS 2	Green	Tube
Poisonous gases	POISON GAS 2	White	Skull and crossbones

***Class 3* Flammable and Combustible Liquids:** Flammable substances are the most common hazard. Flammability of a compound is indicated by flash point. A liquid with flash point less than 15 ºC, is dangerously flammable. The vapour of flammable may drift into a distant ignition and burn back to ignite the bulk source. Organic solvents such as acetone, diethyl ether, ethyl acetate are examples. The flammable liquids should be stored in storage rooms designed.

- ***Flammables:*** Low boiling point compounds such as acetaldehyde, acetone, benzene, carbon disulphide, diethyl ether and ethyl acetate are highly inflammable.
- ***Combustible Liquids:*** Kerosene, diesel oil, engine oil, ethylene glycol and acetic acid are examples of combustible liquid category.

Label	*Background colour*	*Symbol*
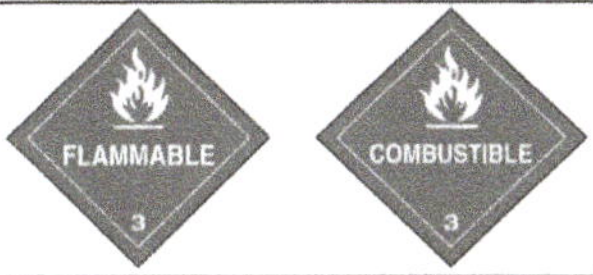	Red	Flame

***Class 4* Flammable Solids:** Flammable solids and spontaneously combustibles are dangerous when they are wet. Examples include metallic hydrides, metallic sodium and potassium, processed metals, nitrocellulose, oily fabrics, etc.

Label	*Background colour*	*Symbol*
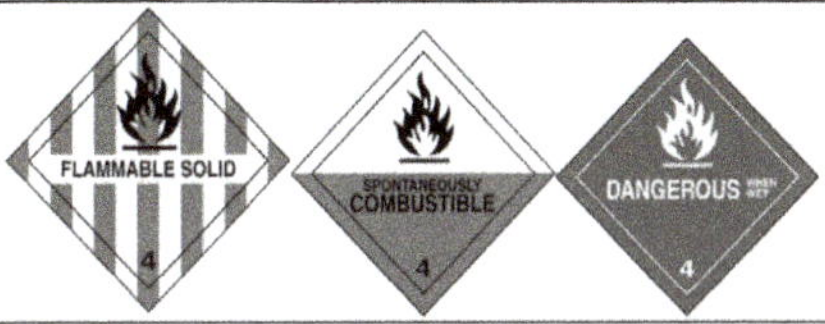	Red and White candy striped Blue if reacts with water	Flame

***Class 5* Oxidizers and Organic Peroxides:** Oxidizers are incompatible with organics, hence oxidizers should be stored separately from organics. Oxidizers promote combustion and produce fire (explosion). Never open an oxidizer container (bottle) with solid formation around the lid. Friction caused by unscrewing the cap leads to an explosion. Organic peroxides, such as Methyl ethyl ketone peroxide (MEKP) and benzoyl peroxide on decomposition produce free radicals and thus useful as initiators of a few polymerization reactions of unsaturated compounds.

Label	*Background colour*	*Symbol*
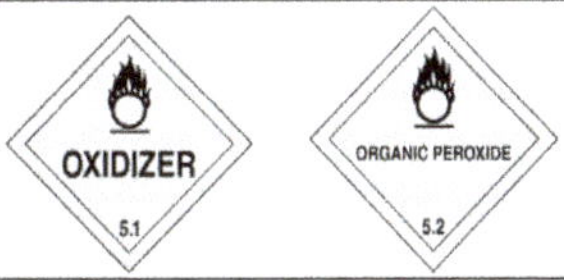	Yellow	Flaming ball

***Class 6* Poisons and Etiologic Materials:** The chemicals which are classified as acute toxicity category 1, 2 and 3 under Globally harmonized system (GHS) of Classification and Labelling belong to class 6. Examples are cyanides, lead compounds, phenol, cresol, a few pesticides, clinical wastes and biological wastes.

Label	*Background colour*	*Symbol*
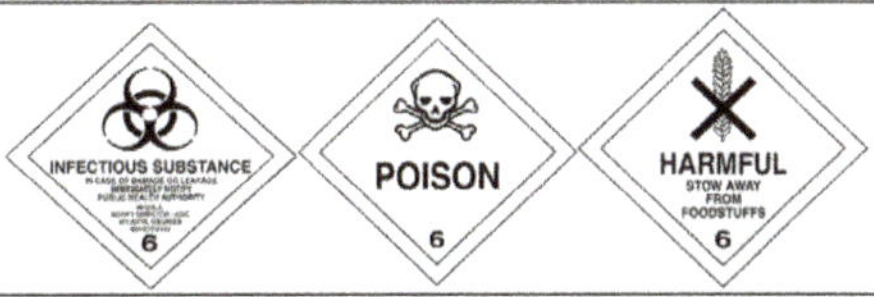	White with black letters	Varies

***Class 7* Radioactive Materials:** Material containing unstable atoms that emit ionizing radiation as they decay are known as radioactive materials. Enriched uranium, radioactive ores, isotopes (Cobalt 60, iodine 131, iridium 131 and hydrogen 3) and some medical equipments are few examples.

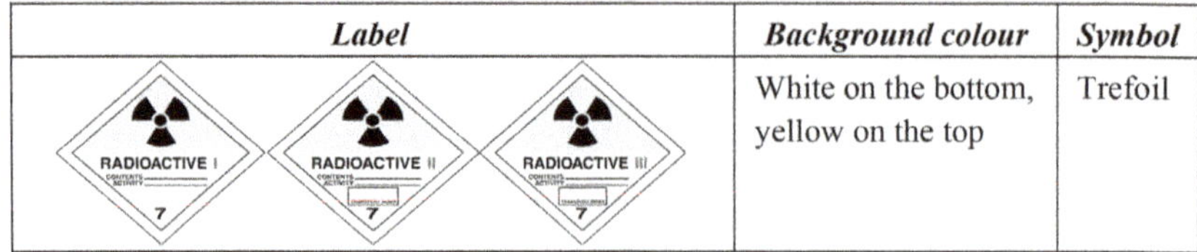

Label	*Background colour*	*Symbol*
RADIOACTIVE I 7 / RADIOACTIVE II 7 / RADIOACTIVE III 7	White on the bottom, yellow on the top	Trefoil

Class 8 **Corrosives:** Materials that are highly reactive and cause damage to living tissue are known as corrosives. Acids and bases are common corrosives. Hydrochloric acid, sulphuric acid and sodium hydroxide and batteries are few examples.

Label	*Background colour*	*Symbol*
CORROSIVE 8	Black on the bottom and white on the top	Piece of metal and a hand damaged by liquid

Class 9 **Miscellaneous:** Hazardous materials which not specified in any other classes are included in this class. Marine pollutants, like zinc oxide, lithium ion batteries, genetically modified organisms, air bag modules and motor engines.

Label	*Background colour*
9	Seven black vertical strips in upper half with white background, figure 9 is underlined.

1.2 Solvents

A solvent (*In Latin*: loosen, untie) is a substance that dissolves a solute and yields a solution. The quantity of solute that can dissolve in a specific volume of solvent varies with temperature. It also depends on rate of interaction between solute and the solvent.

Classification of solvents:

Three broad categories of solvents are known:

1. Protic/aprotic solvents
2. Polar/apolar (non-polar) solvents
3. Donor/non-donor solvents

A protic solvent consists of molecules that can act as hydrogen-bond donors.

e.g., Water, alcohols and carboxylic acids.

Solvents that cannot act as hydrogen-bond donors are termed aprotic solvents.

e.g., Ether, methylene chloride and hexane.

Polar solvents have high dielectric constant and they contain bonds between atoms with different electronegativities, such as oxygen, nitrogen, halogens and hydrogen. Apolar solvent has a low dielectric constant. They contain bonds between atoms with similar electronegativities, such as carbon and hydrogen.

Borderline polar aprotic solvents: These solvents have moderately higher dielectric constants than the nonpolar solvents. Since they have intermediate polarity they are good "general purpose" solvents for a wide range of reactions. They are "aprotic" because they lack -OH or -NH bonds. They generally serve as the medium.

Polar aprotic solvents

These solvents have large dielectric constants (>20) and large dipole moments, but they do not participate in hydrogen bonding (no -OH or -NH bonds). Their high polarity allows them to dissolve charged species such as various anions used as nucleophiles (e.g., $-CN^-$, $-OH^-$, etc.). The lack of hydrogen bonding in the solvent means that these nucleophiles are relatively "free" in solution, making them more reactive. These solvents do not participate in the reactions.

Polar protic solvents

Polar protic solvents tend to have high dielectric constants and high dipole moments. Furthermore, these solvents participate in hydrogen bonding. These solvents can also serve as acids (sources of protons) and weak nucleophiles (forming bonds with strong electrophiles). They are most commonly used as the solvent for their conjugate bases.

- Donor solvents consist of molecules that can donate unshared electron pairs. These molecules can act as Lewis bases.
  e.g., Ether, tetrahydrofuran (THF), methanol.
- Non-donor solvents cannot act as Lewis bases.
  e.g., Pentane, benzene.

Table 1 Properties of some common organic solvents.

Name	Dielectric constant	Dipole moment (μ)
Non-polar solvents		
Pentane	1.8	0.00
Hexane	1.9	0.00
Cyclohexane	2.0	0.00
Benzene	2.4	0.00
Toluene	2.3	0.36
Chloroform	4.8	1.04
Diethyl ether	4.3	1.15
Borderline polar aprotic solvents		
Dichloromethane	9.1	1.60
Tetrahydrofuran (THF)	7.5	1.75
Ethyl acetate	6.0	1.78

Table *Contd...*

Polar aprotic solvents		
Acetone	21	2.88
Dimethylformamide (DMF)	38	3.82
Acetonitrile	37	3.92
Dimethyl sulfoxide (DMSO)	47	3.96
Polar protic solvents		
Ammonia	16.61	1.4
t-Butanol	12	1.7
n-Propanol	20	1.68
Ethanol	25	1.69
Methanol	33	1.70
Acetic acid	6.2	1.74
Water	80	1.85

For the solubility of covalent compounds, *like dissolves the like* is the thumb of rule. Apolar aprotic solvent is good solvent for another apolar aprotic substance. Protic solvent in which significant hydrogen-bonding interactions occur between molecules is likely to dissolve another protic substance.

Among *n*-butane, ethyl chloride, ethyl methyl ether and 1-propanol, the later one is most soluble. A solution is obtained when the alcohol is mixed with water, as it is a protic. The ability to form hydrogen bonds with water is an important factor in water solubility. Ether contains oxygen that can accept hydrogen bonds from water, but it's not a hydrogen-bond donor. Hence it has some water-like characteristics, but less than the alcohol. In case of alkane and alkyl halide, they can neither donate nor accept hydrogen bonds. Therefore they are least soluble in water.

Among the homologous series of alcohols, higher alcohols (with long hydrocarbon chains) are relatively insoluble in water and more soluble in apolar aprotic solvents. Solvents consisting of polar molecules lie between the extremes of water on one hand and hydrocarbons on the other. As it can accept hydrogen bonds, it dissolves water and alcohols. As its dipole moment can interact favourably with other dipoles, it also dissolves polar compounds like alkyl halides. Due to the presence of its hydrocarbon portion, it can take part in van der Waals interactions, hence dissolves hydrocarbons also.

Ionic compounds in solution can exist in several forms, namely *ion pairs* and *dissociated ions*. In an ion pair, each ion is closely associated with an ion of opposite charge. While dissociated ions move more or less independently in solution and are surrounded by several solvent molecules, called collectively the *solvation shell* or *solvent cage* of the ion. Solvation refers to the favourable interaction of a dissolved molecule with solvent. When solvent molecules interact favourably with an ion, they are said to *solvate* the ion.

Applications

Solvent is a liquid used to dissolve a compound. Solvents have many practical applications:

1. For solubilisation of organic compounds
2. As heat transfer medium
3. Recrystallization

1.3 Glassware and Equipments

In general glassware (reaction vessels) are useful in the following purposes:

- for mixing reactants
- for heating/ boiling reaction mixture and solutions
- for distilling the reaction mixture and extracts
- for cooling the hot solutions
- for collecting the products
- for storing the solutions, reagents and isolated products

Flasks

Reaction flasks: The flasks are designed to tolerate the large pressure differences due to vacuum and pressure (applied and generated).

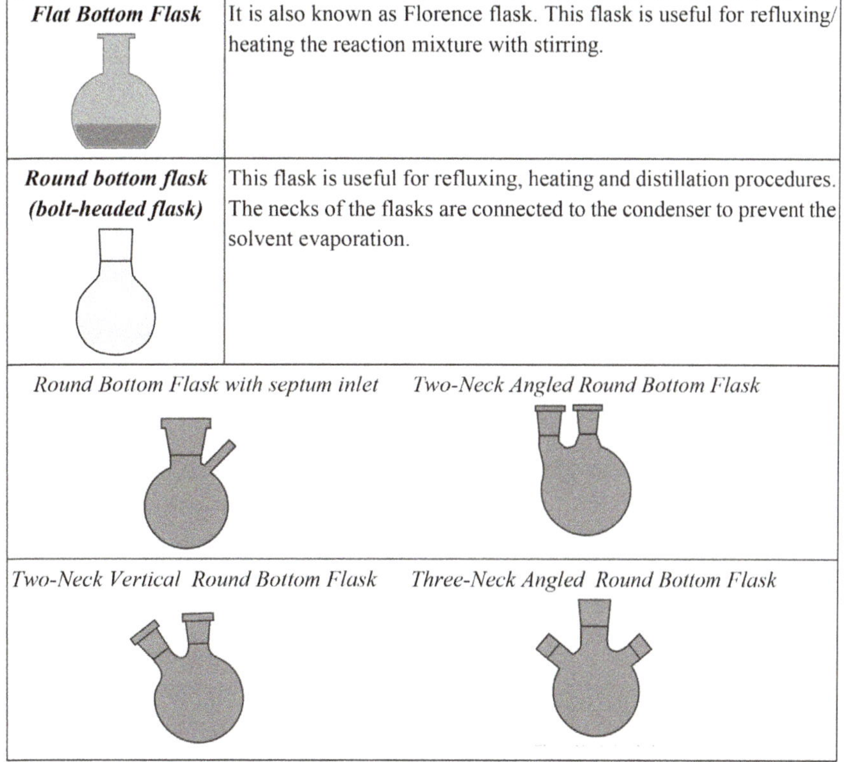

Flat Bottom Flask	It is also known as Florence flask. This flask is useful for refluxing/ heating the reaction mixture with stirring.
Round bottom flask (bolt-headed flask)	This flask is useful for refluxing, heating and distillation procedures. The necks of the flasks are connected to the condenser to prevent the solvent evaporation.
Round Bottom Flask with septum inlet	*Two-Neck Angled Round Bottom Flask*
Two-Neck Vertical Round Bottom Flask	*Three-Neck Angled Round Bottom Flask*

Table ***Contd...***

Erlenmeyer flask (conical flask)	Cone shaped and flat bottomed cylindrical flasks useful in mixing heating, titration and cooling the reaction mixtures.
Volumetric flask	This flask is useful in preparing the liquids with high precision volumes (essential for analysis).
Evaporatory flask	Centered and pear shaped flasks with the socket are useful in solvent recovery (evaporation) procedure in rotary evaporator.
Filtering flask	It is used along with Buchner's funnel. It has a port for connecting to vacuum. This facilitates the filtration under vacuum (enhanced filtration).
Wide necked flask	This flask is useful in conducting semi-micro and macro scale experiments.
Iodine flask	The loss of iodine and other volatile substances (analytes) during the analysis through evaporation is important concern. To overcome this issue Iodine flasks are designed. Iodine flasks differ from Erlenmeyer (conical) flasks, and improve the accuracy of analysis. The difference are: • Ground glass joint: It prevents the evaporation of volatile compounds. • Modified stopper: It provides tight closure. • Funnel shaped top: It prevents the spillage.

Condensers

Condensers are useful in warming, heating, refluxing and distillation process. In heating and reflux process, it condenses the solvent vapours and sends them back to flask thereby reduces the solvent loss. In distillation procedures condenser streamlines the flow of solvent vapour from the flask to the receiver. It provides better separation between the mixture of components.

Types of condensers

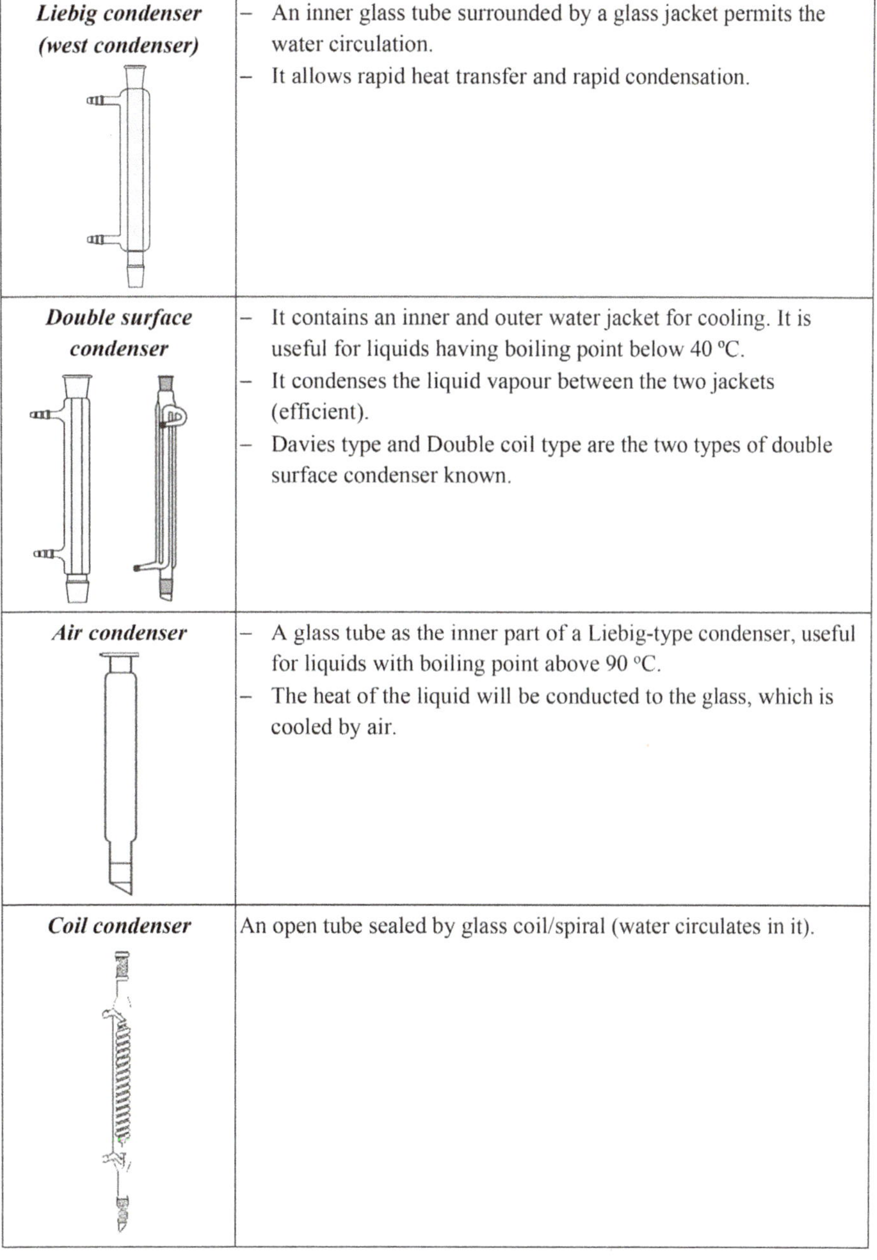

Liebig condenser (west condenser)	– An inner glass tube surrounded by a glass jacket permits the water circulation. – It allows rapid heat transfer and rapid condensation.
Double surface condenser	– It contains an inner and outer water jacket for cooling. It is useful for liquids having boiling point below 40 °C. – It condenses the liquid vapour between the two jackets (efficient). – Davies type and Double coil type are the two types of double surface condenser known.
Air condenser	– A glass tube as the inner part of a Liebig-type condenser, useful for liquids with boiling point above 90 °C. – The heat of the liquid will be conducted to the glass, which is cooled by air.
Coil condenser	An open tube sealed by glass coil/spiral (water circulates in it).

Table ***Contd...***

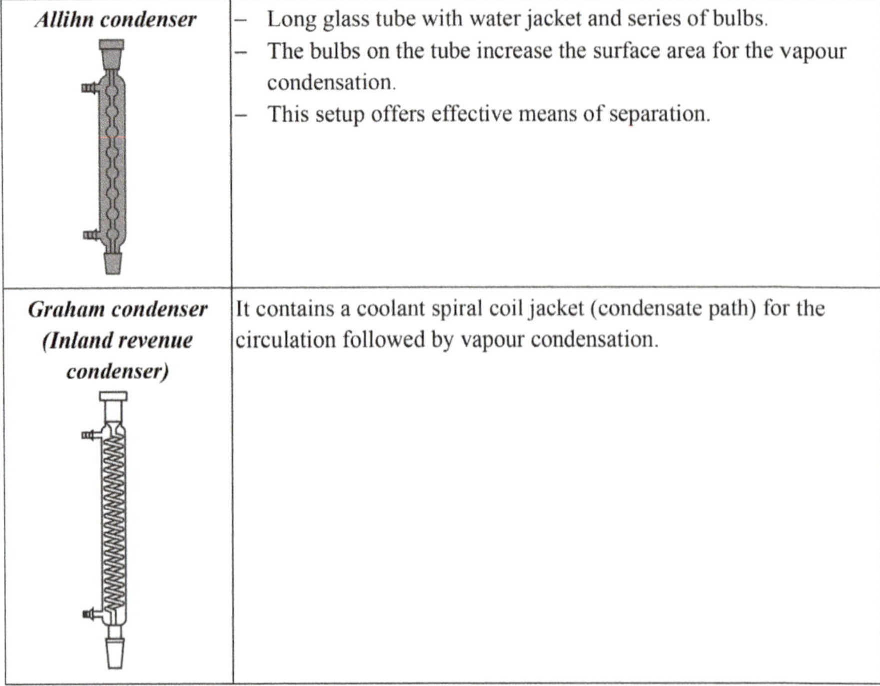

Allihn condenser	– Long glass tube with water jacket and series of bulbs. – The bulbs on the tube increase the surface area for the vapour condensation. – This setup offers effective means of separation.
Graham condenser (Inland revenue condenser)	It contains a coolant spiral coil jacket (condensate path) for the circulation followed by vapour condensation.

Distillation Heads

Knee tube	Mostly utilised in the removal of solvents during distillation.
Claisen distillation head	The left-hand socket accommodates the capillary tube for use in distillation under vacuum. The right-hand socket is for placing suitable thermometer.
Splash-Guard	Employed in rotary evaporators and can be used as splash protection (bubble inhibitor).

Receiver, Adapters/Connectors

Claisen adapter	It is used when the reaction requires both reflux and addition of reactants at the same time. One joint connects to condenser for reflux and the other gets connected with dropping funnel (addition of reactants).
Claisen distillation adapter	This adapter has two connections, one is socket for thermometer and the other one connects to flask.
Vacuum distillation adapter	This adapter provides connection to vacuum pump to facilitate the distillation under reduced pressure (more suitable for thermolabile substances).
Calcium guard tube (drying tube)	It is used to exclude moisture from experimental setup during reflux/ distillation. A tube like structure with one end bend, which connects the tube to reaction vessel. The end contains bulb to pack solid desiccant materials (granular alumina, silica gel, calcium sulphite and calcium chloride). A cotton plug (glass wool plug) to the bottom opening prevents the contact of these desiccants to the reaction vessel.

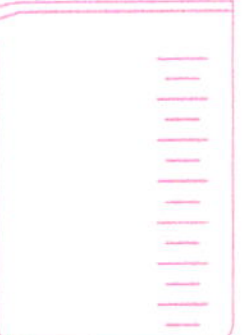

Beakers

Beakers are commonly made up of borosilicate glass, metal (aluminium and stainless steel) but plastic [polythene, polypropylene, polystyrene, polytetrafluoroethylene (PTFE)] beakers are also available for gamma spectral analysis. They are generally graduated, cylindrical with flat bottom and has a spout (beak), which assists in pouring. Griffin with spout and conical beaker are the two common types of beakers in use for stirring, mixing and heating of liquids.

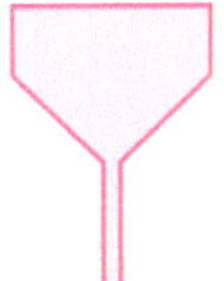

Funnels

Funnels are made up of glass, porcelain or plastics and are useful for the filtration. The hot solution must be rapidly filtered before undue cooling has occurred using fluted filter paper.

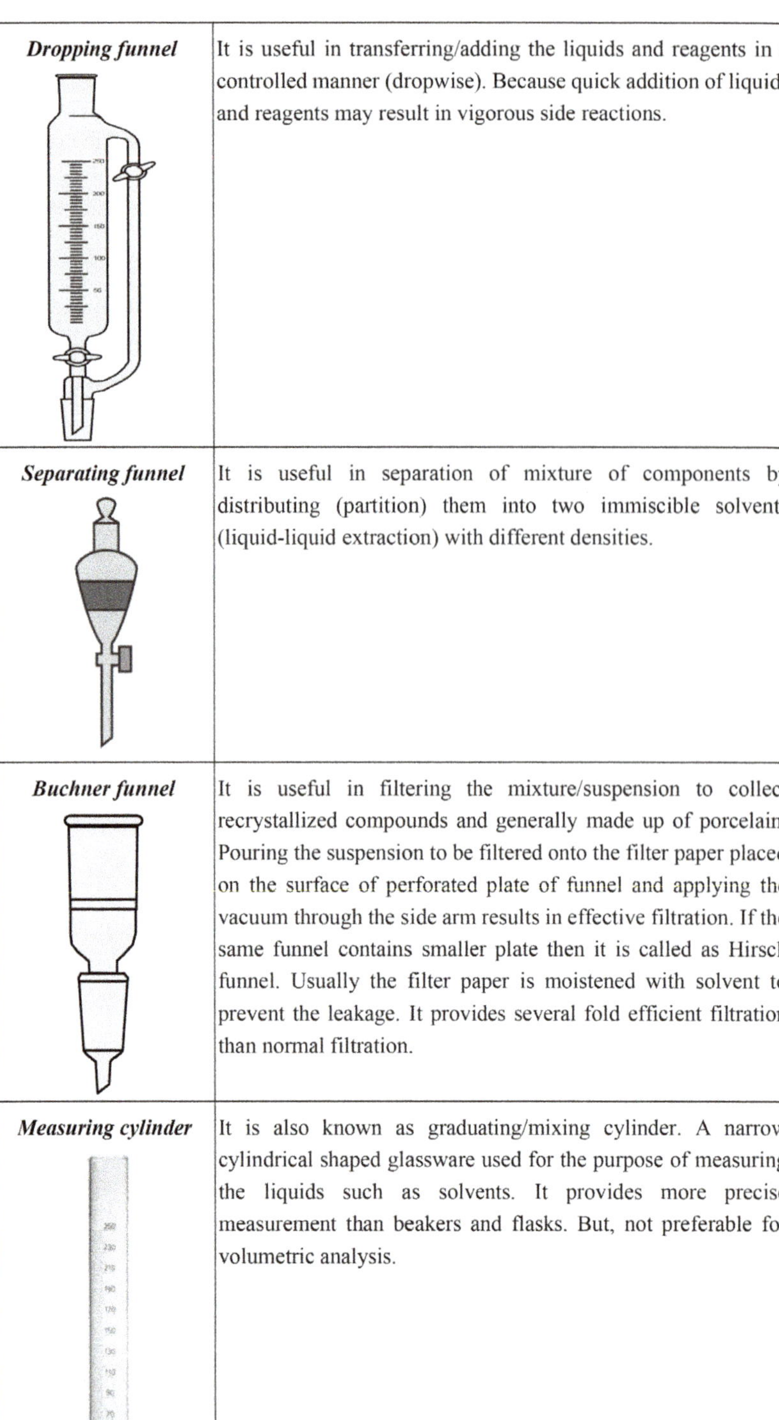

Dropping funnel	It is useful in transferring/adding the liquids and reagents in a controlled manner (dropwise). Because quick addition of liquids and reagents may result in vigorous side reactions.
Separating funnel	It is useful in separation of mixture of components by distributing (partition) them into two immiscible solvents (liquid-liquid extraction) with different densities.
Buchner funnel	It is useful in filtering the mixture/suspension to collect recrystallized compounds and generally made up of porcelain. Pouring the suspension to be filtered onto the filter paper placed on the surface of perforated plate of funnel and applying the vacuum through the side arm results in effective filtration. If the same funnel contains smaller plate then it is called as Hirsch funnel. Usually the filter paper is moistened with solvent to prevent the leakage. It provides several fold efficient filtration than normal filtration.
Measuring cylinder	It is also known as graduating/mixing cylinder. A narrow cylindrical shaped glassware used for the purpose of measuring the liquids such as solvents. It provides more precise measurement than beakers and flasks. But, not preferable for volumetric analysis.

Magnetic Stirrer

Magnetic stirrer	It is a laboratory device that employs rotating magnetic field to cause a stirrer bar immersed in a liquid to spin very quickly. It ensures the uniform and optimum stirring.
Stirring Rod (Stir Bar/Flea) 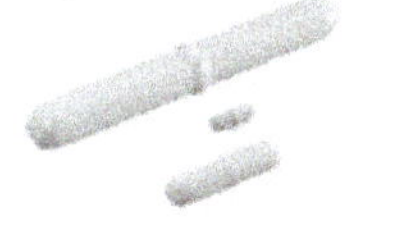	It is a piece of solid glass - magnetic bar generally made up of borosilicate (Pyrex), used for the purpose of mixing chemicals and liquids. The stir bar motion is driven by electromagnets present in the stirrer. They will be coated with Teflon or glass. Glass coating is suitable for the mixing of liquid alkali metals solutions.
Boiling Chips 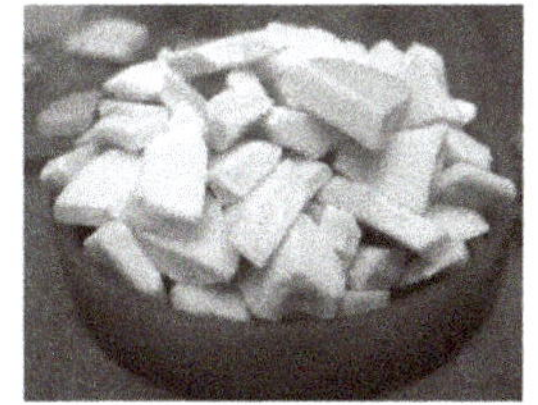	Super heating is a condition in which heat will be trapped around the gas surface and there is no release of energy. This is responsible for the formation of bubbles, which converts into gas phase and can be explosive. Super heated solution results in bumping and causes loss of liquid. Stirring and agitation ensures that the heat is properly distributed in the reaction mixture. Use of porous chips, sticks and wooden splints prevents solvent overheating. Air trapped within the porous chip/ stick/wooden splint initiates the bubble formation to the top of the liquid and allows solution to boil evenly.

Heating Reaction Mixtures

Bunsen burner 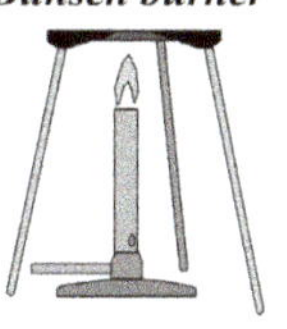	• Supported with tripods and ceramic centred gauze. • Flame should be turned on after ensuring the absence of any fire hazard in the surrounding.
Electrically heated water bath 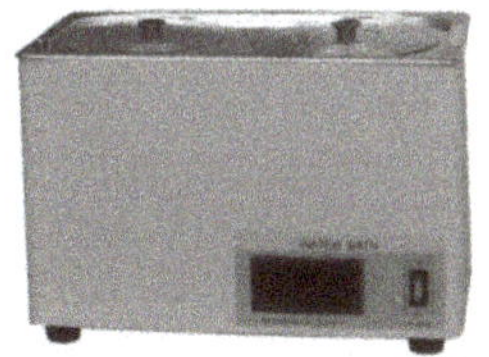	It is useful for boiling liquids with boiling point less than 100 °C.
Steam bath 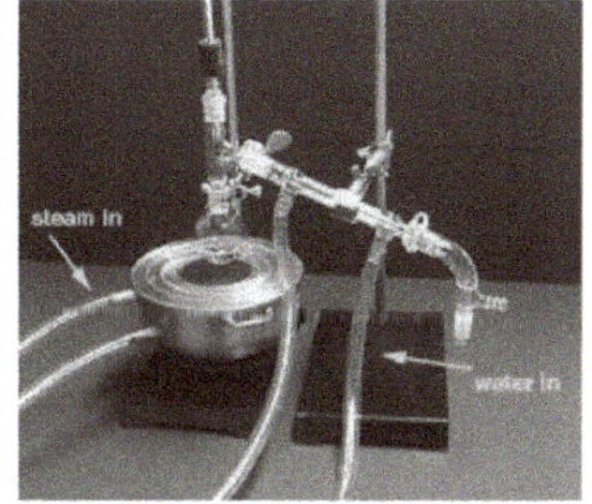	Steam-heated devices are generally preferred whenever temperatures of 100° C or less are required.

Table *Contd...*

Electric heating mantle 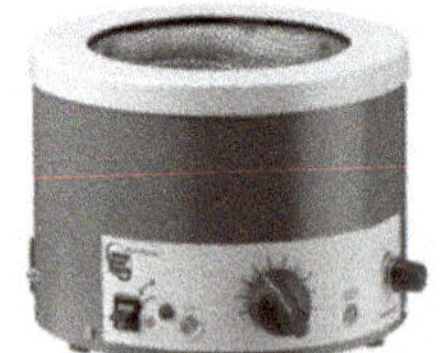	It is also known as isomantle, which supplies heat to the containers and flasks. The heating element is insulated and hence the containers can be directly placed on the mantle. Heating mantle with Rheostat is useful for maintaining the intended temperature. It distributes the heat evenly over the surface of the flask and produces no/less harmful hotspots.
Oil bath 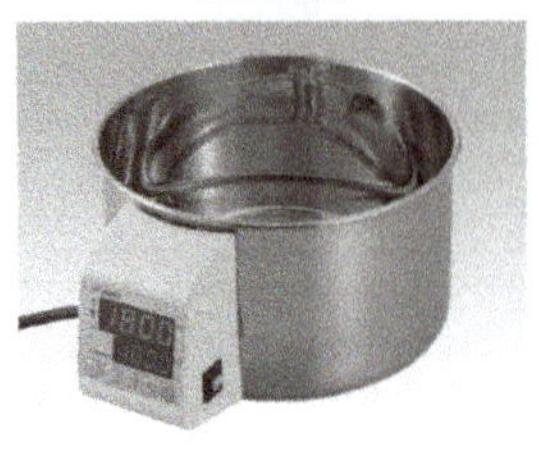	Useful in temperature above 100 °C. The following oils are useful in the heating procedures. - *Hard hydrogenated cotton seed oil:* For temperature up to 250 °C, more advantageous because it is clear, non sticky liquid and solidifies on cooling. - *Medicinal paraffin:* For temperature upto 220 °C. - *Glycerol and dibutyl phthalate:* For temperature up to 140-150 °C. - *Silicone fluids:* Silicone fluids are polymers of inorganic compounds and not derived from petroleum and organics, hence posses unique properties. - (e.g., polydimethylsiloxanes, methylphenyl silicone fluid).

Soxhlet Extractor

Soxhlet extraction is effective in the separation of desired compound with limited solubility than the impurity. Simple filtration is suitable for the separation, if the desired compound has significant solubility in the solvent.

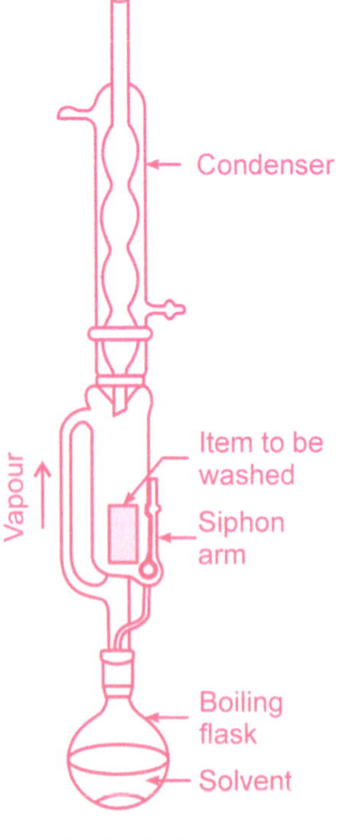

Soxhlet Extractor

SPECIAL APPARATUS

Dean-Stark Apparatus	It is also known as distilling trap used in the continuous removal of liberated water from the reflux mixture (azeotropic distillations). Solvent vapours along with water escapes in to the condenser and then drip into the trap. The two immiscible liquids gets separated into two layers, the high density water flow to the collector through the side arm and low density liquid flows back into flask.
Kipp's Apparatus 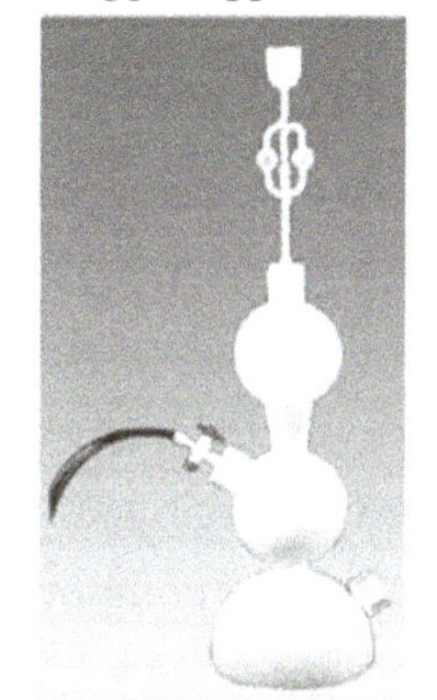	It is also known as Kipp's generator and useful in the preparation of small volume of gases. In general they are made up of glass and polyethylene. The apparatus is made up of three vertically stacked cylinders and the solid material which generates gas will be placed in the middle cylinder. The top cylinder will be loaded with acid which in turn connected to the middle and bottom cylinder through the tube. The middle cylinder has separate tube with stopcork to collect the evolved gas. The closure of the stopcock will raise the pressure of the gas which expels the acid back to the top of the cylinder.

1.4 Glassware Cleaning

Glassware can be cleaned by immersing them in dichromate solution (cleaning solution), followed by draining and rinsing with distilled water.

Preparation of dichromate solution: Dissolve 5 g of potassium/sodium dichromate in 5 mL of water and cool. Add 100 mL of sulphuric acid slowly with stirring (exothermic reaction, hence use fume cupboard).

- Glasswares can be rinsed with acetone and then with petroleum ether or diethyl ether to remove traces of impurities prior to use.
- Alcoholic solution of sodium hydroxide (120 g of sodium hydroxide in 120 mL of water, dilute to 1000 mL with ethanol) can be used for cleaning polyethylene ware.

1.5 Purification Methods

Common methods employed in the purifications are:

- Solvent extraction
- Washing
- Distillation
- Recrystallization
- Sublimation
- Chromatography
- Drying

Solvent Extraction: Organic compounds can be separated from inorganic impurities by shaking the reaction suspension with suitable immiscible solvents (benzene, carbon tetrachloride, diethyl ether, etc). Evaporation of organic layer (containing organic compound) leaves the residue. Addition of electrolytes (ammonium sulphate, calcium chloride and sodium chloride) ensures the organic layer separation and increases organic extraction.

Washing: Phenol impurities can be removed by washing with sodium hydroxide. Organic bases can be removed by adding dilute hydrochloric acid/sulphuric acid. Unsaturated hydrocarbons of alcohols and ethers can be removed by adding concentrated sulphuric acid.

Distillation: Distillation is the method of separating mixtures based on the differences in volatility of components in a boiling liquid mixture.

Simple and fractional distillation: Non-volatile compounds can be separated by simple distillation. Liquids and low melting point solids (volatile compounds) can be purified by fractional distillation. Distillation apparatus consists of distillation flask fitted with fractional column which in turn attached to condenser and thermometer. In case of simple distillation column is not necessary and flask can be attached directly to condenser. Adding boiling chips to the flask reduces the super heating.

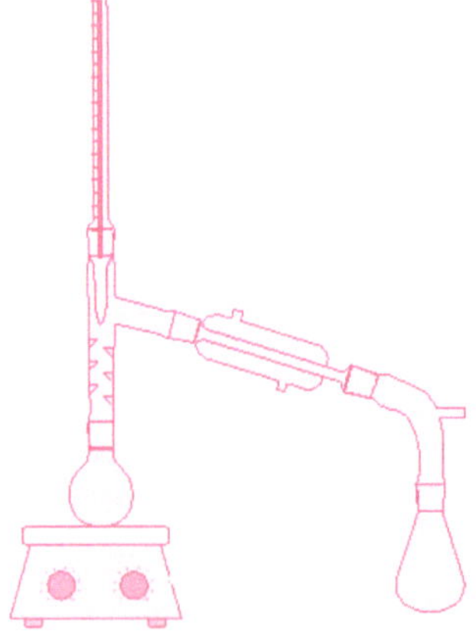

Distillation unit

Upon heating, the contents of the flask vaporizes, passes through the column and condenses back to flask. The vapour passing into the condenser is lowest boiling component of mixture. In fractional distillation the initial and final fractions (lower and higher boiling point components respectively) has to be rejected. Stir the mixture mechanically, in case of suspended insoluble materials present in the mixture to be distilled.

- ***Vacuum distillation:*** Distillation under reduced pressure (lower than atmosphere) is denoted as vacuum distillation. Thermolabile, sensitive and high boiling point liquids can be purified by vacuum distillation.
- ***Steam distillation:*** Temperature sensitive materials (natural aromatics) can be purified by this method.
- ***Isopiestic/isothermal distillation:*** Metal free solutions of volatile acids and bases can be obtained by this method. This can be effected by placing distilled water and solution to be purified in separate beaker in sealed desiccators at room temperature for several days.

Recrystallization: Purification of impure crystalline compounds by crystallization from a suitable solvent or mixture of solvents is known as *recrystallization*. Recrystallization is the effective method for the purification of organic solid compounds. A solid product prepared may contain impurities, and recrystallization separates impurity from product. In this process, the compounds will be crystallized based upon differences in their solubility in a given solvent or mixture of solvents.

The process usually involves following steps:

(a) Dissolving the crude substance in a suitable solvent at its boiling point

(b) Filtering the hot solution from insoluble matter.

(c) Allowing the hot solution to cool. This allows the dissolved substance to crystallize out.

(d) Separating the crystals from the mother-liquor (supernant solution).

The resulting solid is dried and tested for purity by checking its melting point. This process is repeated until pure compound is obtained which is evidenced by its unchanged melting point.

Simplified general procedure for the purification of impure solids

1. Select the right solvent based on the solubility of sample (trial and error method).
2. Place beaker containing known amount of solvent on hot plate.
3. Add small amounts of boiling solvent to the impure solid (partially soluble in solvent) taken in the beaker.
4. Dissolve the solid by heating and stirring if necessary (add more solvent, if necessary to obtain saturated solution).
5. Warm the stemless funnel with the vapours of solvent and filter the hot solution through fluted filter paper placed in funnel.

6. Dissolve the crystals if any formed with adding additional amount of solvent.
7. Cool the clear liquid (collected in the beaker) to room temperature.
8. Place the beaker in an ice-bath (do not disturb) and filter the crystals formed through Buchner funnel (previously wet with solvent).

Steps involved in recrystallization process

- Selection of solvent
- Solubilization of the compound
- Decolorization
- Impurities filtration
- Crystallization
- Filtration
- Drying

Selection of solvent: Solvent can be one or mixture of two liquids. In general solvent with partial solubility will be selected for recrystallization. Solute should be insoluble at room temperature and soluble in high temperature (boiling point). A solvent that can completely dissolve a solid in hot condition gives crystals when the temperature is low. Soluble impurities stay in solution and some of the pure compound may also remain dissolved.

The following are the desired features of a solvent for recrystallization

- It must have high solvent power at elevated temperature and comparatively low power at laboratory temperature.
- It should dissolve the impurities readily to a very small extent.
- It should yield well formed crystals of the purified compound.
- It should not react chemically with the substance to be purified.

If two or more solvents are equally suitable for recrystallization, then the selection depends upon ease of manipulation, toxicity, flammability and cost. If the substance is found to be far too soluble in one solvent and much too insoluble in another solvent to allow of recrystallization, *mixed solvents* or *solvent pairs* may be frequently used. In this case, recrystallization is carried out near the boiling point of the mixture.

Mixture of solvents also can be used when single solvent is not applicable. Second solvent can be added to reduce the strength of first solvent. Most common mixture includes alcohol (strong solvent) and water (weak solvent). For polar molecules (containing oxygen and/nitrogen atom) alcohol-water or alcohol-pentanone is more suitable.

Most commonly used solvent pairs are

- Alcohols and water
- Alcohols and toluene
- Toluene and light petroleum

- Acetone and light petroleum
- Diethyl ether and pentane
- Glacial acetic acid and water
- Dimethylformamide and water
- Dimethylformamide and toluene

Solubilization of the compound: Sample should be dissolved with the aid of solvent by the slow addition of solvent.

Decolourization: The coloured impurities present along with the product can be removed by the treatment with charcoal and filtration. Coloured impurities will adhere to the large surface of charcoal and can be separated by filtration. This step is not necessary, when there is no coloured impurities present.

Impurities filtration: Insoluble impurities will be removed by the filtration through fluted filter paper (provides larger surface area and increase rate of filtration) and stem less funnel (avoids crystallization in the stem during crystallization).

A simple filtration in hot condition separates the product from insoluble impurities. Filtrate upon cooling crystallizes out the pure product and the soluble impurities remain in the solvent. Thus both soluble and insoluble impurities can be removed to obtain the pure solid product.

Crystallization: Solvent upon cooling and/or evaporation initiates crystallization of the solid product.

Filtration: Solid product which crystallizes out can be collected by simple filtration.

Drying: Separated solid may contain some residual solvent in it, so it requires drying to remove solvent completely.

Recrystallization never offer 100% product due to loss while physical handling, impurities and some amount will remain in saturation with solvent. Excess of solvent, inadequate warming and selection of wrong solvent also reduces the yield (crystallization).

Procedure for the purification of benzoic acid

a) Heat the benzoic acid with enough water to dissolve all soluble material.
b) Filter the hot solution to remove insoluble material (if any).
c) Cool the solution to effect crystallization.
d) Filter, wash with water and dry the product.

Procedure for the purification of benzamide

a) Dissolve finely powdered benzamide in boiling water.
b) Filter the insoluble impurities through filtration.
c) Allow it cool to room temperature and collect the crystals through filtration.
d) Wash the crystals with cold water and dry the product.

e) **Sublimation:** The chemical transformation of solids into vapours is known as sublimation. Volatile solids can be converted into vapours on heating and vapours condense as purified solid on cooling. It helps in the purification of volatile solids like naphthalene, iodine, camphor, etc.

Purification of iodine

- Cover the impure iodine placed in the beaker with glass dish.
- Place ice cubes on the glass dish (cover).
- Heat the beaker gently by keeping over the wire gauze.
- The impure iodine vapourizes leaving the impurities.
- Iodine vapours on cooling sublimes in to solid.
- Isolate the pure iodine from glass dish by scratching.

Chromatography: Chromatography is the collective term for the set of techniques applicable for the separation of mixtures. The mixture to be separated is dissolved in mobile phase which carries it through the stationary phase. Column chromatography and thin-layer chromatography (TLC) are the two important separation techniques useful in organic chemistry laboratories.

Column chromatography: Useful in the separation of large quantities of mixtures.

Thin-layer chromatography (TLC): Thin-layer chromatography is a simple, inexpensive analytical and purification technique.

Thin-layer chromatography for salicylic acid and acetyl salicylic acid (aspirin)

- ***Preparation of sample:*** Dissolve the specified quantity of salicylic acid and acetyl salicylic acid in ethanol separately.
- Separately use these solutions for spotting on the TLC plate.
- ***Preparation of developing chamber:*** Prepare mobile phase (hexane: ethyl acetate: acetic acid, 6.5:3:0.5) and load into developing chamber (solvent tank). Cover the chamber with lid to ensure the saturation of chamber with solvent vapour. Line the inside of the beaker with filter paper wet with the mobile phase; this also saturates the chamber with solvent vapour.
- ***Preparation of TLC plate:*** Prepare the silica gel paste, by mixing 5 gm of silica gel with 30 ml of water. Pour this paste onto the glass plate and spread uniformly. [Alternatively aluminium backed precoated plates can be used.] Handle TLC plates by edges only and avoid touching the surface. Draw a line (light) about 1-2 cm from the bottom of the TLC plate.
- ***Loading the TLC plates:*** Dip the capillary into the sample solution and spot on the plate. Touch the tip of the capillary onto the plate, and allow it to dry. Spot the sample for three times and the size should be in between 0.5-1 mm. Use different capillary tube for each sample.

- ***Developing the TLC plates:*** Place the TLC plate into the chamber and make sure that the mobile phase level is below the baseline present in plate. Solvent rises by capillary action and component present in the sample will rise up. Allow the plate to elute until the solvent front is about 1 cm from the top. The rate of sample elution depends upon their partitioning with silica gel. A more polar component spends more time on the polar silica gel surface, move up more slowly than the non-polar component.
- ***Visualizing the TLC plates:*** Remove the plate, mark the solvent front and allow it to dry. Visualize the spots of TLC plate by placing in a UV chamber and keeping in iodine chamber. Different components will appear at distinct locations, and pure sample produces single spot.

  Note: UV light is harmful to eyes and skin, so don't expose hands or eyes to UV light.
- ***Calculation of Retention factor* (R_f):** The ratio of the distance travelled by the sample and distance travelled by the mobile phase (solvent front) is known as R_f.

$$\text{Retention factor } (R_f) = \frac{\text{Distance travelled by the solute}}{\text{Distance travelled by the solvent}}$$

1.6 Drying

Removal of solvents: Removal of solvent from recrystallized compounds can be effected by heating them in an oven above the boiling point of the solvent followed by cooling in a desiccator.

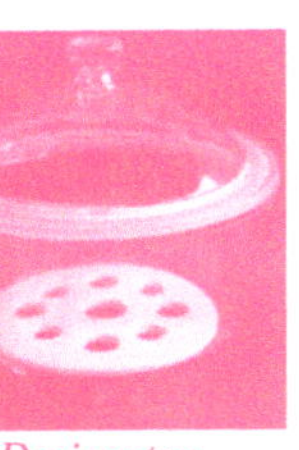
Desiccator

Removal of water: Thermal stability of the compounds determines the method of choice. Direct distillation is suitable for removing organic liquid from solids and liquids. During distillation, guard tube with calcium chloride/silica gel prevents the entry of moisture. Substances with melting point above 100 °C and stable in air can be dried using hot air oven. Drying compounds in vacuum desiccator over sulphuric acid, phosphorous pentoxide, silica gel, calcium chloride and similar desiccants is the safest method of drying water. Water in gases can be removed by adsorption on to a drying agent.

Most common desiccants

- ***Calcium sulphate (anhydrous):*** Very efficient and suitable for most of the organic compounds.
- *Magnesium sulphate (anhydrous).*
- *Sodium sulphate (anhydrous).*
- ***Calcium chloride:*** Absorbs water and becomes hexahydrate below 30 °C (slow in action and less efficient). It is suitable for drying aryl halides, esters, ethers and hydrocarbons. It is unsuitable for drying alcohols, amines, amides, amino acids, ketones and phenols.

- ***Calcium oxide (anhydrous):*** It is suitable for drying alcohols and amines, unsuitable for acids and esters.
- ***Copper (II) chloride (anhydrous):*** It is suitable for esters and alcohols.
- ***Potassium carbonate (anhydrous):*** It is suitable for salting out water soluble alcohols, amines and ketones and unsuitable for phenols, thiols and related compounds.
- ***Granulated silica gel:*** Physical adsorption is the mechanism, which is efficient in room temperature.

1.7 Determination of Melting Point

Melting point is the important physicochemical characteristic of molecules, which can be used for identification purpose. The hydrogen bonding nature of the molecules influence their melting point.

***Definition*:** The temperature at which the highly ordered arrangement of particles in a solid gets converted to more random arrangement that characterizes a liquid is known as melting point. Melting occurs over a temperature range and temperature at which first tiny drop of liquid appears is termed as melting point.

Determination of melting point for organic compounds

Sample filling:

1. Grind the sample, whose melting point has to be determined into fine powder.
2. Seal one end of capillary tube (sealed tubes also can be used). Fill 2-3 mm level of capillary tube with fine powder of sample.
3. Drop the capillary tube through 1 meter length glass tube (broken burette or condenser can be used) several times.

Procedure:

1. Place the capillary tube filled with sample in the melting point apparatus.
2. Switch on the instrument to heat the sample until the contents of the tube melts.
3. Use the knob to set rise of temperature per minute (best set at 2 °C per min).
4. Appearance of first tiny drop indicates the melting of sample and the temperature range should be noted as melting range.
5. Change in crystalline structure, wet appearance and shrinkage of the sample should not be interpret as melting point.

Determination of melting point of mixture of compounds

Sample filling 1: For pure product

1. Grind the pure (recrystallized) sample, whose melting point has to be determined in to fine powder.

2. Seal one end of capillary tube (sealed tubes also can be used). Fill 2-3 mm level of capillary tube with fine powder of sample.
3. Drop the capillary tube through 1 meter length glass tube (broken burette or condenser can be used) several times.

Sample filling 2: **For mixture of pure and impure products**

1. Grind the pure (recrystallized) and impure products, whose melting point has to be determined into fine powder.
2. Seal one end of capillary tube (sealed tubes also can be used). Fill 2-3 mm level of capillary tube with fine powder of sample.
3. Drop the capillary tube through 1 meter length glass tube (broken burette or condenser can be used) several times.

Procedure:

1. Place the capillary tubes filled with pure sample and mixture separately in the melting point apparatus.
2. Switch on the instrument to heat the sample until the contents of the tube melts.
3. Use the knob to set rise of temperature per minute (best set at 2 °C per minute).
4. Appearance of first tiny drop indicates the melting of sample and the temperature range should be noted as melting range.
5. Change in crystalline structure, wet appearance and shrinkage of the sample should not be interpreted as melting point.

Note:

- The determined melting range may differ (small extent) from literature value, if the solid is not completely pure.
- Rapid heating of melting point apparatus and error in the thermometer may also cause to this.

1.8 Determination of Boiling Point

Boiling point reflects the physicochemical characteristic of molecules and can be used for identification purpose. Boiling occurs when the thermal energy of the particles (due to external temperature) is great enough to overcome the cohesive forces that operated in the liquids. Similar to other physical constants of the matter (melting point and solubility) it also depends on nature of bonds in the molecules. The pressure exerted by the surface of the liquid also decides the boiling point of molecules. The atmospheric pressure has the influence on the surface pressure. The presence of volatile impurities increases the boiling point of liquid.

Liquids whose molecules held by hydrogen bonds are known as associated liquids. The energy required to break these bonds will be more, hence their boiling point will be more than others. Among associated liquids, stronger the hydrogen bond, greater will be their boiling point.

Definition: The temperature at which the vapour pressure of the liquid equal to the atmospheric pressure (760 mm) is known as boiling point.

Determination of boiling point for organic compounds (Thiele tube method)

Procedure:

1. Fill a Thiele tube with mineral oil (Liquid paraffin) up to triangle structure.
2. Clamp the Thiele tube in the iron stand placed in the fume cupboard.
3. Insert a Thermometer into the Thiele tube, through a rubber cork.
4. Attach small rubber vial (Durham tube) to the middle of the thermometer bulb with the help of rubber band.
   (a) The rubber band should be on the top, so that its contact with the liquid paraffin bath can be avoided.
   (b) Fill half of the vial with the liquid sample (oil may expand upon heating).
5. Insert the sealed capillary tube into the vial containing sample (open end down and sealed end on the top).
6. Lower the test tube and thermometer set up into a liquid paraffin bath (Thiele tube).
   (Thermometer should not touch the sides)
7. The height of sample should be in the middle of thermometer bulb.
8. Heat the oil gently (oil rises to the trianglular portion of the tube).
9. Continue heating until a stream of bubbles comes out of the capillary tube (individual bubbles can be distinguished.
   (indicates that the vapour pressure inside the tube greater than the atmospheric pressure)
10. Note down the temperature, when there is continuous evolution of bubbles from the capillary tube (**a**).
11. Disconnect the heat supply, and allow the system to cool.
12. Note down the temperature when the evolution of bubbles stops at the end of the capillary tube (**b**).
13. Consider the mean of **a** and **b** as boiling point of the given liquid.

Note: Concentrated sulphuric acid can be used for the liquids with boiling point greater than 200 °C.

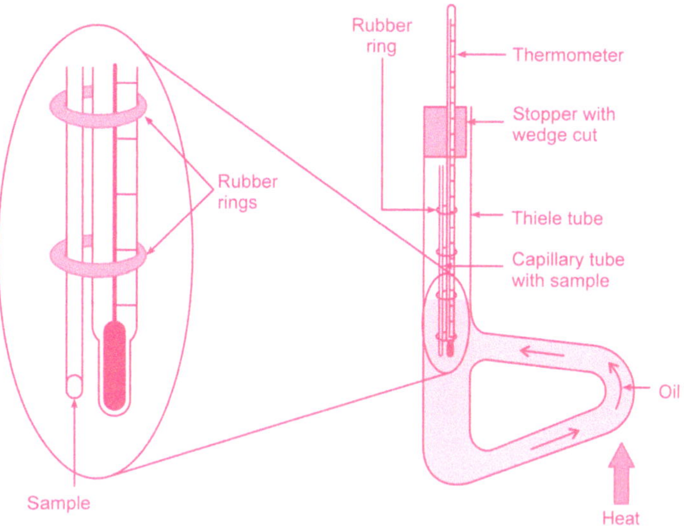

1.9 Yield Calculation

Theoretical yield: The maximum amount of product that results from a chemical reaction is called as theoretical yield. The theoretical yield is based upon the molar quantities of the reactants used. It can be calculated from stoichiometric factors derived from the coefficient of the products and reactants.

Practical yield: The actual yield of the product obtained in the chemical reaction.

Relative yield: The ratio between the practical and theoretical yield is known as relative yield. It is also known as fractional yield. It measures the effectiveness of the synthetic procedure.

$$\text{Relative yield} = \frac{\text{Practical yield}}{\text{Theoretical yield}}$$

Theoretically, the yield of a chemical reaction would be 100%. But in practical it is impossible to achieve. Several experimental factors limit the yield (reaction).
Percentage yield: The percentage yield of the products can be calculated by using the formula given below.

$$\text{Percentage yield} = \frac{\text{Practical yield}}{\text{Theoretical yield}} \times 100$$

Yields can be grouped as follows:

% yield	Description
100	Quantitative yield
>90	Excellent yield
>80	Very good yield
>70	Good yield
>50	Fair yield
<50	Poor yield

The percent yield calculation involves a series of steps

Step 1: Writing a balanced chemical equation for the reaction. The correct ratio of the reactants and the products can be ascertained through the balanced reaction. The stoichiometric coefficients are placed before the reagents and products to equal the number of atoms (or molecules) on both the side.

Unbalanced reaction:

$$\underset{\text{Borax}}{Na_2B_4O_7} + \underset{\text{Sulphuric acid}}{H_2SO_4} + H_2O \longrightarrow \underset{\text{Boric acid}}{H_3BO_3} + \underset{\text{Sodium sulphate}}{Na_2SO_4}$$

Balanced reaction:

$$\underset{\text{Borax}}{Na_2B_4O_7} + \underset{\text{Sulphuric acid}}{H_2SO_4} + 5H_2O \longrightarrow \underset{\text{Boric acid}}{4H_3BO_3} + \underset{\text{Sodium sulphate}}{Na_2SO_4}$$

The differentiation between the reactants (reagents) and other chemical species involved in the reaction are very essential. The chemicals namely, catalysts and solvents are not consumed in the reaction. Hence, they are not considered in the yield calculation.

In case of boric acid preparation, the sulphuric acid is reactant. But in the preparation of benzocaine it acts as a catalyst. Hence it is not considered incase of benzocaine.

$$\underset{\textit{para}\text{-Amino benzoic acid}}{H_2N\text{-}C_6H_4\text{-}COOH} + \underset{\text{Ethanol}}{C_2H_5OH} \xrightarrow{H_2SO_4} \underset{\text{Benzocaine}}{H_2N\text{-}C_6H_4\text{-}C(=O)OC_2H_5} + H_2O$$

Step 2: Calculate the molecular weight of each reactants and product. The sum of the mass of the atoms generate the molecular weight.

Example, Ethanol – C_2H_5OH

Weight of carbon atom	= 2 × 12.01	= 24.02
Weight of hydrogen atom	= 6 × 1.01	= 06.06
Weight of oxygen atom	= 1 × 16.00	= 16.00
Molecular weight		= **44.08**

The volume of liquid (mL) reactants can be converted into weight (g) by using density parameter.

Step 3: Calculate the moles of a product formed from each mole of reactant. In case of boric acid, four moles of product is formed.

Step 4: *Limiting reagent identification*. The completely consumed reagent in the reaction is known as limiting reagent. It limits the amount of product formed. In case of boric acid preparation, borax is limiting reagent (borax runs out first). The amount of limiting reagent is useful in the calculation of the product yield.

The limiting reagent can be identified through two methods.

Method 1- Reactant mole ratio method: Comparison of mole ratio of the reactants is basis for this method.

Method 2- Product method: This method utilizes the weight of the products. The reactant which produces the lowest yield is known as limiting reagent. The reactants which produce the higher yield is known as excess reagent.

Convert the given information of reactants (volume, weight) into moles. Calculate the mole ratio and compare the calculated ratio to the actual ratio.

Step 5: *Theoretical yield calculation*. The reaction stoichiometry, provides the information of about the number of moles of product formed with reference to the number of moles of the reactant. Theoretical yiled can be calculated based on the liming reagent concentration.

Step 6: *Percentage yield calculation*. The below given formula is useful in the percent yield calculation.

$$\text{Percentage yield} = \frac{\text{Practical yield}}{\text{Theoretical yield}} \times 100$$

Problem example 1: Two mole of citric acid react with three moles of sodium carbonate to produce sodium citrate. Calculate the theoretical yield and percentage yield, if 2 g of citric acid reacts with 2.5 g of sodium carbonate and produces 2.2 g (practical yield) of sodium citrate.

Step 1: Writing a balanced chemical equation for the reaction.

$$2\ HO{-}C(CH_2COOH)_2{-}COOH\ (\text{Citric acid}) + 3\ Na_2CO_3\ (\text{Sodium carbonate}) \longrightarrow 2HO{-}C(CH_2COONa)_2{-}COONa\ .2H_2O\ (\text{Sodium citrate}) + 3\ CO_2\uparrow + 3\ H_2O$$

Step 2: Calculate the molecular weight of each reactant and product. The sum of the mass of the atoms generates the molecular weight.

Molecular weight of citric acid = 192.12 g/mol

Molecular weight of sodium carbonate = 105.99 g/mol

Molecular weight of sodium citrate = 294.10 g/mol

Step 3: Calculate the moles of a product formed from each mole of reactant. Convert the mass of reactants in terms of moles.

$$\text{Number of moles of a substance} = \frac{\text{Mass of reactant}}{\text{Molar mass of the reactant}}$$

Number of moles of citric acid = 2 / 192.12 = 0.0104 moles

Number of moles of sodium carbonate = 2.5 / 105.99 = 0.0236 moles

Step 4: Limiting reagent identification. This requires the calculation of theoretical yield of sodium citrate based on the citric acid and sodium carbonate separately.

0.0104 moles of citric acid produces 3.06 g of sodium citrate.

0.0236 moles of sodium carbonate produces 4.62 g of sodium citrate.

Hence, citric acid is the limiting reagent and useful in the percent yield calculation.

Step 5: Theoretical yield calculation.

0.0104 moles citric acid produces 3.06 g of sodium citrate.

Step 6: Percentage yield calculation. It is calculated by the formula given below.

Theoretical yield = 3.06 g

Practical yield = 2.2 g

$$\text{Percentage yield} = \frac{\text{Practical yield}}{\text{Theoretical yield}} \times 100$$

$$= \frac{2.2\ g}{3.06\ g} \times 100 = 71.89\%$$

Problem example 2: One mole aniline reacts with one mole of acetic anhydride to produce acetanilide. Calculate the theoretical yield and percentage yield, if 10 mL of aniline reacts with 15 mL of acetic anhydride and produces 11 g (practical yield) of acetanilide.

- ***Step 1***: Writing a balanced chemical equation for the reaction.

$$\text{Aniline} + \text{Acetic anhydride} \xrightarrow{CH_3COOH} \text{Acetanilide}$$

Aniline ($C_6H_5NH_2$) + Acetic anhydride ($H_3C-CO-O-CO-CH_3$) → Acetanilide ($C_6H_5NHCOCH_3$)

- ***Step 2***: Calculate the molecular weight of each reactant and product. The sum of the mass of the atoms generates the molecular weight.

  Molecular weight of aniline is = 93.13 g/mol

  Molecular weight of acetic anhydride is = 102.09 g/mol

  Molecular weight of acetanilide is = 135.17 g/mol

- ***Step 3***: Calculate the moles of a product formed from each mole of reactant. Convert the mass of reactants in terms of moles.

$$\text{Number of moles of a substance} = \frac{\text{Mass of reactant}}{\text{Molar mass of the reactant}}$$

  Number of moles of aniline = 10 × 1.022 (density) / 93.13 = 0.110 moles

  Number of moles of acetic anhydride = 15 × 1.08 (density) / 102.09 = 0.159 moles

- ***Step 4***: Limiting reagent identification. This requires the calculation of theoretical yield of acetanilide based on the aniline and acetic anhydride separately.

  0.110 moles aniline produces 14.86 g of acetanilide.

  0.159 moles acetic anhydride produces 21.49 g of acetanilide.

  Hence, aniline is the limiting reagent and useful in the percent yield calculation.

- ***Step 5***: Theoretical yield calculation.

  0.110 moles aniline produces 14.86 g of acetanilide.

- ***Step 6***: Percentage yield calculation. The below given formula is useful in the calculation.

  Theoretical yield = 14.86 g

  Practical yield = 11 g

$$\text{Percentage yield} = \frac{\text{Practical yield}}{\text{Theoretical yield}} \times 100$$

$$= \frac{11\text{ g}}{14.86\text{ g}} \times 100 = 74\%$$

Problem example 3: One mole salicylic acid reacts with one mole of acetic anhydride to produce aspirin. Calculate the theoretical yield and percentage yield, if 1 g of salicylic acid reacts with 10 mL of acetic anhydride and produces 1.17 g (practical yield) of aspirin.

- ***Step 1***: Writing a balanced chemical equation for the reaction.

Salicylic acid + Acetic anhydride $\xrightarrow{CH_3COOH}$ Aspirin (acetyl salicylic acid)

- ***Step 2***: Calculate the molecular weight of each reactant and product. The sum of the mass of the atoms generates the molecular weight.

  Molecular weight of salicylic acid is = 138.12 g/mol

  Molecular weight of acetic anhydride is = 102.09 g/mol

  Molecular weight of aspirin is = 180.158 g/mol

- ***Step 3***: Calculate the moles of a product formed from each mole of reactant. Convert the mass of reactants in terms of moles.

$$\text{Number of moles of a substance} = \frac{\text{Mass of reactant}}{\text{Molar mass of the reactant}}$$

  Number of moles of salicylic acid = 1 / 138.12 = 0.0072 moles

  Number of moles of acetic anhydride

  = 10 × 1.08 (density) / 102.09 = 0.106 moles

- ***Step 4***: Limiting reagent identification. This requires the calculation of theoretical yield of aspirin based on the salicylic acid and acetic anhydride separately.

  0.0072 moles salicylic acid produces 1.304 g of aspirin.

  0.106 moles acetic anhydride produces 19.06 g of aspirin.

  Hence, salicylic acid is the limiting reagent and useful in the percent yield calculation.

- ***Step 5***: Theoretical yield calculation.

  0.0072 moles salicylic acid produces 1.304 g of aspirin.

- ***Step 6***: Percentage yield calculation. The below given formula is useful in the calculation.

  Theoretical yield = 1.304 g

  Practical yield = 1.17 g

$$\text{Percentage yield} = \frac{\text{Practical yield}}{\text{Theoretical yield}} \times 100$$

$$= \frac{1.17\ \text{g}}{1.034\ \text{g}} \times 100 = 89.72\%$$

2

Laboratory Safety

2.1 Safety Practices

Chemical experiments are expected to produce danger, if adequate precautions are not taken into consideration. Many potential hazards are known, but caution and precautionary attempts ensures the safety. The majority of chemical hazardous events are due to the hurry in conducting the experiments and negligence in work.

Toxicity and flammability of solvents are major concern in laboratories. Most chemicals are carcinogenic and cause deleterious effect to health.

Safety *is a freedom from danger, injury or damage. The acronym RAMP is a mneumonic guide for laboratory safety.*

R - Recognize hazards

A - Assess the risk of hazards

M - Minimize the risks of hazards

P - Prepare for emergencies

Safety ethics

1) I value safety
2) I learn to recognise the at-risk behaviour
3) I work safety
4) I educate and promote safety
5) I prevent at-risk behaviour
6) I accept responsibility for safety

General requirements

- Water-proof and vapour-proof electric lamps, switches and power points
- Fire resistant doors and walls
- Exhauster fans
- Firc cxtinguishers
- First aid kit
- Safety warning display cards
- Trained lab attender

2.2 Safety Rules

The following specific rules provide adequate guidelines for preventing the hazardous events.

1. ***Good ventilation:*** Adequate ventilation prevents the accumulation of hazardous vapours and flammable vapours. Flammable vapours can travel faster than air and remain in drain troughs and sinks (source for ignition).

   Laboratory should be well ventilated and Personal Protective Equipments (PPEs) should be worn (especially during distillation and operations under reduced pressure/elevated temperature).

2. ***Safety Awareness:***

   (a) ***Personal protective equipments (PPEs):*** Respirators, safety goggles, gloves and lab coats (apron) are examples for PPEs. These PPEs should be available in work place for their use, when required. Plastic or tempered glass safety goggles with side shields and brow bars are useful. A protective glove minimizes the skin contact of chemicals.

   · ***Lab coats (apron):*** Put on laboratory coat, while in the laboratory, handling with hazardous chemicals and hazardous reactions. This provides protection against chemical splashes and potential exposure for both the person and their clothing.

   · ***Respirators:*** It is a form of personal protective equipment (PPE). It filters the contaminated air (airborne contaminants). It provides additional protection along with fume hood and other devices.

   Disposable mask respirator: Mainly useful in hospitals and other clinical areas.

   Cartridge respirator: This forces all inhaled air through a cartridge filled with absorbent material. Different coloured masks are available.

   - *Organic vapour* – Black, brown and yellow
   - *Acid gases* – White, yellow and brown

   Self-contained breathing apparatus (SCBA) – also known as compressed air breathing apparatus (CABA). It is a device that provides breathable air in dangerous atmosphere (fire-fighting/industry). It does not need remote supply of breathing gas hence, known as self-contained.

   Gloves: The thickness of the glove is an important factor. The glove should be removed by reverse peeling (from wrist). This ensures no chemical or hazard transfer to skin.

Glove type	Material	Protection	Caution
Latex glove	Natural rubber	Acids and bases	Latex allergies
Nitrile gloves (blue, purple and green)	Acetonitrile -butadiene (AB)	Hydrocarbons solvents	Hydrocarbons may degrade the glove
Silver shields	Five-layer polyethylene and ethylene vinyl alcohol	Resistant to alcohols, aliphatics, aromatics, chlorines, ketones and esters	-
Mitten	E-glass fabric	Temperature Resistant Gloves	-

(b) ***Safety equipments****:* Gain knowledge on the location and operation of safety equipments. Safety showers, eyewashes, fire extinguishers, first-aid kits and explosion-proof refrigerators are few important safety equipments.

(c) ***Training***: Adequate training should be acquired for operating any laboratory equipment and understanding for safe working. Never attempt to operate equipments/instruments and unfamiliar procedures without training. When performing the new experiments, make sure that the experienced person (instructor) is available for consultation. It is advisable to conduct some experiments under the supervision.

3. ***Personal safety:***
   - ***Physical contact***: Touch, smell, inhalation and taste of chemicals are most dangerous.
   - ***Chemical shield:*** Proper shields must be worn before handling with peroxides.
   - ***Corrosiveness***: Chlorosulphonic acid is more dangerous than sulphuric acid. Picric acid stains the skin. Hence, use rubber gloves, while handling these chemicals.
   - ***Emergency exit***: Knowledge about the emergency exit location is essential.
   - ***Team work***: Never attempt to perform reactions alone in the laboratory.
   - ***Exit safety***: Properly turn-off the gas supply, water supply, power supply, vacuum lines, compression lines and heating apparatus before leaving the laboratory.
   - ***Medical monitoring***: Routine medical monitoring is essential for the workers.
   - ***UV radiation:*** Ultraviolet (UV) lamps and arcs should not be viewed directly. Exposure of eye and skin to UV radiation cause eye damage and skin burns (use goggles and shields).
4. ***Chemical safety:*** Chemical hazardous exposure results in burns, inflammation, allergic responses, eye irritation and dizziness. Hence minimize all chemical exposures, observe exposure limits and institute chemical hygiene plan.

- ***Programs***: Developing and implementing preventative maintenance program and safety awareness for chemical operations provides protection against chemical hazardous exposure. Aware of possible environmental threats and institute environmental protection measures.
- ***Label:*** Label all the reagent/chemical containers to avoid confusion and chemical accidents.
- ***Acids:*** Concentrated acids should be added slowly to the flask containing water under cooling for dilution purpose.
- ***Chemical substituent***: Use prescribed chemicals alone and do not substitute with other similar chemicals. Lithium aluminium hydride (explosive in water) and sodium borohydride should not be substituted.
- ***Chemical disposal:*** The laboratory should be equipped with waste solvent container for collecting waste organic solvents and solutions. Small volume of non-hazardous chemicals can be flushed down (drain) with large volume of water. These chemicals include acids and bases, which can be neutralized and diluted before draining them.
  - Organic solvents are carbon based *(e.g.,* benzene) and are water insoluble (most of them). These solvents are toxic and flammable. Hence require appropriate disposal.
  - Tollen's reagent (oxidising agent for detecting aldehydes and reducing sugar) requires special precaution. The silver nitride (Ag_3N) formed as a by-product is explosive (even by friction). It is hazardous and should be diluted with acid before disposal.
- ***Decontamination:*** This process removes or neutralizes the toxic agents through sterilization and disinfection.
- ***Fume hood***: The reactions with hazardous and toxic substances should be conducted in fume hood. The reaction which produces flammable gases and vapours also requires fume hood environment. Ensure that the exhaust blower is operating and air is entering the fume hood.

  A potentially violent reaction should be conducted on an open bench with safety sides (not on the top). Fume hood is not advisable, because the glass window of fume hood cannot withstand an explosion.

5. ***Compressed Gas Safety:*** Gaseous chemical identity (label and tags) is very important before accessing them. Never use unknown gases. Compressed gas (oxygen, helium and hydrogen) cylinders should be firmly secured at all times. The main valve of the cylinder should be shut off (not the regulator) when the cylinder is not in use. A suspected leak can be confirmed by brushing with 1% Teepol solution.
6. ***Flammable Safety:*** Adequate protection for the inflammable solids and liquids are essential. Diethyl ether (b.p 35 °C) catches fire even from a hot plate (~160 °C).
   - ***Sodium metal safety:*** A contact between water and sodium metal should be avoided. The contact leads to explosions. Hence, it is normally stored in liquid paraffin.

- ***Containers*:** The container should be closed (place lid/cap) immediately after transferring the chemical. Place the containers away from heat, sparks and sources of ignition. Store flammable liquids in the specific cabinets or storage rooms designed for flammables. Bulk solvents should be stored in safety containers for dispensing to prevent the possible flame catching.
- ***Limit*:** The storage of flammable liquids in the laboratory should be limited.
- ***Refrigerator*:** Sparkless "flammable storage" should be installed for storing refrigerator for flammables.
- ***Fire extinguishers*:** The knowledge about the fire extinguishers location and its operation are very essential. Carbon dioxide or dry chemical (ammonium phosphate) fire extinguishers are available.

  ***Dry chemical extinguisher*:** It usually contains ammonium phosphate. Phosphate decomposes into phosphoric acid (on exposure to fire) and seals the burning material from atmospheric oxygen.

  ***Dry powder extinguisher*:** Sand, copper powder, graphite, sodium carbonate.

  ***Halon extinguisher*:** It contains bromochlorodifluoromehane or bromotrifluoromethane. It is very effective and expensive.

Fires

Class A: Ordinary combustibles (e.g., wood, paper).

Class B: Organic flammable liquids (e.g., ether).

Class C: Energised electricity (e.g., hot plate, computer, air conditioner).

Class D: Reactive metals (e.g., sodium, lithium).

Type	A	B	C	D	Colour code of container
Pressurized water	√	-	-	-	Silver
Carbon dioxide	√	√	-	-	Red
Dry chemical (BC)	-	√	√	-	Red
Dry chemical (ABC)	√	√	√	-	Red
Class D (e.g., sand)	-	-	-	√	Red

Easy acronym for the use of fire extinguisher

PASS: **P**ull **A**im **S**queeze **S**weep

- *Pull:* Pull the pin (or ring) at the top of the extinguisher to break the seal.
- *Aim:* Aim the nozzle towards the base of the fire, stand approximately 8 feet away from the fire
- *Squeeze:* Squeeze the handle in short intervals to discharge the extinguisher chemical.
- *Sweep:* Sweep the nozzle back and forth horizontally across the base of the fire.

Do not replace the fire extinguisher, it requires refilling.

A fire in a beaker or flask can be cut-off by covering with flat object (prevents oxygen supply).

7. ***Corrosive Safety:*** Proper personal protective equipments (PPEs) for eyes, face, hands and body should be used while handling corrosive (hazardous) chemicals. Inorganic acids (e.g., concentrated sulphuric acid, concentrated nitric acid, chromic acid and hydrofluoric acid), inorganic bases (e.g., sodium hydroxide, potassium hydroxide) and organic solvents (e.g., acetone) are corrosive chemicals and cause severe burns. They require gloves while handling.
   - Concentrated acids should be poured into the water as a thin stream for dilution. This action prevents acid splash and spray.
   - Chlorosulphonic acid and sodamide reacts very violently with water.
8. ***Toxic Safety:***
   - **Eye toxic:** Sodium hydroxide and potassium hydroxide.
   - **Bronchial irritant:** Ammonium hydroxide.
   - **Lachrymator:** Acid chlorides (benzoyl chloride), inorganic halides and anhydrides.
   - **Lung toxic:** chloroform, hydrogen sulphide
   - **Mucous membrane toxic:** Ammonium sulphide, ammonium chromate, chromic acid, benzoyl peroxide, chromic acid and formaldehyde.
   - **Teratogenic chemicals:** These chemicals are toxic to embryo (cause abnormalities in fetus). It includes benzene, toluene, xylene, phenol, nitrobenzene, dimethyl formamide (DMF) dimethyl sulphoxide (DMSO), formaldehyde, hydrogen sulphide (H_2S), carbon disulphide (CS_2), carbon monoxide, nitrites, nitrous oxide, heavy metals and polyphenols.
   - **CNS toxic:** The inhalation of dimethyl sulphate vapours leads to giddiness and more toxic effects. Hydrazine vapours cause CNS toxicity. Mercury, phenol, benzene, carbon disulfide, chloroform, methylene chloride and sodium fluoride. Liquid and vapours of benzene are potentially carcinogenic and can be replaced with less toxic toluene.
9. ***Glassware Safety:*** Borosilicate is recommended for all laboratory glassware and never use cracked or chipped glassware. Pyrex and shatterproof glassware can be used for special applications.
10. ***Electrical Safety:*** The following guidelines should be verified before switching on the electrical instrument.
    - Good operating condition.
    - Absence of loose wires or connections.
    - Correct type of plug, good quality cable with insulation.

    The flammable vapour may remain in thermostat vacuum pumps, drying ovens and gets ignited by electrical spark.

2.3 First Aid

First-aid is the very first (immediate) assistance given to an ill or injured person. It also includes calling emergency medical services. It provides a simple reassurance after a small accident to dealing with a life threatening emergency. The very important aspect of the first aid is to create comfort, reassurance and not to create panic. A speedy (in-time) attempt is very important.

The best response is to take a deep breath to calm down (overcomes panic) and then decide the actual response.

First-aid box: Each laboratory must be equipped with first-aid box. Wall chart should be located near the first-aid box.

Health, safety & environment (HSE) guidelines

- **Assessment of first aid needs:** It depends on the type of work in that laboratory, hazards and the likely risk, size of the workforce, working patterns of the staff and history of the previous accidents.
- **Appointment of in charge of first aid:** A person has to be appointed to take care of first aid arrangements, such as monitoring of equipement, facilities and calling emergency services. Incharge must be always available when staffs/students are at work.
- **Contents of first aid kit:** The contents of a first aid kit vary according to the work activities at low, moderate/high-risk areas. The minimum requirements include a leaflet with first aid guidelines, individually wrapped sterile plasters, sterile eye pads, triangular sterile bandages, safety pins, wound dressings of different sizes and disposable gloves. The kit should be checked regularly and replace the items as per their expiry date.

Trained first-aider: First aiders should be trained in two areas

- ***First aid at work (FAW):*** Training to address a range of specific injuries and illnesses.
- ***Emergency first aid at work (EFAW):*** Training to give emergency first aid to someone who injured or ill while at work.

The ABC (Airway, Breathing and Circulation) support is the top priority of first aid.

Airway: Opening the airway with a head tilt chin lift maneuver.

Breathing: Looking, listening and feeling for breathing.

Circulation: Perform chest compression to support circulation in case of non-responsive individuals.

The major first aid activities applicable to the laboratory are

- Cleaning minor cuts, scrapes and scratches
- Treating minor burns
- Applying bandages and dressings
- Cold compress, cold pack ice bag
- Splint

All injuries that are a result of a spill must be attended immediately.

(1) ***Cuts and bleeding:*** Flush the wound thoroughly with water, apply antiseptic and bandage to prevent contamination. If the bleeding is uncontrollable then rise the bleeding part and apply pressure to the wound with sterile gauze.

- ***Minor cut:*** Wash the cut with water, remove any visible pieces of glass (causative) or other objectives. Apply pressure to arrest the bleeding. Medical attention is required based on the severity.
- ***Major cut:*** Never use tourniquet. Place a pad directly on the cut (wound), apply pressure. Do not create panic.

(2) ***Inhalation:*** Move to fresh air.

(3) ***Swallowing:*** Get emergency medical assistance.

(4) ***Burns***

- ***Thermal burns:*** Flush the burned area with cool running water at least for 15 minutes (can be continued, if required). Do not try to blisters or rub the skin. Place a dry, sterile dressing over the burn are to keep clean.
- ***Chemical burns:*** Flush the affected area with plenty of water for several minutes (at least 15 minutes). Acid or minor bromine burns may be treated with sodium bicarbonate (5%) solution. Alkali burns may be washed with 5% acetic acid or saturated boric acid. Wrap the burned area loosely. Skin burns requires immediate medical attention.
- ***Cloth burning:*** Prevent the person from running and fanning the flames. Roll the person on the floor (clean). This prevents the inhalation of flames and extinguishes the flame. Remove the contaminated clothing and move the person under safety shower for extinguishing the flames. Medical attention is required.
- ***Dimethyl sulphate burns***: Wash the spills and splash of dimethyl sulphate (DMS) immediately with ammonium hydroxide and then rub gently by cotton wool soaked in ammonia solution.

(5) ***Eye injury:*** Flush the eye immediately with copious amount of water in the water wash fountain for about 15 minutes. Alternatively the person can be positioned on the floor and water can be sprayed. Medical attention is required.

- Irritation in eyes can be treated with thorough water washing.
- Acid/alkali in eyes can be removed by thorough water washing.
- In case, glass pieces in eyes, glass should be removed gently without rubbing eyes and immediately consult doctor.

(6) ***Chemical spills on skin:*** The treatment of skin in case spills depends on the type of spill. Use safety shower for large amount of chemical slipped on the body.

- ***Acidic spills:*** Wash with water followed by ice-cold water, then treated with saturated sodium bicarbonate solution and then again with ice-cold water. Apply disinfectant, dry the skin and cover with antiseptic cream

- ***Basic spills:*** Wash with water followed by ice-cold water, then treated with acetic acid (1%) solution and then again with ice-cold water. Apply disinfectant, dry the skin and cover with antiseptic cream.
- ***Bromine spills:*** Treated liberally with ammonia solution (2%) and then with ice-cold water. Wipe gently with glycerine and apply antiseptic cream.

(7) ***Fainting and shock:*** Place the victim in a prone position with head lower than the feet.

DOs and DONT's		
	DO'S	DON'TS
Lab coats must be worn in this area	Wear laboratory coat (apron).	Never conduct experiment without wearing laboratory coats (apron).
	Wear safety gloves.	Do not touch objectives like computer and doors, when wearing gloves.
Eye protection must be worn	Wear safety goggles. Keep a warning board about the importance of goggles.	Do not expose to hazardous reaction environment without putting eye shield. Do not wear contact lenses during laboratory work. But, contact lenses along with safety goggles can be used
	Legs should be covered with closed-toe shoes. Feet must be completely covered. Shoes with soles are advisable.	Do not wear open toed shoes. Shoes with heels and sneakers are not advisable.
	Use fume hood for cautious reactions.	Do not introduce face inside the fume hood and ensure the minimum storage of chemicals in the fume hood.
	Confine long hair and loose clothing.	Don't leave hair uncovered. Avoid tight clothing, as it creates breathing problem while handling strong acids and alkalies in lab.

Table *Contd...*

DOs and DONT's		
	DO'S	DON'TS
	Wash hands before (especially before eating) and after handling contaminated material.	Do not eat anything while working in lab.
	Use bulb pipette/micro pipette for measuring harmful liquid chemicals.	Do not attempt to pipette through mouth suction.
	Wash off spilled and splashed chemicals on skin and cloths with water immediately.	Do not use solvent to remove chemical from skin.
	Return reagent continers to proper locations.	Do not leave any chemical/ solvent bottles on platform after completion of experimentation.
No Food or Drink	Practice the habit of not having water and food in the laboratory.	Drinking and eating in the laboratory is forbidden.
CAUTION CHEMICAL STORAGE ONLY NO FOOD OR DRINK IN THIS UNIT; BIOHAZARDS NO FOOD OR DRINK STORAGE IN THIS REFRIGERATOR	Laboratory refrigerator is meant for chemicals and related substance. Keep a label on the refrigerator stating not to keep food inside.	Do not store food and beverages in the lab refrigerator.
Wash your hands before handling food	After the laboratory experiment, immediately clean hands with soap solution.	Do not touch anything (food, clean surfaces, clothes, etc) without cleaning hands after laboratory work/experiment.

3

Acylation

Acylation process involves the introduction (addition) of an acyl group (R_2-C=O) into the aromatic compounds. The acylation is an intermediate step in the synthesis of several pharmaceuticals. The most important acylation reactions are listed below.

1. **Friedel-Crafts acylation:** It involves the reaction between arenes and acylchlorides/anhydrides in presence of Lewis acid catalyst ($AlCl_3$). This reaction produces ketones and can be converted into corresponding alkanes by reduction (Clemmenson/Wolff-Kishner reduction).
2. **C-Acylation:** Attachment of acyl group (substitution) to aromatic rings forms ketone.
3. **N-Acylation:** It involves the reaction between amines (ammonia, primary and secondary amines) and acylating agents to form amides (primary, secondary and tertiary amides).
4. **O-Acylation:** It involves the reaction between phenolic–OH group and acylating agents to form esters.
5. **S-Acylation:** It involves the reaction between thiol group and acylating agents to form thioesters.

General Reaction Mechanism

$$R-\overset{O}{\overset{\|}{C}}-Cl + AlCl_3 \longrightarrow R-C\overset{+}{\equiv}O + \overset{-}{AlCl_4}$$

Acid chloride → Acylium ion

Arene + Acylium ion ($R-C\overset{+}{\equiv}O$) → [arenium intermediate] $\xrightarrow{\overset{-}{AlCl_4}}$ Acylated arene + $AlCl_3$ + HCl

Reaction mechanism for Friedel-Crafts acylation

Step 1: Complex formation between acyl halide and Lewis acid

$$R-\overset{O}{\overset{\|}{C}}-Cl + AlCl_3 \longrightarrow R-\overset{O}{\overset{\|}{C}}-\overset{+}{Cl}-\overset{-}{Al}Cl_3$$

Acid chloride — Acyl chloride-aluminium chloride complex

Step 2: Formation of acylium ion

$$R-\overset{O}{\overset{\|}{C}}-\overset{+}{Cl}-\overset{-}{Al}Cl_3 \longrightarrow R-\overset{+}{C}\equiv O + Al\overset{-}{Cl_4}$$

Acyl chloride - aluminium chloride complex — Acylium ion

Step 3: Nucleophilic attack on electrophilic carbon of acylium ion

Acylium ion $R-\overset{+}{C}\equiv O$

H

O

H

R

+

Arene

Step 4: Removal of proton from aromatic compound and regeneration of catalyst

H O

R $Al\overset{-}{Cl_4}$

+

O

R

$+ AlCl_3 + HCl$

Acylated arene (aryl ketone)

Acylating agents

Acyalting agents contain activated acyl group. Acyl group is a cation formed from the corresponding carboxylic acid by the removal of hydroxyl group. The compounds which provide acyl groups are known as acylating agents (e.g., acyl halides, R-CO-X). The R group can be aliphatic, alicylic and aromatic.

- **Acyl halides:** The acyl halides names are derived from the corresponding carboxylic acid by incorporating the suffix 'oyl'. In case of acetyl chloride (ethanoyl chloride), the name is derived from ethanoic acid with the suffix 'oyl'.
  - **(a)** ***Acetyl chloride*:** Acetyl chloride in pyridine is the most common acetylating agent. Acetyl chloride in combinations with $ZrOCl_2.8H_2O$,

zinc dust and thermally decomposed Ni-Fe-hydrotalcite also can be used. The high reactivity and water instability (explosive) limits the use of acetyl chloride.

(b) ***Benzoyl chloride:*** This acylating agent attaches benzoyl group into the aromatic compounds. It is useful in the Schotten-Baumman reaction and Friedel-crafts reactions. It is useful in the manufacture of benzophenone, which is intermediate in the synthesis of pharmaceuticals.

- **Acetic anhydride:** In view of the above mentioned limitations of acetyl chloride, acetic anhydride is preferred for acetylation. Generally acetylation with acetic anhydride will be carried out in presence of bases, such as triethylamine, pyridine and 4-dimethyl amino pyridine (DMAP). Acetylation by acetic anhydride proceeds very well in aqueous medium, such as acetic acid and sodium bicarbonate solution.
- **Miscellaneous:** Isocyanate, isothiocynates, imidoesters, *N*-hydroxysuccinimidyl esters, sulphonyl chlorides and ketenes.

Catalysts in acylation

Acylation process can be catalyzed by acidic, basic and organo metallic compounds.

Acidic catalysts: The majority of acylation reactions are catalyzed by acidic catalysts. These catalysts increase the electrophilic character of the acylating agents.

- ***Acidic halides*:** Aluminium chloride ($AlCl_3$), ferric chloride ($FeCl_3$), boron trifluoride (BF_3), cadmium chloride ($CdCl_3$), zinc chloride ($ZnCl_2$), stannous chloride ($SnCl_2$), rutherium (III) chloride ($RuCl_3$), Lanthanide nitrate ($LaNO_3$), niobium (v) chloride ($NbCl_5$), sodium bisulphate ($NaHSO_4$) and silicon *di*-oxide (SiO_2).
- ***Proton acids*:** Sulphuric acid (H_2SO_4), anhydrous hydrogen fluoride (HF), hydrogen chloride (HCl) and phosphoric acid (H_3PO_4). Combination of proton acids and Lewis acids such as hydrochloric acid-aluminium chloride (HCl-$AlCl_3$) hydrochloric acid-boron trifluoride (HCl-BF_3) and acid-borontrifluoride (H_2SO_4- BF_3).
- ***Liquid super acid*:** Sulphuric acid (100%), antimony pentafluoride (SbF_5), niobium (v) fluoride (NbF_5), arsenic pentafluoride (AsF_5) and tantalum pentafluoride (TaF_5).
- ***Supported acids*:** Solid phosphoric acid (phosphoric acid adsorbed on Kiselguhr), graphite-intercalated aluminium chloride.
- ***Heteropolyacids*:** Vanado, Molibdo and tungsto polyacids.
- ***Ionic liquids*:** Chloroaluminate (III) liquids namely 1-butylpyridinium chloride-aluminium (III) chloride and 1-butyl-3-methylimidazolium chloride-aluminium (III) chloride.
- ***Solid super acids*:** Sulphated oxides

- ***Alkoxides*:** Aluminium phenoxide.
- ***Miscellaneous*:** Ethyl acetate, ammonium acetate in acetic acid and acetic acid with ferric-monomorillonite.

Basic catalysts: These catalysts increase the nucleophilicity of the substrates.

- Sodium alkoxides, sodium amide, sodium hydride (NaH), tributylphosphines, 4-pyrrolidinopyridine and *N,N*-dimethyl amino pyridine (DMAP).
- ***Basic oxides*:** Magnesium oxide (MgO), zirconium dioxide (ZrO_2) and lanthanum oxide (La_2O_3).

Important acylation reactions

Schotten-Baumann reaction: The reaction between aliphatic amine, alcohol and acid chloride in aqueous alkali generates an amides /esters.

$$\underset{\text{Amine}}{R{-}NH_2} + \underset{\text{Acid chloride}}{R_1{-}\overset{O}{\overset{\|}{C}}{-}Cl} \xrightarrow{NaOH} \underset{\text{Amide}}{R_1{-}\overset{O}{\overset{\|}{C}}{-}NH{-}R}$$

$$\underset{\text{Alcohol}}{R{-}OH} + \underset{\text{Acid chloride}}{R_1{-}\overset{O}{\overset{\|}{C}}{-}Cl} \xrightarrow{NaOH} \underset{\text{Ester}}{R_1{-}\overset{O}{\overset{\|}{C}}{-}O{-}R}$$

Kostanecki reaction: The acylation of *ortho*-hydroxyaryl ketones with aliphatic anhydrides and subsequent cyclization forms chromones and coumarins.

OH, CH_3, O — o-Hydroxy acetophenone + R, O, O, O, R — Aliphatic anhydride → O, CH_3, O — Chromone; O, O, R — Coumarin

Houben Hoesch reaction: The nitrile group reacts with an arene group and forms an arylketone. This reaction can be catalyzed by the mixture of hydrochloric acid and aluminium chloride.

HO, OH — Resorcinol $\xrightarrow[HCl,\ AlCl_3]{R\text{-}CN}$ HO, OH, NH.HCl, R → HO, OH, O, R — Arylketone

Acetylation: Acylation of functional group by acetyl chloride and/acetic anhydride is known as acetylation. It is also known as ethanoylation. The alcohols (R-OH), phenols (Ar-OH), primary amines (R-NH_2) and secondary amines (R-NH-R) can be directly acetylated. This reaction replaces the active hydrogen of hydroxyl and amino (1° & 2°) groups by an acetyl group of acetylating agent.

Acetic anhydride

Acid chloride

Substituted arene
X = OH, NH_2

Acetylated arene
X = O, NH

- ***O-Acetylation:*** Acetylation of alcohol and phenols offer acetyl esters. It is an efficient method for the characterization and protection of amines.
- ***N-Acetylation:*** Acetylation of primary and secondary amines offer amides. It is an efficient method for the characterization and protection of amines.

Pharmaceutical Applications

1. Friedel-Crafts acylation

(a) The C-acylation of 3-methoxynaphthalene offers 2-acyl-6-methoxynaphthalene, the precursor of anti-inflammatory drug naproxen.

CH_3COCl, $AlCl_3$

3-Methoxynaphthalene

2-Acyl-6-methoxy naphthalene

Naproxen

2. C-Acylation

(a) Acetophenone, an acylation product of benzene is useful in the synthesis of perfumes and pharmaceuticals.

Acetic anhydride

Acetyl chloride

Benzene

Acetophenone (acylated benzene)

(b) The *para* acylated (C-acylated) veratrole is an intermediate for the synthesis of cardiotonic drug vesnarinone.

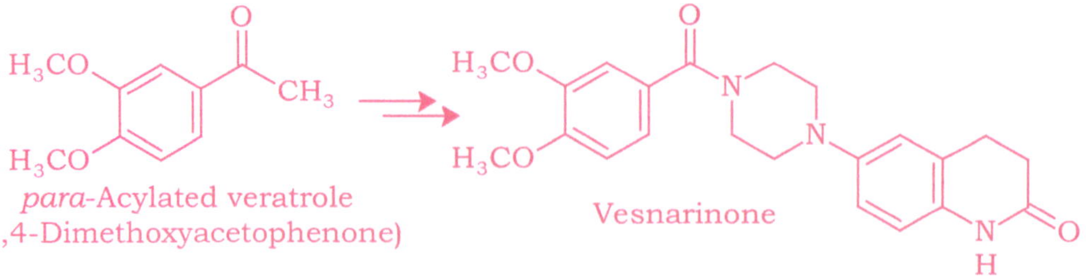

para-Acylated veratrole
(3,4-Dimethoxyacetophenone)

Vesnarinone

(c) Tolmetin (anti-inflammatory drug) preparation involves the Friedel-Crafts acylation. The acylation between (1-methyl-1*H*-pyrrol-2-yl)acetonitrile and *para*-toluoyl chloride forms the intermediate for the generation of tolmetin.

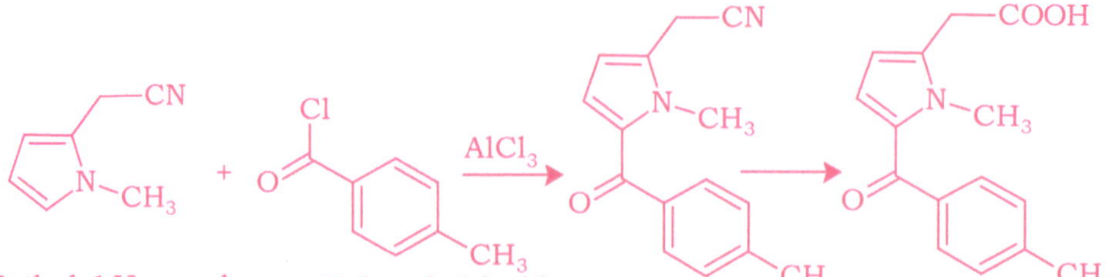

$AlCl_3$

(1-Methyl-1*H*-pyrrol-2-yl) acetonitrile

para-Toluoyl chloride

Tolmetin

(d) The *para* acylated (C-acylated) anisole is an intermediate in the preparation of sweetening agent 2-(4-methoxy benzoyl) benzoic acid.

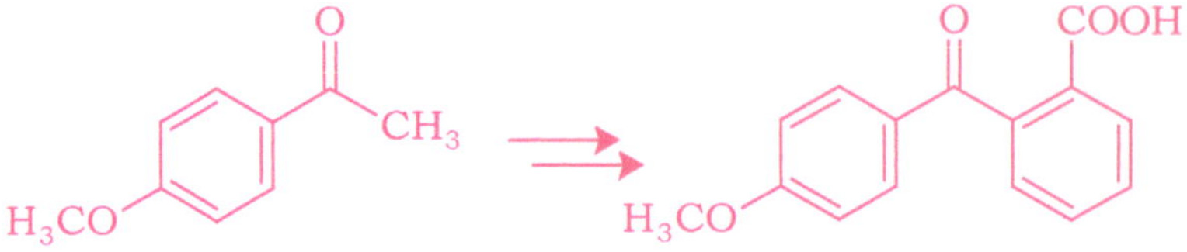

para-Acylated anisole
(4-Methoxyacetophenone)

2-(4-Methoxy-benzoyl) benzoic acid

3. N-Acylation

(a) The N-acylation of 5-methoxy-2-methyl-*1H*-indol-3-yl acetic acid with *para*-chlorobenzoyl chloride offers the indomethacin, an anti-inflammatory agent.

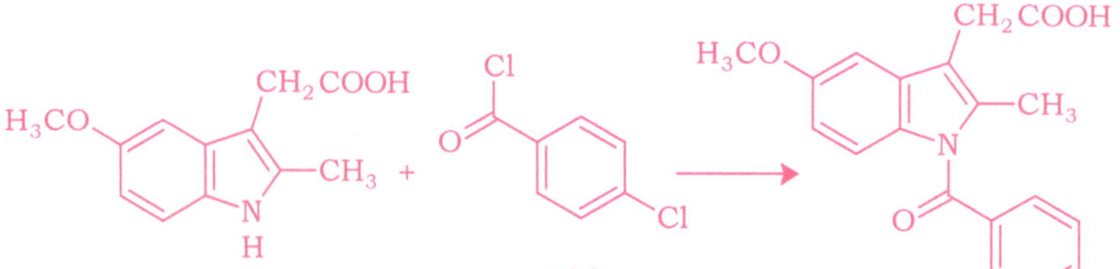

5-Methoxy-2-methyl-1*H*-indol-3yl-acetic acid

4-Chloro benzoyl chloride

Indomethacin

(b) The N-acylation of 3,5-diamino-2,4,6-triiodo benzoic acid offers amidotrizoic acid (X-ray contrast agent).

COOH, I, I, H_2N, NH_2, I — $(CH_3CO)_2O$ → COOH, I, I, O, O, H_3C, N, H, N, H, CH_3, I

3,5-Diamino-2,4,6-triiodo benzoic acid — Amidotrizoic acid

(c) Acetylation of 4-aminophenol (N-acetylation) offers antipyretic drug paracetamol (4-hydroxyacetanilide).

HO—C₆H₄—NH_2 $\xrightarrow{(CH_3CO)_2O}$ HO—C₆H₄—NH—C(=O)—CH_3

para-Aminophenol (4-Aminophenol) — Paracetamol

(d) The acetylation (N-acetylation) of 4-amino-5-chloro-2-methoxy benzoic acid produces metoclopramide (anti-histaminergic and anti-emetic drug).

COOH, H_3CO, Cl, NH_2 — $(CH_3CO)_2O$ → COOH, H_3CO, Cl, $NHCOCH_3$ — $SOCl_2$, $NH_2(CH_2)_2N(C_2H_5)_2$ → O, $NH(CH_2)_2N(C_2H_5)_2$, H_3CO, Cl, $NHCOCH_3$

4-Amino-5-chloro-2-methoxybenzoic acid — Acetylated intermediate — Metoclopramide

(e) The N-acetylation of salicylamide produces salacetamide (anti-pyretic, anti-inflammatory).

OH, O, NH_2 — $(CH_3CO)_2O$ → OH, O, $NHCOCH_3$

Salicylamide — Salacetamide

(f) Cinapazet (anti-hypercholesteremic) can be prepared by the N-acylation between piperazine ethyl acetate and 3,4,5-cinnamoyl chloride.

4. **O-Acylation:** The acetylation of alcohols and phenols are special case of esterification.

(a) Aspirin, an anti-inflammatory and antiplatelet drug can be prepared by the acetylation (*O*-acylation) of salicylic acid.

PREPARATION OF DRUG INTERMEDIATES

3.1 Preparation of Acetanilide

Traditional Name: Antifebrin, Acetyl aniline, Acetyl amino benzene

IUPAC Name: N-Phenylacetamide **Mol wt**: 135.17 g/mol

History of acetanilide: The acetanilide was discovered serendipitously in 1886 and introduced as medicine in the name of antifebrin for the analgesic and antipyretic effects. The toxic effects namely cyanosis and methemoglobinemia made their use obsolete. The structural modifications generated alternative for acetanilide, namely paracatamol and phenacetin.

Method-1

Principle: Acetanilide can be prepared by N-acetylation of aniline. The replacement of active hydrogen of amino group of aniline by an acetyl group (N-acetylation) of acetylating reagent (acetic anhydride/acetyl chloride) produces acetanilide. The reaction occurs readily in the presence of acetic acid.

$$C_6H_5NH_2 + (CH_3CO)_2O \xrightarrow{\text{Gla } CH_3COOH} C_6H_5NHCOCH_3$$

Aniline Acetic anhydride Acetanilide

Reaction Mechanism

The movement of carbonyl group electrons towards oxygen make carbonyl carbon positive (electron deficient). The unpaired electrons in nitrogen attaches to positively charged carbon. Elimination of hydrogen atom from the amino group removes the positive charge present on it. Movement of electrons from carbonyl oxygen reestablishes π bond between carbon and oxygen. This facilitates the bond breaking between carbonyl carbon and acetoxy oxygen of acetic anhydride and generates acetanilide.

H_3C O CH_3 Acetic anhydride :NH_2 Aniline → H_3C O CH_3 H–$\overset{+}{N}$–H → – CH_3COOH → HN CH_3 Acetanilide

Procedure:

Chemicals Required: Aniline, Acetic anhydride, Glacial acetic acid, Charcoal.

1. Place acetic anhydride (5 mL, 53 mmol) and glacial acetic acid (5 mL, 87 mmol) to the flask containing aniline (5 mL, 55 mmol).
2. Swirl the flask gently to dissolve the contents completely.
   (If it is in brown colour, decolorize the solution by boiling with charcoal and filter).
3. Attach condenser to the flask and boil it gently for 10 min.
4. Pour the hot reaction mixture into beaker containing cold water (100 mL) with stirring.
5. Isolate the crude acetanilide crystals by filtration under suction, wash with water and dry.
6. Purify the crude acetanilide by recrystallization with hot water.
7. The melting range of pure acetanilide is 113 to 115 °C.

Method-2

Principle: N-acetylation in aniline occurs readily in the presence of hydrochloric acid. The hydrochloric acid enhances the solubility of aniline by converting it into anilinium ion. Anhydrous sodium acetate converts the anilinium ion (*in situ*) into aniline which then undergoes acetylation to produce acetanilide. This process offers improved reaction rate and product yield.

$$C_6H_5NH_2 + (CH_3CO)_2O \xrightarrow[CH_3COONa]{HCl} C_6H_5NHCOCH_3$$

Aniline Acetic anhydride Acetanilide

Reaction Mechanism

Acetic anhydride

NH_2, Aniline $\xrightarrow{HCl}$ $^{+}NH_3Cl$, Anilinium ion $\xrightarrow{CH_3COONa}$ $:NH_2$, Aniline $\rightarrow$ H_3C, O^-, O, CH_3, $H-\overset{+}{N}-H$ $\xrightarrow{-CH_3COOH}$ HN, O, CH_3, Acetanilide

Procedure:

Chemicals Required: Aniline, Acetic anhydride, Hydrochloric acid, Charcoal, Sodium acetate.

1. Dilute hydrochloric acid (4.6 mL) using water (125 mL) with swirling.
2. Add aniline (5 mL, 55 mmol) to the resulting dilute acid containing beaker with swirling (swirling facilitates the solubilization).

   (If it is in brown colour, decolorize the solution by boiling with charcoal and filter).
3. Warm the aniline hydrochloride solution (~50 °C), and add redistilled acetic anhydride (6.4 mL, 68 mmol).
4. Swirl the flask vigorously and pour the contents immediately into the sodium acetate solution (crystallized sodium acetate (8.3 g) in water (25 mL)) containing beaker.
5. Cool the reaction mixture by placing in an ice- bath and continue swirling, until crystals separates out.
6. Filter the crystals under suction, wash with water (10 mL) and dry.
7. Purify the crude acetanilide by recrystallization with hot water.
8. The melting range of pure acetanilide is 113 to 115 °C.

PREPARATION OF DRUGS

3.2 Preparation of Paracetamol

Traditional Name: Acetaminophen

IUPAC ***Name:*** N-(4-Hydroxy phenyl) acetanilide **Mol wt**: 151.17 g/mol

Principle: Paracetamol can be prepared by acetylating the 4-aminophenol. The replacement of active hydrogen of amino group of 4-aminophenol by an acetyl group (electrophile) of the acetylaing agent (e.g., acetic anhydride) generates paracetamol. The acetylation reaction utilizes hydrochloric acid as a catalyst.

4-Aminophenol + $(CH_3CO)_2O$ (Acetic anhydride) $\xrightarrow[-CH_3COOH]{HCl}$ Paracetamol (4-acetamido phenol)

Reaction Mechanism

The lone pair of electrons of amino group of 4-aminophenol attacks the electropositive carbonyl carbon (due to inductive effect) of acetic anhydride. Elimination of hydrogen atom from the amino group of 4-aminophenol removes the positive charge present on it. Movement of electrons from carbonyl oxygen reestablishes π bond between carbon and oxygen. This facilitates the bond breaking between carbonyl carbon and acetoxy oxygen of acetic anhydride and generates paracetamol.

Acetic anhydride + 4 Aminophenol → [tetrahedral intermediate] $\xrightarrow{-CH_3COOH}$ Paracetamol (4-acetamidophenol)

Procedure:

***Chemicals Required*:** 4-Aminophenol, Acetic anhydride, Water

1. Place 4-aminophenol (1.1 g, 10 mmol) and water (3 mL) in a conical flask.
2. Stir the mixture vigorously at room temperature to suspend the solid in the water.
3. Add acetic anhydride (1.2 mL, 13 mmol) to the stirred suspension.
4. Stir the reaction mixture (*warm by placing in water bath, if necessary*) to dissolve the solid and continue until it reprecipitate.
5. Isolate the precipitate under vacuum filtration, wash with cold water and dry it.
6. Purify the crude paracetamol by recrystallization with hot water (10 mL).
7. The melting range of pure paracetamol is 168 to 170 °C.

Note:

- Though $-NH_2$ is more nucleophilic than –OH, excess acetic anhydride should be avoided as there is chance of double acetylation of 4-aminophenol.
- High temperature may also facilitate the double acetylation, hence it should be avoided.

3.3 Preparation of Aspirin

Traditional Name: Acetylsalicylic acid, Spiraeic acid.

IUPAC Name: 2-Acetyloxybenzoic acid **Mol wt**: 180.16 g/mol

History of aspirin: Aspirin was developed from the observations that willow bark could cure malarial fever and its extracts act as a remedy for acute rheumatism. Later it is identified that the salicin (β-glycoside), an active constituent present in the bark is responsible for the therapeutic effect. In the biological system, salicin transforms into salicylic acid and produces therapeutic effect. This made medicinal chemists to prescribe salicylic acid for the relief of fever and pain. Severe gastric irritations produced by salicylic acid prompted the need for the alternative. Thus aspirin, a prodrug of salicylic acid was developed. The name ASPIRIN is derived from Acetylated SPIRaeic acid.

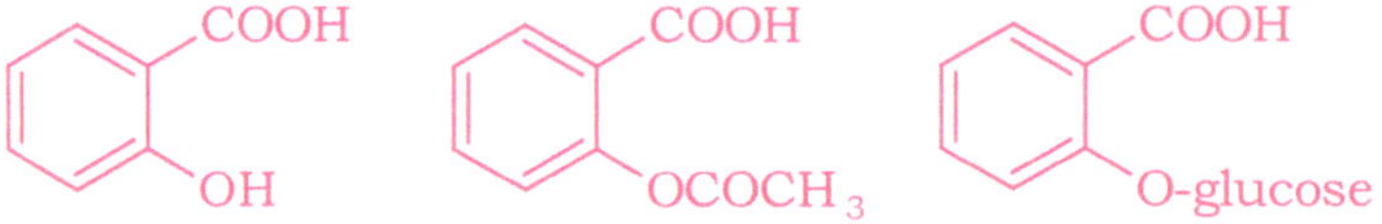

COOH, OH — Salicylic acid

COOH, $OCOCH_3$ — Aspirin (Acetylsalicylic acid)

COOH, O-glucose — Salicin

Principle: The *O*-acetylation of salicyclic acid with the mixture of acetic anhydride in glacial acetic acid produces aspirin (acetylsalicylic acid). In place of glacial acetic acid, sulphuric acid or phosphoric acid also can be used. The reaction takes place by the replacement of active hydrogen of phenolic group of salicylic acid by an acetyl group of acetylating agent (e.g., acetic anhydride). The acetylsalicylic acid can be prepared using acetyl chloride in pyridine. Pyridine absorbs the formed hydrogen chloride.

Reaction Mechanism

The lone pair of electrons of oxygen present in hydroxy group of salicylic acid attacks the electropositive carbonyl carbon (due to inductive effect) of acetic anhydride. Elimination of hydrogen atom from the hydroxy group of salicylic acid removes the positive charge present on it. Movement of electrons from carbonyl oxygen reestablishes π bond between carbon and oxygen. This facilitates the bond breaking between carbonyl carbon and acetoxy oxygen of acetic anhydride and generates aspirin.

Procedure:

Method 1

Chemicals Required: Salicylic acid, Acetic anhydride, Glacial acetic acid, Ethanol.

1. Place distilled acetic anhydride (10 mL, 106 mmol) and glacial acetic acid (10 mL, 174 mmol) in a dry beaker.
2. Add salicyclic acid (1 g, 7 mmol) to the mixture and condense for 45 min.
3. Pour the hot mixture into beaker containing cold water (100 mL).
4. Stir vigourously until shiny white crystals of Acetylsalicylic acid (aspirin) separates out.
5. Filter and wash the product with cold water for several times.
6. Purify the product by recrystallization with ethanol.
7. The melting range of pure aspirin is 135 to 137 °C.

Method 2

Chemicals Required: Salicylic acid, Acetyl chloride, Dry pyridine and Acetic acid.

1. Place salicylic acid (1.3 g, 9.4 mmol) to the flask containing dry pyridine (1.5 mL, 18.6 mmol).
2. Mix the contents of the flask and add acetyl chloride (1 mL, 14 mmol) immediately to the mixture with shaking (maintain the temperature between 50 to 60 °C).
3. Heat the mixture by placing on a water bath for 5 min.
4. Cool the reaction mixture and pour into the beaker containing cold water with vigorous stirring.

   (*Aspirin separates as oil. But continuous and rapid stirring converts oil into crystals*).
5. Filter the solid and wash with water.
6. Purify the crude aspirin (acetyl salicylic acid) by recrystallization with the mixture of water and acetic acid (1:1).
7. The melting point of pure aspirin is 135 to 137 °C.

Method 3

Chemicals Required: Salicylic acid, Acetic anhydride, Concentrated sulphuric acid / Phosphoric acid (85%) and Ethanol.

1. Place salicylic acid (1 g, 7 mmol) into the beaker and add concentrated sulphuric acid (4 drops) / phosphoric acid (200 mg, 85%).
2. Add acetic anhydride (1 mL, 10.6 mmol) and mix thoroughly.
3. Heat the mixture gently by placing on a water bath for 15 min (maintain the temperature between 50-60 °C).
4. Cool the reaction mixture and pour into the beaker containing cold water (10 mL) with stirring (decomposes the excess of acetic anhydride).
5. Stir the mixture and collect the crystals by vacuum filtration.
6. Purify the crude aspirin (acetylsalicylic acid) by recrystallization with ethanol.
7. The melting point of pure aspirin is 135 to 137 °C.

PREPARATION OF PHARMACEUTICAL AIDS

3.4 Preparation of N-Acetylglycine

Traditional Name: Acetyl glycocoll, Aceturic acid

IUPAC Name: 2-Acetamidoacetic acid **Mol wt**: 117.10 g/mol

Principle: Glycine undergoes N-acetylation readily with acetic anhydride to form *N*-acetylglycine.

$$HOOC-CH_2-NH_2 + (CH_3CO)_2O \xrightarrow[-CH_3COOH]{} HOOC-CH_2-NHCOCH_3$$

Glycine Acetic anhydride N-Acetylglycine

Reaction Mechanism

The lone pair of electrons of amino group nitrogen of glycine attack the electropositive carbonyl carbon (due to inductive effect) of acetic anhydride. The movement of π electrons of carbonyl group of acetic anhydride towards carbonyl oxygen (negative inductive effect) makes carbonyl carbon positive. Elimination of hydrogen atom from the amino group nitrogen of glycine removes the positive charge present on it. Movement of electrons from carbonyl oxygen reestablishes π bond between carbon and oxygen. This facilitates the bond breaking between carbonyl carbon and acetoxy oxygen of acetic anhydride and generates N-acetylglycine.

$H_3C-CO-O-CO-CH_3$ (Acetic anhydride) + $HOOC-CH_2-\ddot{N}H_2$ (Glycine) $\longrightarrow$ $HOOC-CH_2-N^{+}H(H)-C(O^{-})(CH_3)-O-CO-CH_3$ $\xrightarrow[-CH_3COOH]{}$ $HOOC-CH_2-NHCOCH_3$ (N-Acetyl glycine)

Procedure:

Chemicals Required: Glycine, Acetic anhydride and Distilled water.

1. Place glycine (1 g, 13 mmol) and water (4 mL) into a 50 mL conical flask.
2. Stir vigorously using mechanical stirrer until solid dissolves completely.
3. Add acetic anhydride (2.5 mL, 26 mmol) in one portion and continue stirring for 20 min.
4. Cool the reaction mixture in a refrigerator overnight to crystallize the N-acetylglycine.
5. Filter, wash the crude N-acetylglycine with ice-cold water and dry at 100 °C.
6. Evaporate the combined filtrate and washings to dryness under reduced pressure on a water bath at 50 to 60 °C.
7. Purify the crude *N*-acetylglycine by recrystallization with boiling water.
8. The melting range of pure *N*-acetylglycine is 207 to 208 °C.

3.5 Preparation of Hippuric Acid

Traditional Name: Benzoylglycine, Hippurate

IUPAC Name: 2-Benzamidoacetic acid **Mol wt**: 179.18 g/mol

Principle: Acylation of glycine with benzoyl chloride in basic medium generates hippuric acid (*N*-benzoylglycine).

Benzoyl chloride + NH_2CH_2COOH (Glycine) $\xrightarrow{NaOH,\ HCl}$ Hiuppuric acid (N-benzoylglycine)

Reaction Mechanism

Benzoyl chloride + $\ddot{N}H_2CH_2COOH$ (Glycine) $\longrightarrow$ tetrahedral intermediate (O^-, $N^+H_2-CH_2-COOH$) $\xrightarrow{-H^+}$ Hiuppuric acid (N-benzoylglycine)

Procedure:

Chemicals Required: Benzoyl chloride, Glycine, Sodium hydroxide, Hydrochloric acid, Carbon tetrachloride, Charcoal.

1. Transfer glycine (1 g, 13 mmol) into the flask containing cold sodium hydroxide (10 mL, 10%).
2. Add benzoyl chloride (2 mL 17 mmol) to the flasks in small portions.
3. Shake the flask to dissolve the contents after each addition.
4. Cool the mixture and acidify with hydrochloric acid (10%).
5. Hippuric acid separates out upon acidification (benzoic acid may present in small amounts).
6. Filter the separated hippuric acid, wash with cold water and dry.
7. Heat the precipitate with carbon tetrachloride (5 mL) for 10 min and filter.
8. Purify the crude hippuric acid by recrystallization with boiling water. (treat with charcoal to remove colouring impurities, if any present).
9. The melting range of pure hippuric acid is 187 to 188 ºC.

KEYPOINTS

- Acylation introduces acyl group (R_2-C=O) into the aromatic compounds.
- Majority of acylation reactions are catalyzed by acidic catalysts.
- Friedel-Crafts acylation, C-Acylation, N-acylation and O-acylation are the pharmaceutically important acylations.
- Anti-inflammatory drugs namely, naproxen, tolmetin, indomethacin, paracetamol and aspirin can be synthesized through acylation.

4

Alkylation

The replacement of active hydrogen of the hydroxyl, amino (1° and 2°) and sulfhydryl group by an alkyl group (R^+) of alkylating agent is called as alkylation. Alkyl group can be transfered as a free radical, carbanion, carbene and electrophile. Alkylation with one carbon containing alkylating agent is called as methylation and it founds major utility in synthetic organic chemistry. The most important alkylation reactions are listed below.

1. **Friedel-Crafts alkylation:** The most important alkylation reaction is called as Friedel-Crafts alkylation. It involves the alkylation of arenes with alkyl halides in presence of Lewis acid catalyst ($AlCl_3$).
2. Alkylation can be grouped based on the hydrogen bearing group, which undergoes replacement with alkylating agent.
   - **N-Alkylation:** Alkylation of amino group is known as *N*-alkylation.
   - **O-Alkylation:** Alkylation of hydroxy group is named as *O*-alkylation.
   - **S-Alkylation:** Alkylation of sulfhydryl group is known as *S*-alkylation.
3. **Friedel-Crafts sulphonylation:** It involves the reaction between the arenes and sulphonyl chlorides/sulphonic acid anhydrides in presence of Lewis acid catalyst ($AlCl_3$).

General reaction mechanism

Reaction mechanism for Friedel-Crafts alkylation

Step 1: Complex formation between alkyl halide and Lewis acid

$$\underset{\text{Alkyl halide}}{R-X} + \underset{\text{Aluminium chloride}}{AlCl_3} \longrightarrow \underset{\text{Alkyl halide -aluminium chloride complex}}{R-\overset{+}{X}-\overset{-}{Al}Cl_3}$$

Step 2: Formation of alkyl carbocation

$$\underset{\text{Alkyl halide - aluminium chloride complex}}{R-\overset{+}{X}-\overset{-}{Al}Cl_3} \longrightarrow \underset{\text{Carbocation}}{R^+} + AlCl_3 + X^-$$

Step 3: Nucleophilic attack on electrophilic carbon of alkyl carbocation.

Carbocation

R^+

Arene

Step 4: Formation of alkylated arene.

$AlCl_4^-$ + $AlCl_3$ + HCl

Alkylated arene

Alkylating agents: Alkylating agents are grouped as:

1. ***Nucleophilic alkylating agent:*** These alkylating agents displace halide substitutents on carbon (alkyl and aryl halides).
   - **Alkyl halides**: Methyl chloride, methyl iodide, ethyl chloride, isopropyl chloride, *tert*-butyl chloride and benzyl chloride. Alkyl halides finction effectively with Lewis acid catalysts.

     Aryl halides: Benzyl chloride.
   - This category includes Grignard reagent, organolithium reagent, organocopper reagent, organo sodium reagent and methanol acidified with hydrochloric acid and boron trifluride.
2. ***Electrophilic alkylating agent:*** These agents alkylate aromatic compounds (Friedel-Crafts alkylation), amines (N-alkylation), hydroxyl and carboxylic (o-alkylation) and thiol groups (S-alkylation). Electrophilic alkylating agents are very toxic in nature.

   ***Alkylating agents for acidic conditions*:** Methyl iodide, methyl tosylate, dimethyl sulphate and methoxy acetate.
3. ***Carbene (neutral) alkylating agent:*** Carbenes are extremely reactive and attack even unactivated C-H bonds. Diazo group upon elimination produces carbenes. It includes diazo methane, triazene, dimethyl formamide acetal, isourea and orthoacetal.
4. ***Olefins:*** Ethylene, propene, dodecane and linear olifines.
5. ***Miscellaneous:*** Alcohols, ethers, esters, epoxides, aldehydes, ketones, dimethyl sulphate, diethyl sulphate, ethyl-*p*-toluene-sulphonate, trifluoromethanesulfonic acid, aliphatic diazo compounds and triethyloxonium tetrafluoroborate.

Pharmaceutical Applications

1. N-Alkylation

(a) Cetrizine (antihistamine) can be prepared by the N-alkylation reaction between 1-[4-chlorophenyl-p)phenylmethyl]-piperazine and 2-chloroethoxyacetamide.

1-[(4-Chlorophenyl) phenylmethyl]-piperazine + 2-Chloroethoxy acetamide $\xrightarrow{H^+}$ Cetrizine

(b) Cinepazet (anti-hypercholesteremic) can be prepared from 1-benzyl piperazine ethyl acetate (N-alkylation product of 1-benzylpiperazine).

1-Benzyl-piperazine + $Cl—CH_2COOC_2H_5$ (Ethyl chloroacetate) → Piperazine ethyl acetate $\xrightarrow{\text{3,4,5-Cinnamoyl chloride}}$ Cinepazet

2. O-Alkylation

(a) Paracetamol can be converted into phenacetin (antipyretic) through O-alkylation.

Paracetamol $\xrightarrow{C_2H_5I}$ Phenacetin

(b) Tolimidone (anti-diabetic) can be prepared through O-alkylation of *meta*-cresol.

meta-Cresol + Dimethyl acetal → → Tolimidone

3. **Clarke-Eschweiler methylation:** The mixture of formaldehyde and formic acid selectively methylates the primary and secondary amines. This approach is useful in the synthesis of adrenaline.

H_3CO / H_3CO — NH_2 —(HCHO, HCOOH)→ H_3CO / H_3CO — NH CH_3 ⇒ HO / HO — NH CH_3, OH

2-Amino-1-(3,5-dimethoxy phenyl)ethan-1-one   Adrenaline precursor   Adrenaline

PREPARATION OF DRUG INTERMEDIATES

4.1 Preparation of Methyl-2-Naphthyl Ether

Traditional Name: Nerolin

IUPAC Name: 2-Methoxynaphthalene **Mol wt**: 158.2 g/mol

Principle: Methyl-2-naphthyl ether can be prepared by methylation (*O*-alkylation) reaction. Dimethyl sulphate in alkaline medium (sodium hydroxide) acts as alkylating agent. Alkali (sodium hydroxide) abstracts hydrogen from 2-naphthol and generates sodium-2-naphthoxide (nucleophile). Sodium 2-naphthoxide upon alkylation with dimethyl sulphate forms methyl-2-naphthyl ether.

OH —($(CH_3)_2SO_4$, NaOH)→ OCH_3

2-Naphthol   Methyl-2-naphthyl ether

Reaction Mechanism:

Step 1: Formation of nucleophile

O-H, OH^- —($-H_2O$)→ O^-

2-Naphthol   2-Naphthoxide (nucleophile)

Step 2: Nucleophilic attack on dimethyl sulphate

2-Naphthoxide (nucleophile) + Dimethyl sulphate ⟶ Methyl-2-naphthyl ether

Procedure:

Chemicals Required: 2-Naphthol, Dimethyl sulphate, Sodium hydroxide (10%), Ethanol.

1. Dissolve 2-naphthol (1 g, 6.9 mmol) in aqueous solution of sodium hydroxide (0.3 g in 5 mL of water) contained in the flask with stirring (stirring facilitates solubilization).
2. Cool the warm mixture to about 10 °C by placing the flask in an ice-bath.
3. Add dimethyl sulphate (0.65 mL, 6.9 mmol) from burette dropwise cautiously, with vigorous stirring.
4. Warm the mixture for 1 h at 70 to 80 °C with vigorous stirring.
5. Cool the reaction mixture and filter the crude methyl-2-naphthyl ether under suction.
6. Wash the residue with sodium hydroxide (10%), followed by water to remove unreacted reactants and dry.
7. Purify the crude methyl-2-naphthyl ether by recrystallization with ethanol.
8. The melting point of the pure methyl-2-naphthyl ether is 72 °C.

Precautions:

- Dimethyl sulphate in liquid and vapour form is very corrosive. Hence, rubber gloves should be worn and it should be used in fume cupboard.
- Dimethyl sulphate inhalation leads to CNS disturbances (giddiness).
- Wash the accidental liquid splash on the skin with ammonium hydroxide (neutralization), followed by gentle rubbing with ammonia soaked cotton wool.

4.2 Preparation of 7-Methoxy-4-Methyl-Coumarin

IUPAC Name: 7-Methoxy-4-methyl-*2H*-1-benzopyran-2-one

Mol wt: 190.20 g/mol

Principle: The methylation (*O*-alkylation) of 7-hydroxy-4-methyl coumarin with dimethyl sulphate under alkaline condition forms 7-methoxy-4-methyl coumarin. In this conversion anhydrous potassium carbonate is useful. Alkali (potassium carbonate) abstracts hydrogen from 7-hydroxy-4-methyl coumarin and generates nucleophile. The nucleophile upon alkylation with dimethyl sulphate forms 7-methoxy-4-methyl coumarin.

Reaction Mechanism:

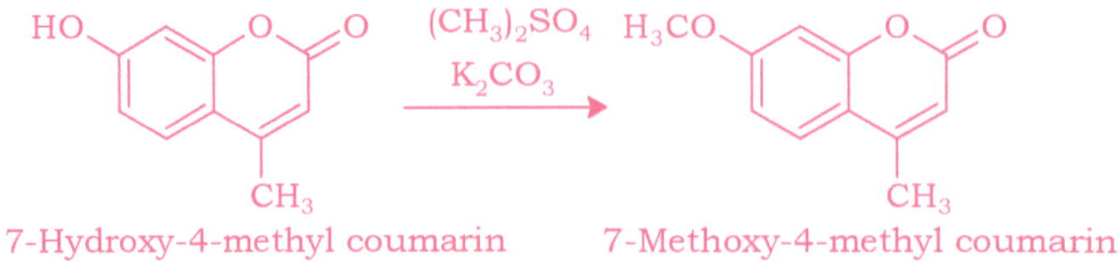

$(CH_3)_2SO_4$, K_2CO_3

7-Hydroxy-4-methyl coumarin → 7-Methoxy-4-methyl coumarin

Step 1: Formation of nucleophile

Step 2: Nucleophilic attack on dimethyl sulphate

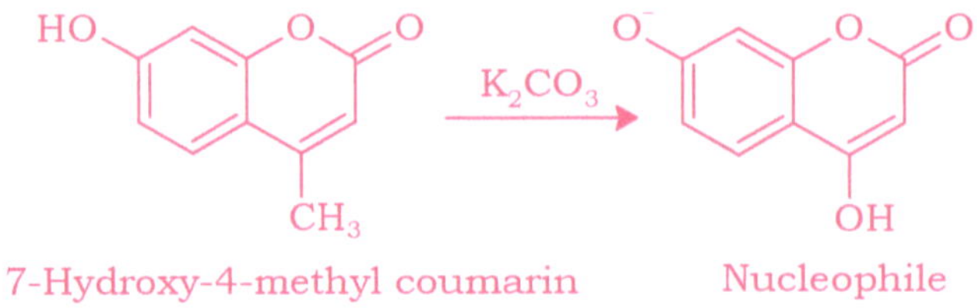

K_2CO_3

7-Hydroxy-4-methyl coumarin → Nucleophile

Procedure:

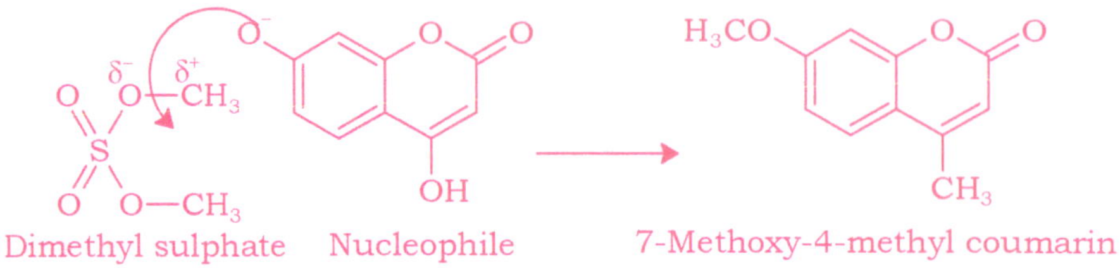

Dimethyl sulphate + Nucleophile → 7-Methoxy-4-methyl coumarin

Chemicals Required:7-Hydroxy-4-methyl coumarin, Dimethyl sulphate, Potassium carbonate, Acetone, Ethanol.

1. Place 7-hydroxy-4-methyl coumarin (5.53 g, 31 mmol) into the round bottom flask containing acetone (75 mL).
2. Add dimethyl sulphate (3.55 mL, 38 mmol) and ignited potassium carbonate (12 g) to the flask.
3. Reflux the reaction mixture for 4 h under anhydrous condition.
4. Filter the acetone solution and wash the residue with hot acetone (25 mL).
5. Distil the combined acetone fractions.
6. Add crushed ice into the oily residue and allow it to macerate.
7. Isolate the separated product and wash with ethanol.
8. Purify the crude product by recrystallization with ethanol.
9. The melting range of pure 7-methoxy-4-methyl coumarin is 216 to 218 °C.

Note:

1. **Refer 26.1 (page 196)** for the preparation of 7-hydroxy-4-methyl coumarin.

PREPARATION OF DRUGS

4.3 Preparation of Antipyrine

Traditional Name: Phenazone, Phenozone, Analgesine

IUPAC Name: 1,5-dimethyl-2-phenyl-1,2-dihydropyrazole-3-one

Mol wt: 188.23 g/mol

Principle: Antipyrine is an antipyretic and anti-inflammatory agent. The condensation of ethyl acetoacetate and phenyl hydrazine produces 5-methyl-2-phenyl-pyrazole-5-one. This upon methylation (*N*-alkylation) with dimethyl sulphate forms antipyrine.

Phenylhydrazine + Ethyl acetoacetate → 5-Methyl-2-phenyl-1, 2-dihydro-3*H*-pyrazol -3-one —$(CH_3)_2SO_4$, NaOH→ Antipyrine

Reaction Mechanism

Keto-enol tautomerism in ethyl acetoacetate: Inductive effect on the two carbonyl group (keto and carboxylic) of the ethyl acetoacetate, increases the acidity of the carbon-hydrogen (C-H) bond of active methylene group. This favours the dissociation of hydrogen atom from active methylene group and abstraction of the hydrogen by keto group. Hence, ethyl acetoacetate exisits in *keto-enol* forms (*keto-enol* tauotomerism).

The *enol* form of the ethyl acetoacetate readily condenses with phenyl hydrazine and forms 5-methyl-2-phenyl-1,2-dihydro-pyrazol-3-one. This upon methylation with dimethyl sulphate gives antipyrine (1,5-dimethyl-2-phenyl-1,3-dihydro-pyrazol-3-one).

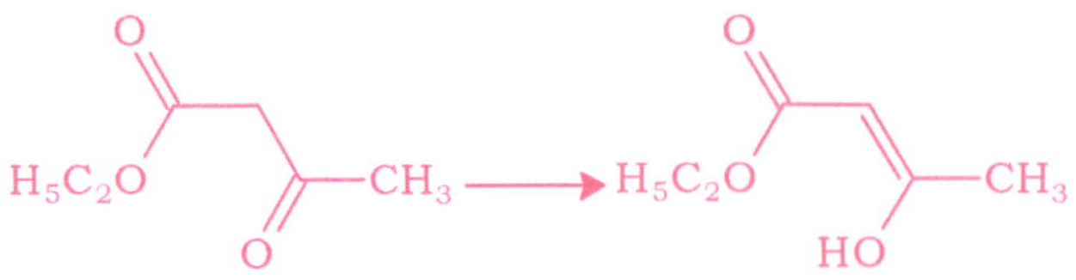

Ethyl acetoacetate (keto form) — Ethyl acetoacetate (enol form)

Step 1: **Formation of 5-methyl-2-phenyl-1,2-dihydro-3*H*-pyrazol-3-one**

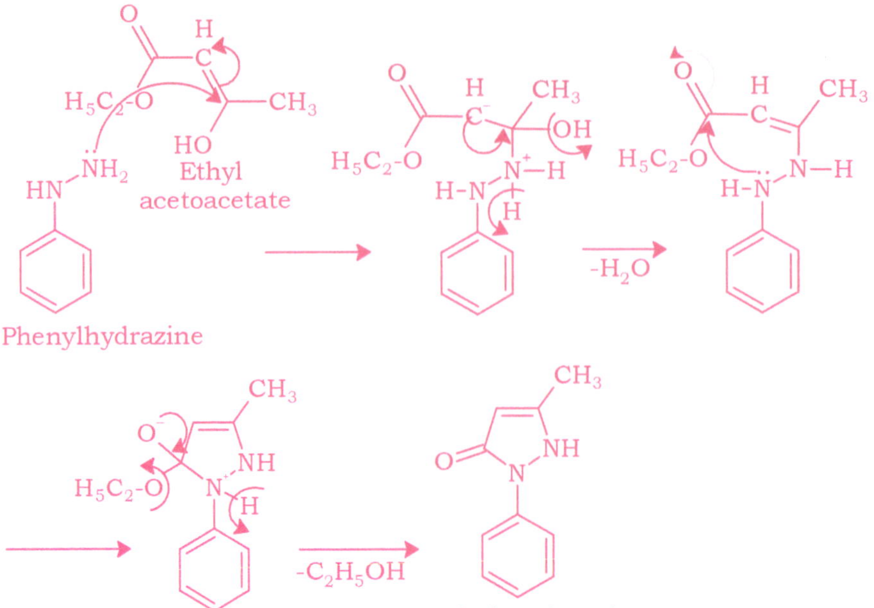

5-Methyl-2-phenyl-1,2-dihydro-3*H*-pyrazol-3-one

Step 2: **Methylation of 5-methyl-2-phenyl-1,2-dihydro-3*H*-pyrazol-3-one (formation of antipyrine)**

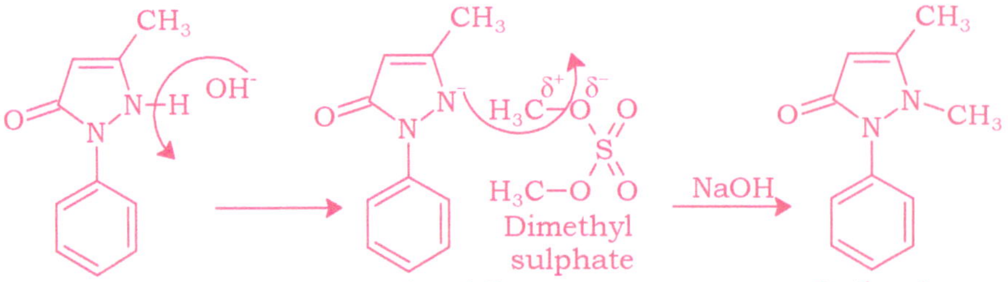

5-Methyl-2-phenyl-1,2-dihydro-3*H*-pyrazol-3-one — Nucleophile — Antipyrine

Procedure:

Chemicals Required: Ethyl acetoacetate, Phenylhydrazine, Diethyl ether, Sulphuric acid, Sodium hydroxide, Dimethyl sulphate.

Step 1: Preparation of 5-methyl-2-phenyl-1,2-dihydro-3H-pyrazol-3-one

1. Mix distilled ethyl acetoacetate (2 mL, 16 mmol) and phenylhydrazine (1.5 mL, 15 mmol) in a china dish.
2. Heat the mixture in a fume cupboard for 2 h (stir with glass rod).
3. Cool the red syrup, add diethyl ether (4 mL) and stir the mixture vigorously.
4. Keep the mixture aside for 15 min and filter the solid (vacuum filtration).
5. Wash the filtered solid with ditethyl ether (to remove unreacted reactants and impurities) and dry.
6. Purify the crude product by recrystallization with hot water (or ethanol-water mixture (1:1)).
7. The melting point of pure 5-methyl-2-phenyl-1,2-dihydro-3*H*-pyrazol-3-one is 127 °C.

Step 2: Preparation of antipyrine

1. Transfer the aqueous solution of sodium hydroxide (0.23 g in 3 mL of water) and the solution of 5-methyl-2-phenyl-1,2-dihydro-3*H*-pyrazol-3-one (1 g, 6 mmol) in methanol (1 mL) into a round bottom flask, set in a fume hood.
2. Warm the reaction mixture and add dimethyl sulphate (0.66 mL, 7 mmol) from dropping funnel or burette.
3. Reflux the mixture for 1 h with stirring.
4. Cool the reaction mixture to room temperature, evaporate and add hot water to the crude residue.
5. Filter and extract the filtrate with benzene.
6. Evaporate the solvent and recrystallize the antipyrine with hot water/benzene.
7. The melting point of pure antipyrine is 113 °C.

KEYPOINTS

- Replacement of active hydrogen of the hydroxyl, amino (1° and 2°) and sulfhydryl group by an alkyl group (R^+) is called as a alkylation.
- Friedel-Crafts alkylation, Friedel-Crafts sulphonylation, N-Alkylation, O-Alkylation and S-Alkylation are most important alkylation reactions.
- Cetrizine (antihistamine), Cinepazet (antihistamine), phenacetin (analgesic and antipyretic) and tolimidone (antidiabetic) can be synthesized through alkylation.
- Clarke-Eschweiler methylation is a special type of alkylation and is useful in the synthesis of adrenaline.

5

Aromatic Electrophilic Subsitution

Aromatic substitution refers to the replacement of an atom (generally hydrogen) or a group attached to the benzene by another atom or group. This includes electrophilic, nucleophilic and free radical substitution reactions. Aromatic compounds most often undergo electrophilic substitution reaction. The aromatic electrophilic substitution can be depicted as follows.

Benzene + E^+ (Electrophile) ⟶ Electrophile substituted benzene + H^+

The five-membered heterocyclic systems, such as pyrrole, furan and thiophene are highly activated towards electrophilic attack compared to benzene. The hetero atoms (nitrogen, oxygen, sulphur) with lone pair of electrons increase the stability of the cationic intermediate (Meisenheimer complex).

General reaction mechanism

Benzene ring with its delocalization of six π electrons in a cyclic conjucated system (above and below the plane) provides site for the attack of electrophiles. The benzene ring acts as an electron donor (Lewis base, Nucleophile) and reacts with electron acceptors (Lewis acid, Electrophile). The ability of the compound to undergo electrophilic substitution is a good test for unsaturation (bromine test). In general, these reactions occur through two steps:

1. ***Addition***: The π electrons of the aromatic ring system attack the electrophile and form addition product called as cationic intermediate (Meisenheimer complex).
2. ***Elimination***: The complex eliminates proton and forms substituted product.

The general reaction mechanism involved in the aromatic electrophilic substitution can be explained through following steps.

Step **1: Generation of an electrophile (E^+):** Dissociation of the reagent suitable reaction conditions.

E - B (Electrophile reagent) ⟶ E^+ (Electrophile) + B^-

Step 2: **Attack of ring electrons on electrophile:** The aromatic ring π electrons attack the positively charged (electron deficient) electrophile. The temporary disruption of the aromatic π system forms resonance-stabilized carbocation (rate determining step).

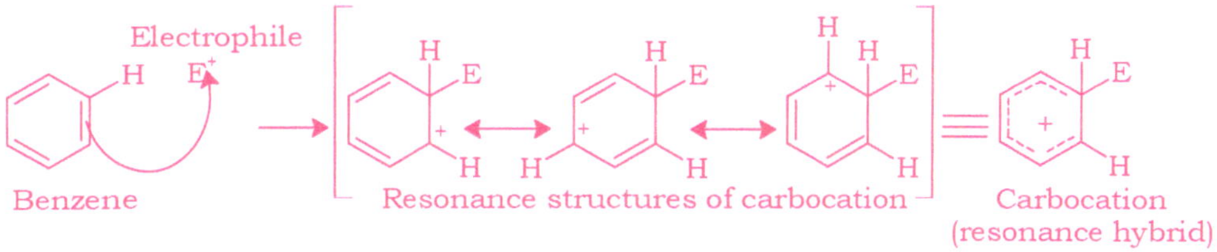

Electrophile

Benzene

Resonance structures of carbocation

Carbocation (resonance hybrid)

Step 3: The base (released from the reagent) abstracts the ring proton (deprotonation) and generates electrophile substituted benzene.

Base

Carbocation

-BH

Electrophile substituted benzene

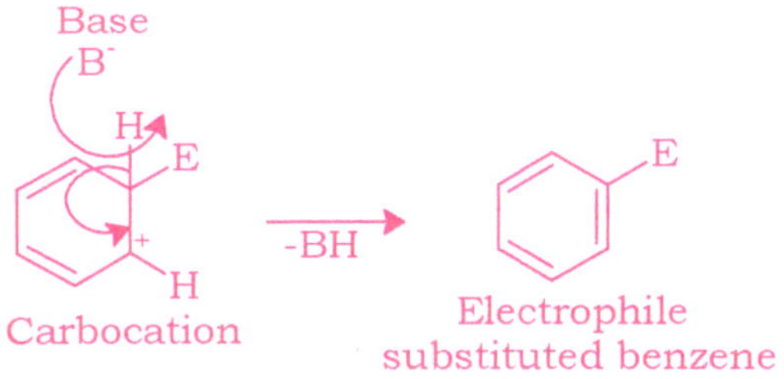

Ipso **substitution**: A special kind of electrophilic aromatic substitution is called as *ipso* substitution. In this case, the leaving group is not hydrogen. Synthesis of picric acid is an example for *ipso substitution* reaction. In salicylic acid, one of the leaving group is carboxylic acid (-COOH), which is not hydrogen.

Effect of Groups on Aromatic Electrophilic Substitution

The nature of substituent group present in the aromatic ring system decides the position for electrophilic attack. These substituted groups are broadly divided into following categories:

1) **Ring activating groups:** *Ortho and para* director: A substituent group which makes the substituted benzene *more* reactive than benzene itself is called as ring activating group. The substituent group favours the electrophilic attack chiefly at *ortho* and *para* positions of the ring system (*ortho* and *para* director). The electron releasing/donating substituent group (designated as X) makes *ortho and para* positions of the ring electron rich. This makes *ortho-* and *para-*positions as reactive site for electrophile. The resonance stabilization of positive charge will be optimized at *ortho and para* position.

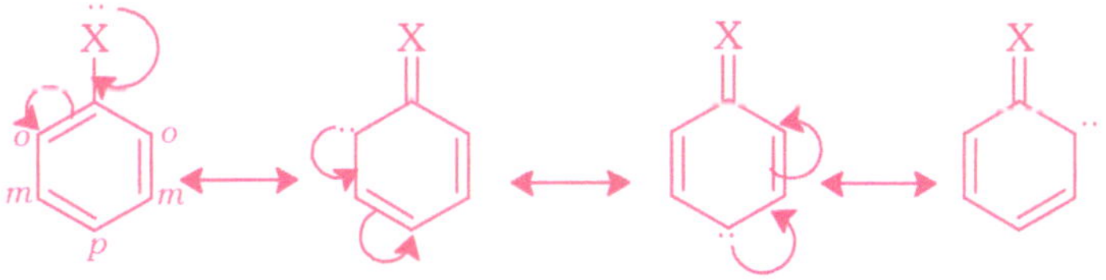

Friedel-Crafts acylation of anisole (methoxy benzene) is much *faster* (~3,00, 000 times) than the reaction on benzene.

Ring activating groups (*Ortho and para* directors)

- *Strongly activating* : $-NH_2$, -NHR, $-NR_2$, -OH
- *Moderately activating* : $-OCH_3$, $-OC_2H_5$, $-NHCOCH_3$
- *Weakly activating* : $-C_6H_5$, $-CH_3$, $-C_2H_5$, etc

2) **Ring deactivating groups:** A substituent group which makes the substituted benzene *less* reactive than benzene itself is called as ring deactivating group.

- ***meta* directors:** These groups favour the electrophilic substitution chiefly at *meta* position. The electron withdrawing substituent (designated as Y) deactivates the ring in all positions, but its deactivation is less prominent at *meta* position. The electron withdrawing groups stabilize resonance charge at *meta* position, hence the preferred position for electrophilic substitution is *meta* position.

The bromination of nitrobenzene is much *slower* (10^{-5} times) than the benzene.

Meta directors: $-NO_2$, $-N(CH_3)_3^+$, -CN, -COOH, -COOR, $-SO_3H$, -CHO, -COR.

- ***Ortho, para* directors**: Halogens bear both electron releasing and electron withdrawing effects and show unusual effects on electrophilic aromatic substitution. The electron withdrawing inductive effect of halogen causes the ring deactivation. But the electron-releasing nature through resonance cause ring activation, and this promotes the *ortho* and *para* substitions. The electron-withdrawing inductive effect of halogen intensifies the ring positive charge and destabilizes the ring. This is responsible for the low reactivity when compared with other *ortho* and *para* directors.

  Ortho, para director: -F, -Cl, -Br, -I

Ortho attack

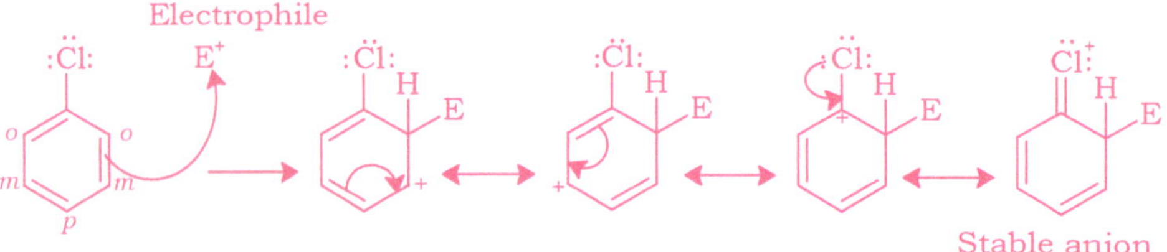

Meta attack

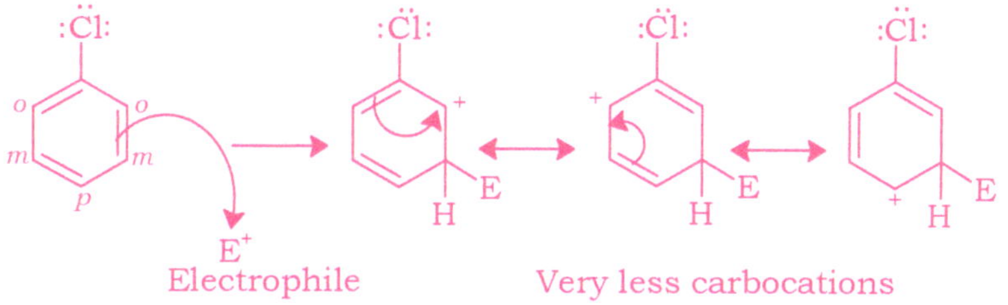

Para attack

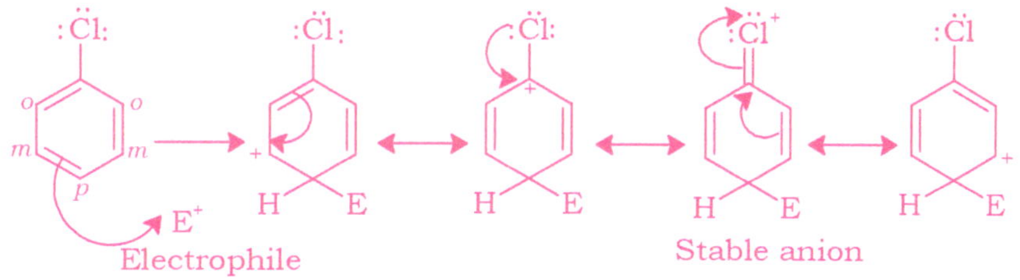

Role of Catalysts in Aromatic Electrophilic Substitution

Lewis acids (anhydrous $AlCl_3$ and $FeCl_3$) and mineral acids (HCl, HNO_3, H_2SO_4) catalyzes the generation of electrophile in aromatic electrophilic substitution reactions. The electron deficient catalyst causes polarization on the attacking molecule. Anhydrous $FeCl_3$, and $FeBr_3$ are catalysts for halogenation reactions.

- Anhydrous $FeCl_3$ (and $FeBr_3$) takes up Cl^- ion from the Cl_2 and gives Cl^+ (electrophile).

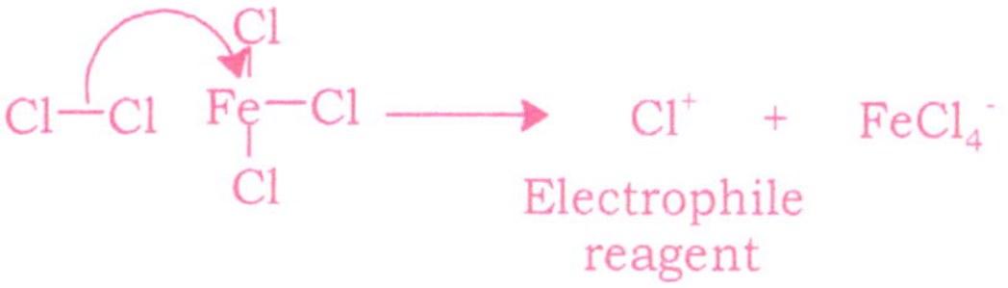

- Anhydrous $AlCl_3$, is catalyst for Friedel-Crafts alkylation and Friedel-Crafts acylation.

Pharmaceutical Applications

Nitration, halogenation, sulphonation, Friedel-Crafts alkylation and Friedel-Crafts acylation reaction are the typical examples of aromatic electrophilic substitution reactions.

1. Nitration

(a) The intermediate for the metronidazole (antiprotozoal drug) can be prepared through nitration reaction.

2-Methylimidazole —(HNO_3)→ [nitro intermediate] —(ethylene oxide)→ Metronidazole

2. Friedel-Crafts acylation

- In the synthesis of anti-inflammatory drug naproxen.

2-Methoxynaphthalene —(CH_3COCl, $AlCl_3$)→ 2-Acyl-6-methoxy naphthalene → → Naproxen

- In the synthesis of anti-inflammatory drug ibuprofen.

Isobutylbenzene —(CH_3COCl, $AlCl_3$)→ [acylated intermediate] → → Ibuprofen

PREPARATION OF DRUG INTERMEDIATES

5.1 Preparation of Nitrobenzene

Traditional Name: Oil of mirbane

IUPAC Name: Nitrobenzene **Mol wt**: 123.11 g/mol

Principle: Aromatic electrophilic substitution of benzene with mixed acid reagent generates nitrobenzene. Mixture of concentrated nitric acid and sulphuric acid is called as a mixed acid reagent, which generates nitronium ion. Concentrated nitric acid generates nitronium ion, NO_2^+ (an effective nitrating agent) using sulphuric acid as a catalyst. Nitronium ion (electrophile) substitutes the proton (H^+) of benzene (electrophilic substitution) and forms nitrobenzene. Nitrobenzene is an important drug intermediate used in the manufacture of paracetamol, phenacetin and sulphonamides. This nitration reaction is involved in the preparation of drugs namely, mebendazole, primaquine, pamaquine and metronidazole.

Benzene + Con HNO_3 $\xrightarrow[55-60\ °C]{Con\ H_2SO_4}$ Nitrobenzene (NO_2)

Reaction Mechanism

Step 1: Generation of electrophile: Sulphuric acid protonates the nitric acid to generate nitronium ion (NO_2^+, electrophile) with the elimination of water molecule.

$HO_3S-\ddot{O}-H$ (Sulphuric acid) + $H-\ddot{O}-NO_2$ (Nitric acid) $\xrightarrow{-OSO_3H}$ $H-\overset{+}{O}(H)-NO_2$ $\xrightarrow{-H_2O}$ $O=\overset{+}{N}=O$ Nitronium ion (electrophile)

Step 2: Attack of ring electrons on electrophile**:** The aromatic ring π electrons attack the positively charged (electron deficient) nitronium ion (electrophile). The temporary disruption of the aromatic π system forms resonance-stabilized carbocation (rate determining step).

Nitronium ion (electrophile) $O=\overset{+}{N}=O$

Benzene → Resonance structures of carbocation ≡ Carbocation (resonance hybrid)

Step 3: Deprotonation of carbocation**:** Loss of proton (H^+) from the carbocation generates nitrobenzene.

Base $-OSO_3H$

Carbocation $\xrightarrow{-H_2SO_4}$ Nitrobenzene

Procedure:

Chemicals Required: Benzene, Concentrated nitric acid, Concentrated sulphuric acid, Sodium hydroxide (1 N).

1. Load concentrated nitric acid (3.5 mL, 50 mmol) to the round bottom flask.
2. Add concentrated sulphuric acid (4 mL) dropwise to the flask with shaking. *(ensure the cold environment during the addition of concentrated sulphuric acid by placing the flask in an ice bath)*

3. Keep the mixture in cool condition during the addition by immersing the flask in ice bath (to ensure the temperature below 55 °C).
4. Add benzene (3 mL, 33 mmol) in small portions with shaking (ensure thorough mixing after each addition and maintain the temperature below 55 °C).
5. Attach the reflux condenser to the flask and reflux the mixture, maintaining the temperature between 55-60 °C for 45 min.
6. Shake the flask occasionally to ensure mixing of two immiscible (benzene and acid mixture) layers.
7. Pour the contents of the flask into beaker containing cold water (50 mL).
8. Stir the reaction mixture to remove the acid and then decant the aqueous layer.
9. Add sodium hydroxide (3 mL) to the reaction mixture and collect the organic layer (benzene layer) using separating funnel.
10. Transfer the organic layer into a conical flask containing anhydrous calcium chloride (1.25 g)
11. Warm the mixture to get clear solution if necessary.
12. Filter and distill the organic layer at 210 °C to collect the pure form of nitrobenzene.

Precautions: The temperature should not exceed 55 °C, as it favors the polynitration (e.g., formation of dinitrobenzene) and oxidative breakdown of aromatic ring.

5.2 Preparation of *meta*-Dinitrobenzene

IUPAC Name: 1,3-Dinitrobenzene **Mol wt**: 168.11 g/mol

Principle: Aromatic electrophilic substitution of nitrobenzene with nitronium ion (NO_2^+, an effective nitrating agent) generates *meta*-dinitrobenzene. Nitric acid component of mixed acid generates nitronium ion using sulphuric acid as a catalyst. Nitronium ion substitutes the hydrogen of nitrobenzene ring (aromatic electrophilic substitution) and forms *meta*-dinitrobenzene. Nitro group directs the incoming electrophile (NO_2^+) into *meta* position (*m*-directing group) and generates *meta*-dinitrobenzene.

NO_2 + Con HNO_3 —(Con H_2SO_4, 55 - 60 °C)→ NO_2, NO_2

Nitrobenzene

meta-Dinitrobenzene

Reaction Mechanism

Step 1: Generation of the electrophile: Sulphuric acid protonates the nitric acid to generate nitronium ion (NO_2^+, electrophile) with the elimination of water molecule.

$HO_3S-\ddot{O}-H$ (Sulphuric acid) + $H-\ddot{O}-NO_2$ (Nitric acid) $\xrightarrow{-OSO_3H}$ $H-\overset{+}{O}(H)-NO_2$ $\xrightarrow{-H_2O}$ $O=\overset{+}{N}=O$ Nitronium ion (electrophile)

Step 2: Attack of ring electrons on electrophile: The aromatic ring (nitrobenzene) π electrons attack the positively charged (electron deficient) nitronium ion (electrophile). The temporary disruption of the aromatic π system forms resonance-stabilized carbocation (rate determining step).

Nitrobenzene (o, m, p positions marked) + Nitronium ion (electrophile) $O=\overset{+}{N}=O$ ⟶ Carbocation

Step 3: Deprotonation of carbocation: Loss of proton (H^+) from the carbocation generates nitrobenzene.

Carbocation + $^{-}OSO_3H$ (Base) $\xrightarrow{-H_2SO_4}$ *meta*-Dinitrobenzene

Procedure:

Chemicals Required: Nitrobenzene, Concentrated nitric acid, Concentrated sulphuric acid.

1. Load concentrated sulphuric acid (7 mL) and fuming nitric acid (5 mL) into the round bottom flask.
2. Add nitrobenzene (4.2 mL) in small portions to ensure thorough mixing to the flask.
3. Add few boiling chips to the flask, attach reflux condenser and heat the mixture with occasional shaking for 30 min.

   (*continue heating until the evolution of brown nitric oxide gas ceases, ~30 min*).
4. Cool the reaction mixture to the room temperature and pour into the beaker containing cold water (170 mL) with vigorous shaking.
5. Isolate the solid precipitated by vacuum filtration and wash with cold water.
6. Transfer the solid into the flask and add rectified spirit (30 mL).

7. Attach reflux condenser and heat the contents to dissolve the solid product. (*filter if necessary through preheated Buchner funnel to obtain clear solution*).
8. The colourless crystals of *meta*-dinitrobenzene deposits upon cooling.
9. The melting range of pure *meta*-dinitrobenzene is 89 to 90 °C.

5.3 Preparation of *Para*-Bromoacetanilide

Traditional Name: Antisepsin, Asepsin, Bromoanilide, Bromoantifebrin

***IUPAC Name*:** N-(4-Bromophenyl)acetamide **Mol wt**: 214.06 g/mol

Principle: Acetanilide reacts with bromine in glacial acetic acid and forms *para*-bromoacetanilide. Acetanilide (acylated aniline) favours the selective aromatic electrophilic substitution at *para* position . The *ortho*-bromoacetanilide population is very small and is more soluble in ethanol than *para*-bromoacetanilide. Hence *ortho*-bromoacetanilide can be readily eliminated by recrystallization. In case of aniline (highly reactive), the bromination favours the formation of 2,4,6-tribromoaniline (bromination at three sites). In phenol, the solvent carbon disulphide and temperature at 55 ºC produces the *para*-bromophenol exclusively.

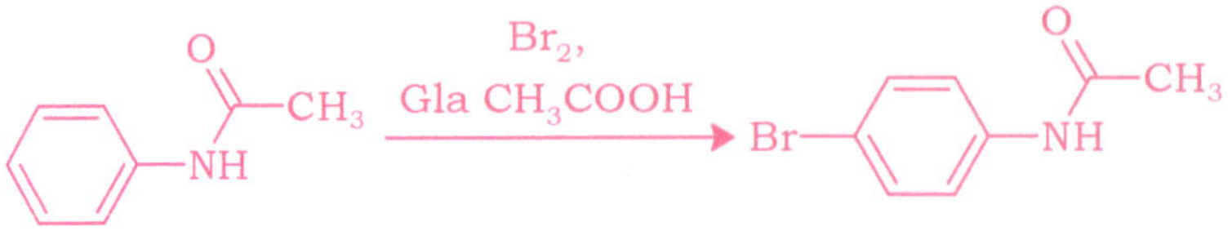

Acetanilide $\xrightarrow{Br_2,\ Gla\ CH_3COOH}$ *para*-Bromo acetanilide

The lone pair of electrons on the nitrogen atom of the amide (acetanilide) is conjugated with the carbonyl group. The electrons are weakly delocalized into the benzene ring, compared with aniline. This resonance controls the aromatic electrophilic substitution (bromination) in the *ortho* and *para* postions (it occurs chiefly in one position). Theoretically, the possibility of *ortho* product is twise as *para* product because there are two ortho positions. But steric hindrance produced by acetyl amino group inhibits *ortho* substitution and favours *para* substitution (*para*-bromoacetanilide).

Steric hindrance

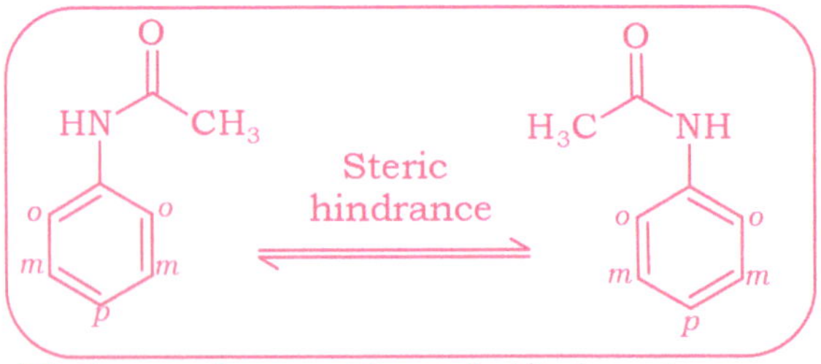

Steric hindrance favours the substituion at *para* position

Reaction Mechanism

Step 1: *Generation of the electrophile*

$Br_2 \longrightarrow Br^+ + Br^-$

Step 2: Attack of ring electrons (acetanilide) on electrophile

Step 3: *Deprotonation of carbocation*

Procedure:

Chemicals Required: Acetanilide, Bromine, Glacial acetic acid, Sodium metabisulphite.

1. Place acetanilide (1.35 g, 10 mmol) into a flask and dissolve with cold glacial acetic acid (4.5 mL).

   Bromine solution can be prepared by mixing bromine (0.53 mL, 11 mmol) with glacial acetic acid (2.5 mL).
2. Add the bromine solution from dropping funnel or burette slowly to the flask placed in a cold water with constant shaking to ensure thorough mixing.
3. An orange yellow colour will appear after the complete addition of bromine due to excess of bromine.

   If the orange yellow colour is strong, add sodium metabisulphite to the mixture to remove the colour.
4. Allow the reaction mixture to stand at room temperature (~30 min).
5. Pour the mixture into the beaker containing cold water (40 mL).
6. Filter the resulting precipitate under suction, wash with cold water and dry.
7. Purify the crude *para*-bromoacetanilide by recrystallization with ethanol.
8. The melting point of pure *para*-bromoacetanilide is 167 °C.

Precautions:

1. Bromine produces painful burns and the vapors are unpleasant. Hence it should be handled in the fume cupboard with great care.
2. Bromine burns should be treated immediately with glycerin.
3. If the vapour is inhaled relief may be obtained by holding hand kerchief soaked in alcohol near to the nose.

KEYPOINTS

- Replacement of an atom (generally hydrogen) or a group of benzene through electrophilic, nucleophilic and free radical substitution reactions are known as aromatic substitution.
- Aromatic compounds most often undergo electrophilic substitution reaction.
- The ability of the compound to undergo electrophilic substitution is a good test for unsaturation.
- A special kind of electrophilic aromatic substitution is called as ipso substitution. In this case, the leaving group is not hydrogen.
- Synthesis of metronidazole (antiprotozoal), naproxen (anti-inflammatory) and ibuprofen (anti-inflammatory) follows aromatic electrophilic substitution reaction.

6

Beckmann Rearrangement

Migration of chemical unit (an atom, an ion, a group of atoms) or a bond from one location to another location is known as rearrangement reaction. Most commonly known rearrangement is Whitmore 1,2-shift, where one group migrates to adjacent atom.

$$\underset{\text{A}-\text{B}}{\overset{\text{G}}{|}} \xrightarrow[\text{(rearrangement)}]{\text{1,2-Shift}} \text{A}-\overset{\text{G}}{\underset{\text{B}}{|}}$$

G = *migrating group*

The catalytic chemical conversion of ketoxime into more stable N-substituted amide is known as Beckmann rearrangement. This reaction is named after the German chemist Ernst otto Beckman (1886). The rearrangement requires acid catalysts or acidic catalysts. Cyclic ketoximes forms amides, where as acyclic ketoximes such as cyclohexanoxime forms lactam.

$$\underset{\text{Ketoxime}}{(R^1)(R)C{=}N{-}OH} \xrightarrow{\text{Catalyst}} \underset{\text{N-Subtituted amide}}{R{-}C({=}O){-}NH{-}R^1}$$

Catalysts

- ***Acid catalysts***: Sulphuric acid, hydrochloric acid, acetic acid and formic acid.
- ***Acidic catalysts***: Phosphorous pentachloride (PCl_5), phosphorous pentaoxide (P_2O_5), Liquid sulphur dioxide (SO_2), hexamethylphosphoramide (HMPA), thionyl chloride ($SOCl_2$), benzenesulphonyl chloride, methanesulphonic acid and acetic anhydride.
- ***Beckmann mixture***: A solution of acetic acid and acetic anhydride saturated with gaseous hydrogen chloride.
- ***Oleum solution***: A mixture of sulphuric acid and sulphur trioxide.

Reaction mechanism

Step 1: Protonation of oximes: Catalysts converts the hydroxyl group (-OH) attached to the nitrogen of the ketoxime into better leaving group.

- Acid catalysts protonates the hydroxyl group (-OH) into proton acid ($^{+}OH_2$), which is better leaving group.
- Phosphorous pentachloride (PCl_5) forms ester leaving group ($OPCl_4$).
- Benzene sulphonylchloride also forms an ester leaving group ($C_6H_5SO_2$-O).

Step 2: Formation of protonated oximes: The leaving group detaches from the nitrogen atom and generates electron deficient nitrogen species. It releases water or anionic group from the nitrogen atom and introduces positive charge (electron deficiency) on nitrogen atom.

Step 3: Formation of carbocation: The transfer of 'R^1' to the electron-deficient nitrogen facilitates the formation of carbocation.

Step 4: Formation of amide precursor intermediate: Water molecules attack on carbocation followed by the loss of proton forms the intermediate (precursor for amide).

Step 5: Formation of amide: The intermediate upon tautomerization generate amide.

Acid catalyst mediated Beckmann rearrangement

Formation of carbocation

Ketoxime $\xrightarrow{H^+}$ $\xrightarrow{-H_2O}$ $\longrightarrow$ Carbocation

Formation of amide

Carbocation $\xrightarrow{H_2O}$ $\xrightarrow{-H^+}$ Amide precursor (intermediate) $\rightleftharpoons$ N-Subtituted amide

Phosphorous pentachloride mediated Beckmann rearrangement

Formation of carbocation

Ketoxime $\xrightarrow[-HCl]{PCl_5}$ $\xrightarrow{-POCl_3, -Cl^-}$ $\longrightarrow$ Carbocation

Formation of amide

Carbocation → (H_2O) → → ($-H^+$) → Amide precursor (intermediate) ⇌ N-Subtituted amide

Pharmaceutical applications

1. **Stereospecificity:** *Anti* (*trans*) group migration strategy is used in the determination of the configuration of ketoximes. The group orientation decides the migration of the group. The group which is anti- to the ketoxime hydroxyl group migrates to the nitrogen (stereospecific).
   - In case of 2-bromo-5-nitroacetophenone oxime, the *isomer*-1 has both the hydroxyl (-OH) and bromo (-Br) groups close enough. This permits the cyclization in cold sodium hydroxide and generates the cyclic product 1. The migration of *anti*-CH_3 group to the nitrogen atom (Beckmann rearrangement) forms the benzamide derivative (product 2).

Isomer 1 → Beckmann rearrangement → Benzamide derivative (Product 2) (Beckmann rearrangement product)

Isomer 1 → Cold NaOH → Cyclized product (Product 1)

   - In case of 2-bromo-5-nitroacetophenone oxime, the *isomer*-2 has both the hydroxyl (-OH) and bromo (-Br) groups far away and hence no cyclization results. The migration of anti aryl group to the nitrogen atom generates Beckmann rearrangement product-2.

Isomer 1 → Beckman rearrangement → Beckman rearrangement product-2

Isomer 1 → Cold NaOH ✗ → No product

The oximes with two alkyl groups at positions R and R_1 forms the mixture of two amides. The unsymmetrical ketones produce two *geometrical isomers* of unsymmetrical oximes (*cis/trans* isomers of C=N bond) and generate mixture of amides. But the ratio of the products is exactly the ratio of geometrical isomers in the starting materials. The amides are equal in population and the *trans* group migrate each case.

2. The Beckmann rearrangement strategy was utilized in the synthesis of natural product isocryptolepine (antimalarial).

Methanone $\xrightarrow{NH_2OH.HCl}$ (oxime) $\xrightarrow{\text{Ammonium persulphate}}$ Beckman rearrangement product → → Isocryptolepine

3. Preparation of paracetamol

4-Hydroxy acetophenone $\xrightarrow{NH_2OH.HCl}$ Ketoxime $\xrightarrow{CF_3COOH,\ SOCl_2}$ Paracetamol

4. Isoquinoline synthesis involves the Beckmann rearrangement strategy.

Cinnamaldehyde $\xrightarrow{NH_2OH.HCl}$ Cinnamaldehyde oxime $\xrightarrow{P_2O_5}$ Beckman rearrangement product → Isoquinoline

6.1 Preparation of Benzanilide

Traditional Name: Benzanilid, Benzoylanilide

IUPAC Name: N-Phenylbenzamide **Mol wt**: 197.24 g/mol

Principle: Benzanilide can be prepared from benzophenone oxime via Beckmann rearrangement. Benzophenone condenses with hydroxylamine hydrochloride in presence of sodium hydroxide and forms benzophenone oxime. Benzophenone oxime gets converted into benzanilide (amide) by Beckmann rearrangement.

Benzophenone $\xrightarrow{NH_2OH.HCl}$ Benzophenone oxime $\xrightarrow{PCl_5}$ Benzanilide

Reaction mechanism

The carbonyl carbons of benzophenone bear partial positive charge (polarization). The electron rich nitrogen of hydroxylamine (nucleophile) attacks positively charged carbonyl carbon (electrophile) and forms an intermediate. The optimum pH for this reaction is 7. Strong acidity converts the hydroxylamine into conjugate acid, reduces the concentration of nucleophilic hydroxyl amine and results in no reaction.

Phosphorous pentachloride (PCl_5) in anhydrous ether is a useful catalyst for the benzanilide formation. Phosphorous pentachloride (PCl_5) converts -OH group into better leaving group -$OPCl_4$ (ester). Detachment of leaving group generates electron deficient nitrogen species (loss of water or anion). Migration of the phenyl group to the electron deficient nitrogen occurs and forms carbocation. Addition of water on carbocation, loss of proton from the intermediate and tautomerisation yields benzanilide.

Step 1: Formation of Benzophenone oxime

Benzophenone + $NH_2OH.HCl$ ⟶ (intermediate: OH, NH–OH) $\xrightarrow{-H_2O}$ Benzophenone oxime

***Step 2*:** Formation of carbocation

***Step 3*:** Formation of amide

Procedure:

Chemicals Required: Benzophenone, Hydroxylamine hydrochloride, Sodium hydroxide pellets, Hydrochloric acid (dilute), Rectified spirit, Methanol.

***Step* 1: Preparation of Benzophenone oxime**

1. Place benzophenone (2.5 g, 13.7 mmol), hydroxylamine hydrochloride (1.5 mg, 22 mmol), rectified spirit (4 mL) and water (5 mL) into a round bottom flask.
2. Add sodium hydroxide pellets (2.8 g, 70 mmol) in small portions with shaking. (Cool the flask, if the reaction becomes too vigorous).
3. Attach the reflux condenser to the flask and reflux for 10 min.
4. Cool the reaction mixture and pour the contents into the beaker containing dilute hydrochloric acid (7.5 mL in water (50 mL)).
5. Filter the precipitate, wash with cold water and dry in an oven at 40 °C (or in a desiccator).
6. Purify the crude benzophenone oxime by recrystallization with methanol.
7. The melting point of pure benzophenone oxime is 142 °C.

Precautions:

(a) Hydroxylamine hydrochloride is skin irritant and requires caution and precaution.

(b) Traces of oxygen or moisture convert oxime into benzophenone and nitric acid.

Hence, it should be stored in vacuum desiccator filled with dry carbon dioxide or nitrogen.

***Step* 2: Preparation of Benzanilide**

1. Load benzophenone oxime (1 g, 5 mmol) into the conical flask containing anhydrous diethyl ether (10 mL) and stir it to dissolve.
2. Add powdered phosphorous pentachloride (1.5 g, 7.2 mmol). (*alternatively thionyl chloride (1.5 mL) can be used*)
3. Distil off the solvent ether and other volatile products.
4. Filter the solid and dry.
5. Add water (15 mL) to the flask and boil to break up any lumps.
6. Decant the supernatant liquid.
7. Purify the crude benzanilide by recrystallization with boiling ethanol.
8. The melting point of pure benzanilide is 163 °C.

6.2 Preparation of Acetanilide

Traditional Name: Antifebrin, Acetyl aniline, Acetylamino benzene

IUPAC Name: N-Phenylacetamide. **Mol wt**: 135.17 g/mol

Principle: Acetanilide can be prepared from acetophenone oxime. Acetophenone on condensation with hydroxylamine hydrochloride in presence of sodium acetate yields acetophenone oxime. Polarization of carbonyl group of acetophenone allows protonation. The positively charged carbonyl carbon (electrophile) will be attacked by electron rich nitrogen of hydroxylamine (nucleophile) and forms an intermediate. Removal of hydrogen from nitrogen followed by the dehydration generates acetophenone oxime.

CH_3 $NH_2OH.HCl$ CH_3 H_2SO_4 O $-CH_3$
O N–OH NH
Acetophenone Acetophenone oxime Acetanilide

Acetophenone oxime can be converted into acetanilide (amide) by Beckmann rearrangement. Concentrated sulphuric acid (H_2SO_4) converts the hydroxyl (-OH) group into better leaving group. Detachment of leaving group generates electron deficient nitrogen species (loss of water or anion). Migration of the phenyl group to the electron deficient nitrogen occurs and forms carbocation. Addition of water on carbocation, loss of proton from the intermediate and tautomerization yields acetanilide.

Step 1**:** Formation of Acetophenone oxime

$NH_2OH.HCl$ OH
CH_3 HN CH_3 CH_3
O OH $-H_2O$ N–OH
Acetophenone Acetophenone oxime

***Step 2*:** Formation of carbocation

***Step 3*:** Formation of Acetanilide

Procedure:

Chemicals Required: Acetophenone, Sodium acetate dihydrate, Hydroxylamine hydrochloride, Concentrated sulphuric acid, Methanol.

***Step* 1: Preparation of Acetophenone oxime**

1. Dissolve acetophenone (3 mL, 26 mmol) in a mixture of methanol (8 mL) and water (28 mL) loaded in the flask.
2. Add sodium acetate dihydrate (3 g, 37 mmol) and hydroxylamine hydrochloride (3 g, 44 mmol) to the flask.
3. Heat the reaction mixture in a water bath for 10 min.
4. Cool the hot mixture by placing on ice-bath.
5. Isolate the crude acetophenone oxime by filtration.
6. Purify the crude acetophenone oxime by recrystallization with hot water.
7. The melting point of the pure acetophenone oxime is 59 °C.

***Step* 2: Preparation of Acetanilide**

1. Load concentrated sulphuric acid (6 mL) into the beaker and heat it . (*thionyl chloride is an alternative it requires heating upto 70-80 °C*).
2. Add acetophenone oxime (3 g, 22 mmol) slowly with stirring to the hot sulphuric acid and continue the stirring for 15 min.
3. Cool the hot mixture and pour into crushed ice with stirring.
4. Isolate the crude acetanilide by filtration and wash with water.
5. Purify the crude acetanilide by recrystallization with boiling water.
6. The melting range of the pure acetanilide is 113 to 115 °C.

KEYPOINTS

- Migration of chemical unit (an atom, an ion, a group of atoms) or bond from one location to another location is known as rearrangement reaction.
- The catalytic chemical conversion of ketoxime into more stable N-substituted amide is known as Beckmann rearrangement.
- Beckmann rearrangement used in the determination of the configuration of ketoximes.
- Paracetamol (analgesic, antipyretic) can be synthezised by applying Beckmann rearrangement.

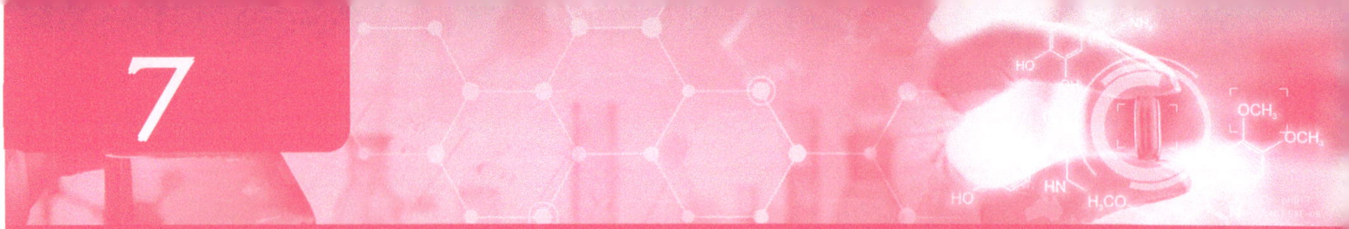

7

Bernthsen Synthesis

7a Bernthsen Acridine Synthesis

Acridine based drugs have antimalarial, anticancer and antifungal properties. The anticancer functions of acridine alkaloids namely cystodytin A and acronycine are demonstrated. Bernthsen (1878) reported the synthesis of acridine. It involves the heating of diphenylamine hydrochloride with benzonitrile to generate acridine molecule. In the modified method, diphenylamine is heated with a carboxylic (aromatic or aliphatic) acid at 200 to 270 °C for 24 h. This reaction is catalyzed by zinc chloride.

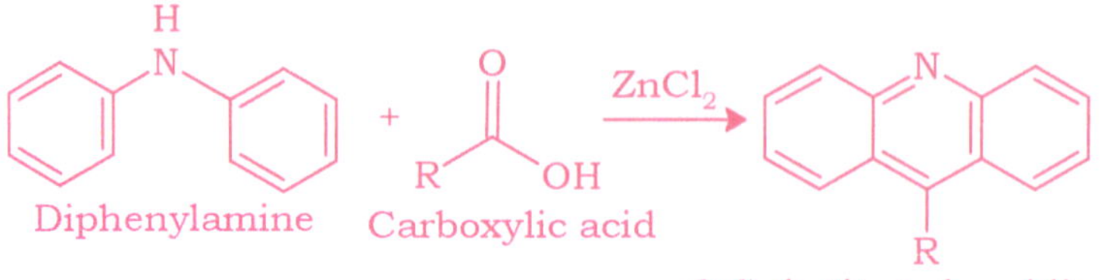

Diphenylamine + Carboxylic acid $\xrightarrow{ZnCl_2}$ 9-Substituted acridine

Polyphosphoric acid also catalyzes the reaction. It reduces the reaction temperature (195 to 205 °C from 200 to 270 °C) and reaction time (15 min from 24 h). But the polyphosphoric acid catalyzed reaction produces relatively lower yields when compared with zinc chloride catalyzed reactions.

General reaction mechanism

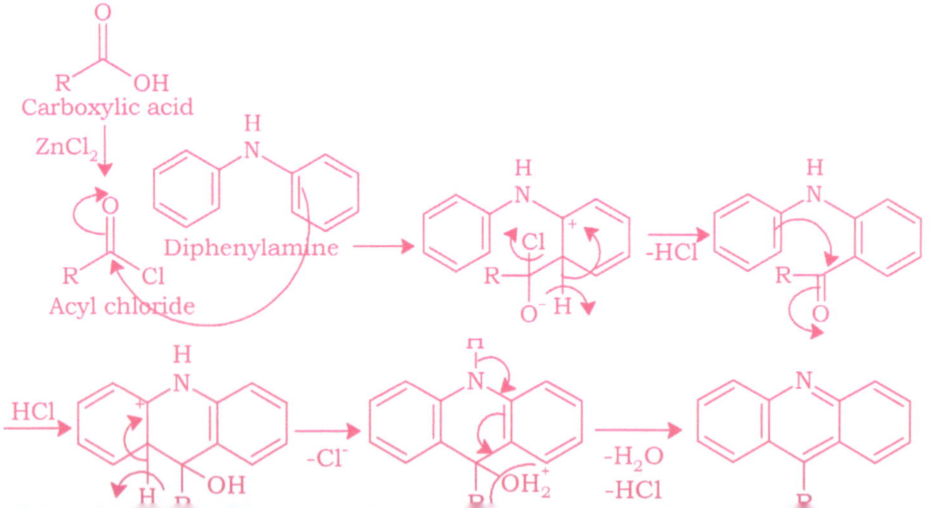

Carboxylic acid $\xrightarrow{ZnCl_2}$ Acyl chloride + Diphenylamine → $\xrightarrow{-HCl}$ → $\xrightarrow{HCl}$ → $\xrightarrow{-Cl^-}$ → $\xrightarrow{-H_2O,\ -HCl}$

Acridine containing drugs

1) Antimalarial drugs

Quinacrine	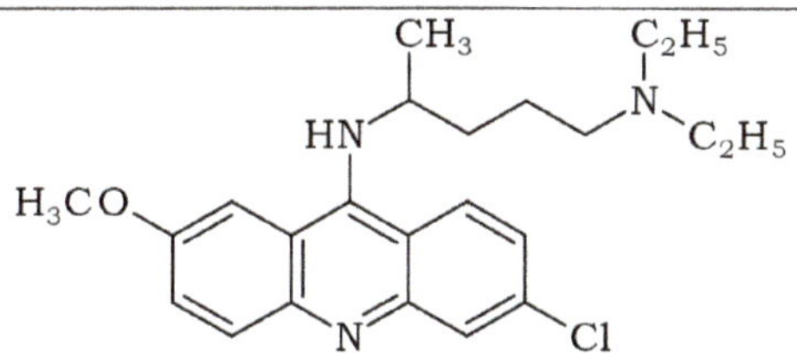
Mepacrine (acriquine)	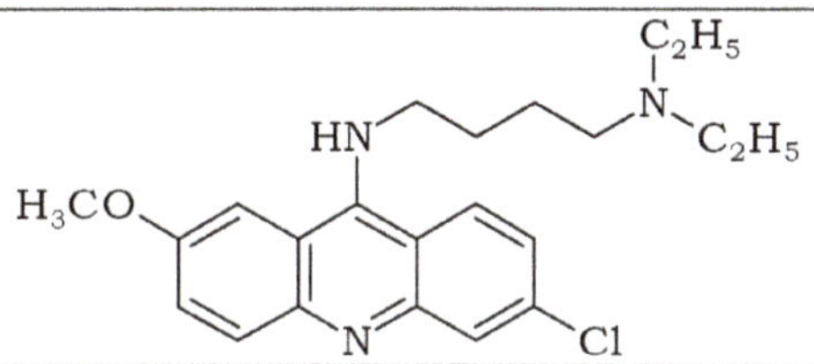

2) Anticancer drugs

Amsacrine	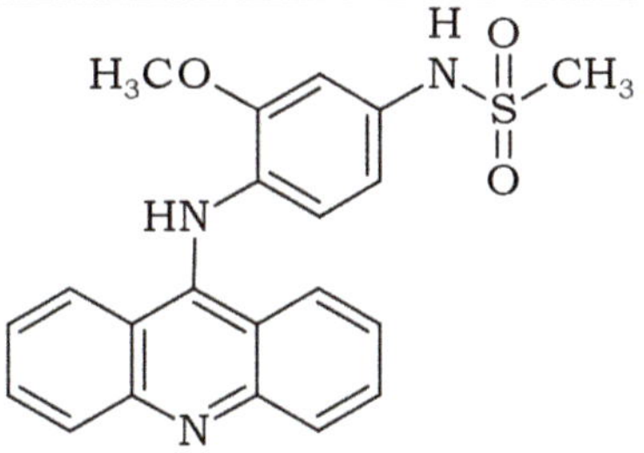

3) Antiprotozoal drugs

Quinacrine	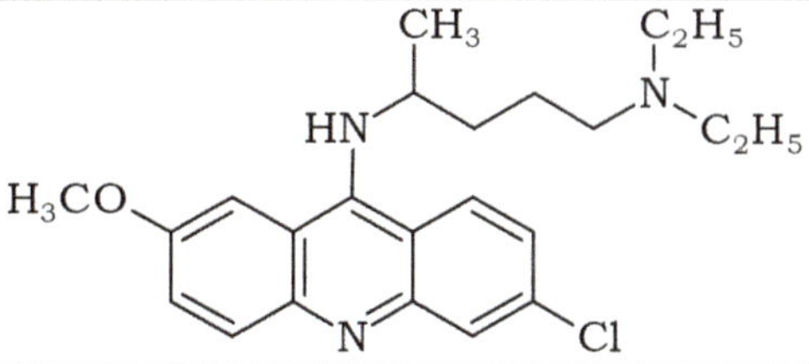
Mepacrine (acriquine)	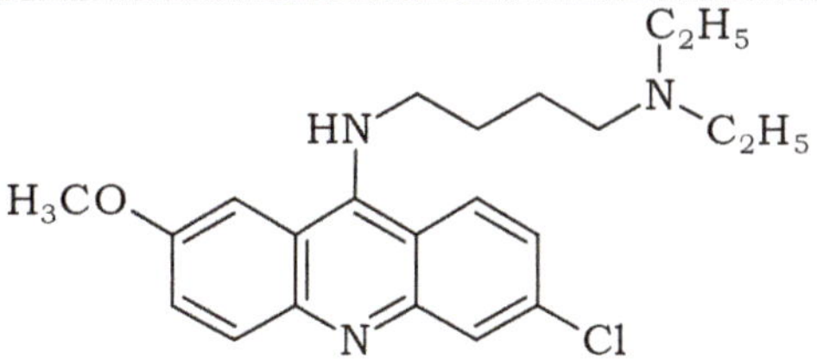

4) Antifungal drug

Aminocrine	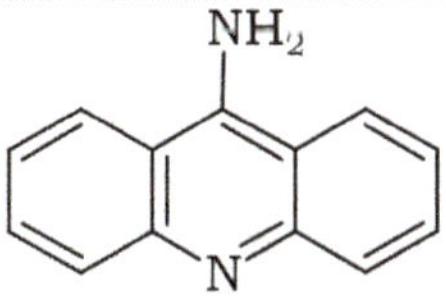

7.1 Preparation of 9-Phenylacridine

IUPAC Name: 9-Phenylacridine **Mol wt**: 255.32 g/mol

Principle: 9-Phenylacridine can be prepared from Bernthsen synthesis. The reaction involves condensation of diphenylamine and benzoic acid in presence of polyphosphoric acid as a catalyst. Polyphosphoric acid is replaced with zinc chloride (original catalyst) in order to reduce the reaction temperature and reaction time.

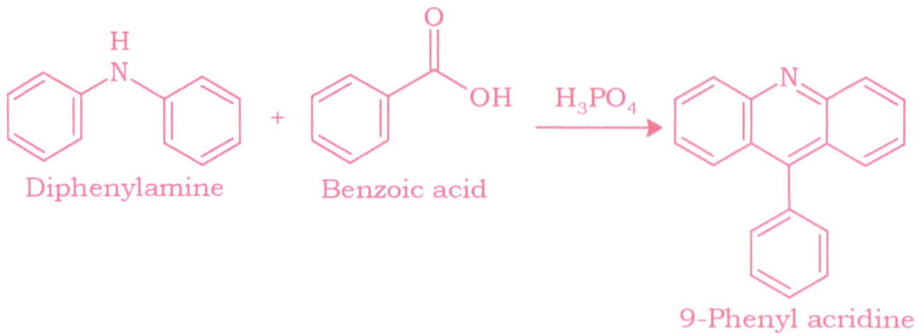

Diphenylamine + Benzoic acid $\xrightarrow{H_3PO_4}$ 9-Phenyl acridine

Reaction Mechanism

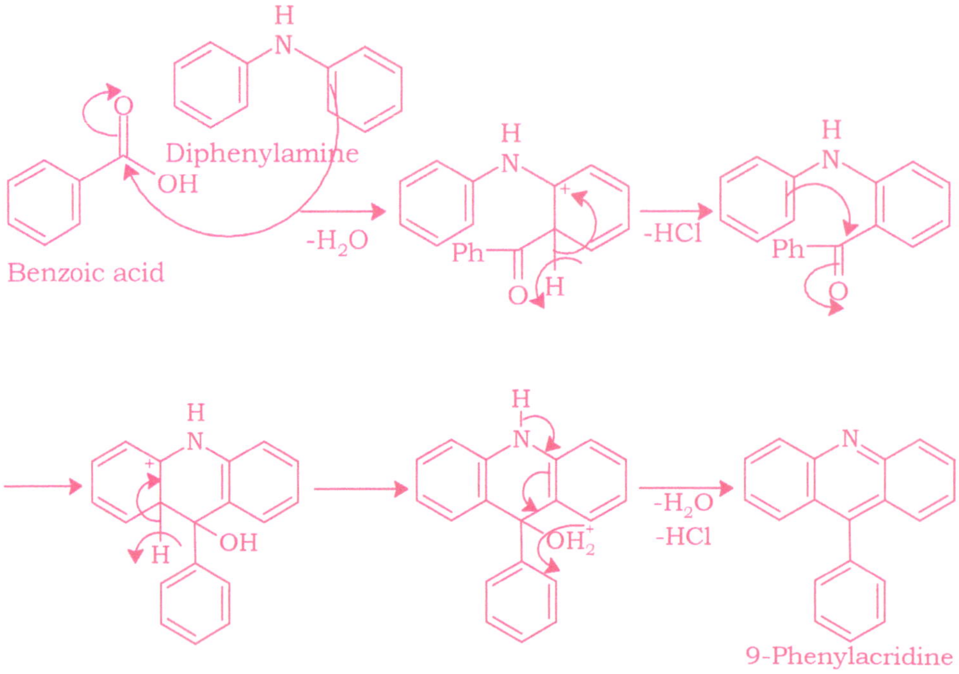

Diphenylamine

Benzoic acid

$-H_2O$

$-HCl$

$-H_2O$

$-HCl$

9-Phenylacridine

Procedure:

Chemicals Required: Diphenylamine, Benzoic acid, Polyphosphoric acid, Sodium hydroxide (25%), Ethanol.

1. Load diphenylamine (1 g, 6 mmol), benzoic acid (1 g, 30 mmol) and polyphosophoric acid (250 g) into the flask.
2. Heat the reaction mixture with stirring at 195 to 205 °C for 15 min.
3. Cool the warm mixture and pour into the beaker containing crushed ice.
4. Filter and add sodium hydroxide (25% w/v) to the filtrate.
5. Wash the white precipitate of crude 9-phenylacridine with water and ethanol.
6. Recrystallize the crude 9-phenylacridine from ethanol.
7. The melting point of the pure 9-phenylacridine is 184 to 185°C.

7b Bernthsen Phenothiazine Synthesis

Phenothiazine is an important pharmacophore present in many centrally (CNS) acting drugs. It includes antiemetics (promethazine), antihistamines (trimeprazine), antipsychotics (chlorpromazine), and antimigraines (prochlorperazine). Heinrich August Bernthsen (1883) reported the synthesis of phenothiazine. It involves the heating of diphenylamine hydrochloride with elemental sulphur at 250 °C. Hence this reaction is known as Bernthsen phenothiazine synthesis. Metal halides, aluminium chloride, zinc chloride and elemental iodine are the catalysts used in the preparation.

N H Diphenylamine $\xrightarrow[I_2]{S}$ S N H Phenothiazine

Phenothiazine containing drugs

1) Antihistamines

Promethazine	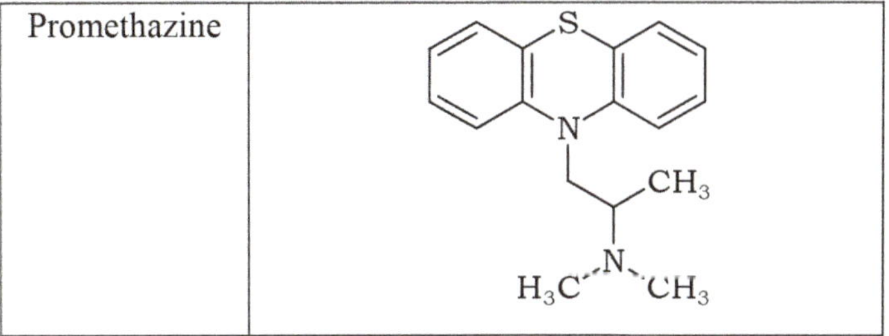

Table *Contd...*

Trimeprazine	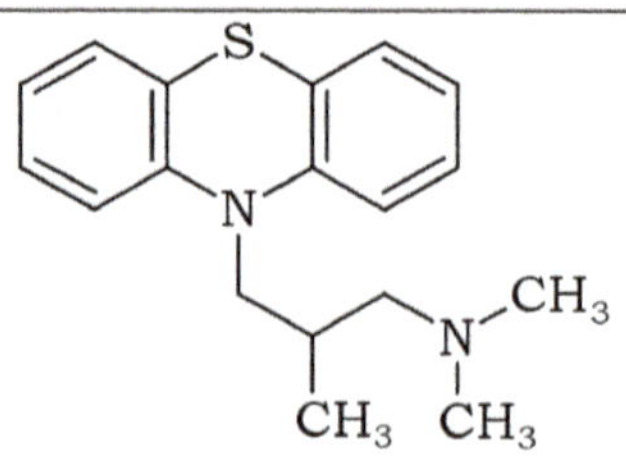
Methdilazine	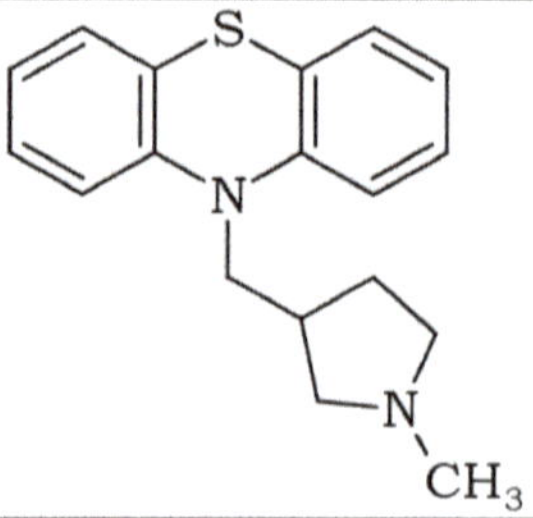
Dimetothiazine	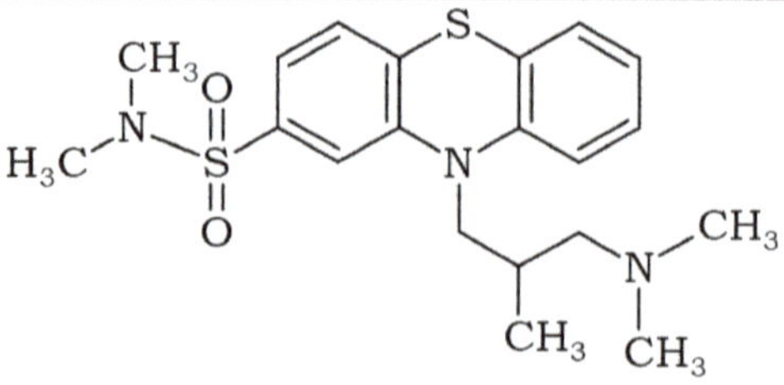

2) Antipsychotics

Chlorpromazine	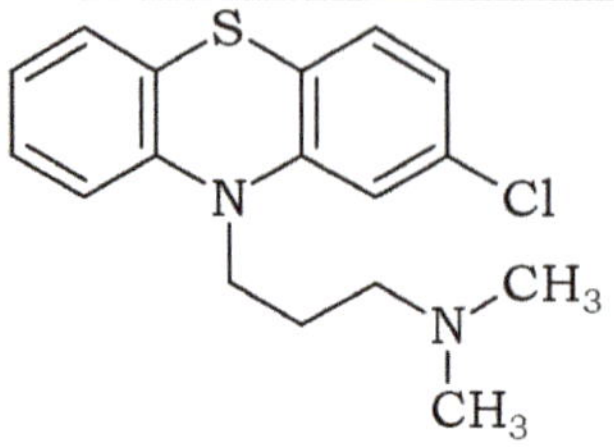
Prochlorperazine	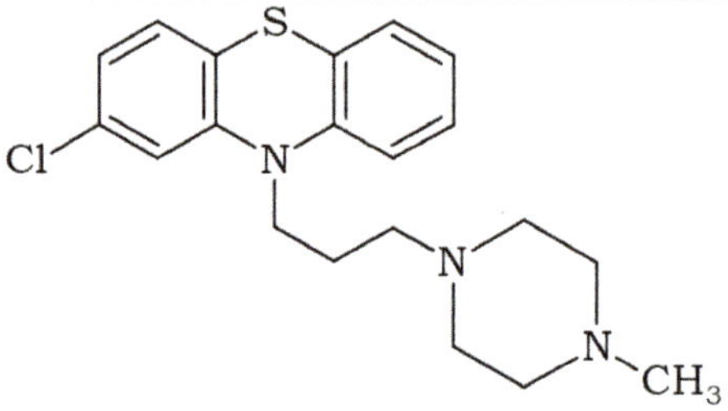

3) Antiparkinsonism drugs

Diethazine	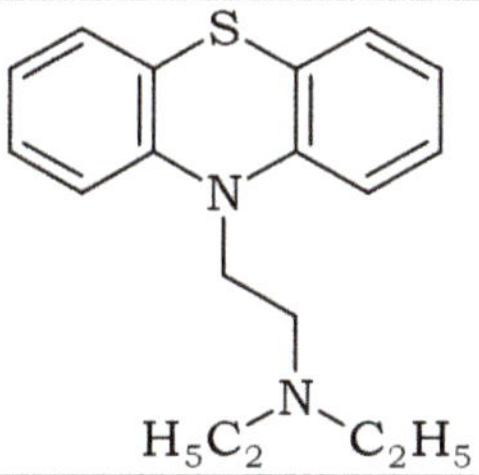
Ethopromazine	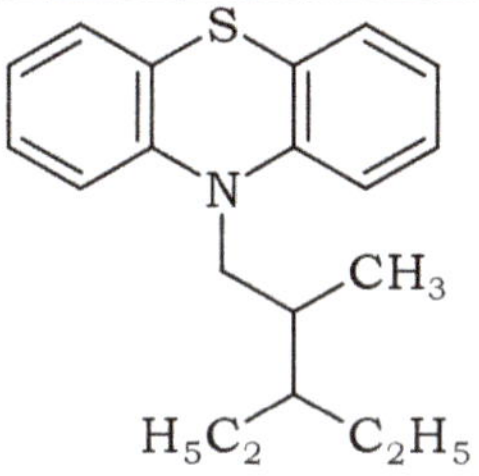

4) Muscle relaxant

Chlorproethazine	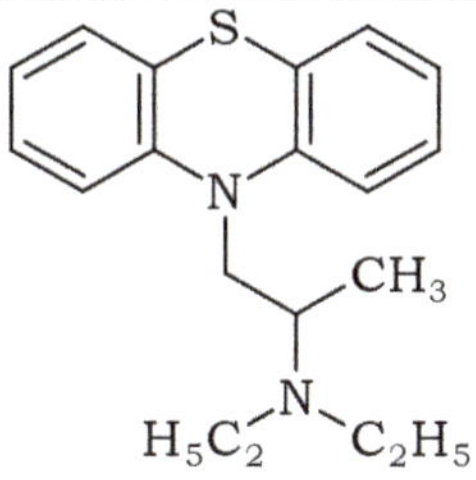

5) Vasodiltor

Chlorazine	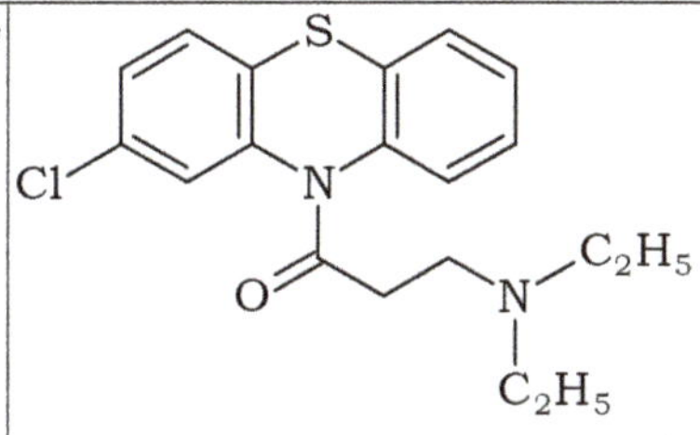

7.2 Preparation of Phenothiazine

Traditional Name: Thiodiphenylamine, Phenthiazine, Phenoverm

IUPAC Name: Dibenzo-[b,e]-1,4-thiazine **Mol wt**: 199.27 g/mol

Principle: Phenothiazine is the central molecular framework of a number of antihistamines, antipsychotics and antiemetics. It can be prepared by melting diphenylamine with elemental sulphur. This reaction can be catalyzed by metal halides (e.g., $AlCl_3$ and $ZnCl_2$) and elemental iodine. But the elemental iodine catalyzed reaction gives better yields.

Diphenylamine $\xrightarrow[I_2]{S}$ Phenothiazine

Method 1

Chemicals Required: Diphenylamine, Sulphur, Resublimed iodine, Ethanol.

1. Place diphenylamine (8.4 g, 50 mmol) and elemental sulphur (3.2 g) in a round bottom flask.
2. Add resublimed iodine (0.15 g) to the flask as a catalyst.
3. Melt the mixture by keeping in an oil bath at 190-200 °C for 30 min, until the evolution of hydrogen sulphide (H_2S) gas ceases.
4. Cool the molten solid and powder it using mortor and pestle.
5. Recrystallize the product from ethanol.
6. The melting range of pure phenothiazine is 184 to 185 °C.

Method 2

Chemicals Required: Diphenylamine, Sulphur, Anhydrous aluminum chloride, Ethanol.

1. Place diphenylamine (22 g, 131 mmol) and elemental sulphur (8.2 g) in a round bottom flask.
2. Add anhydrous aluminum chloride (3.2 g, 24 mmol) to the flask as a catalyst.
3. Melt the mixture by keeping in an oil bath at 190-200 °C for 30 min.
4. The reaction release hydrogen sulphide (H_2S) gas at 140 to 150 °C, it can be reduced by lowering the temperature for a few min.
5. Cool the molten solid and powder it using mortor and pestle.
6. Wash with water and ethanol.
7. Recrystallize the yellowish leaflets from ethanol.
8. The melting range of pure phenothiazine is 184 to 185 °C.

KEYPOINTS

- Heating of diphenylamine hydrochloride with benzonitrile to generate acridine molecule is known as Bernthsen acridine synthesis.
- Mepacrine (antimalarial), amacrine (anticancer), quinacrine (antiprotozoal) and aminocrine (antifungal) contains acridine nucleus.

- Heating of diphenylamine hydrochloride with elemental sulphur generates phenothiazine and the reaction is known as Bernthsen phenothiazine synthesis.
- Antiemetics (promethazine), antihistamines (trimeprazine), antipsychotics (chlorpromazine), and antimigraines (prochlorperazine) contain pehnothiazine nucleus.

8

Biginelli Synthesis

The one pot condensation of an aryl aldehyde, β ketoester and urea/thiourea under acid catalysis forms dihydropyrimidinones (3,4-dihydro pyrimidn-2-ones/ 2-thiones, DHPMs). This reaction is first reported by Pietro Biginelli (1893), hence referred as Biginelli synthesis.

Ar
O H
Aryl aldehyde
+
O
R_1-O
R O
NH$_2$
H$_2$N X
H^+, Δ
-H_2O
O Ar
R_1-O NH
R N X
H

β-Keto ester

Urea (X=O) / Thiourea (X=S)

3,4-Dihydropyrimidin-2-one/ 2-thione

Urea (X=O) / Thiourea (X=S)

Reaction mechanism

Three plausible reaction mechanism for the Biginelli reaction was reported and are namely Kappe mechanism, Folkers and Johnson mechanism, and Sweet and Fissekis mechanism. Kappe mechanism is widely accepted on various scientific aspects. Kappe explored the reaction mechanism using NMR spectroscopy, X-ray crystallographic analysis and trapping experiments. According to Kappe hypothesis, aryl aldehyde reacts with urea (or thiourea) and forms an *N*-acyliminium intermediate. The intermediate *N*-acyliminium reacts with ethyl acetoacetate (enol tautomer) and forms precursor for the 3,4-dihydropyrimidine. The precursor upon cyclization gives 3,4-dihydro pyrimidinone-2-ones/2-thione. Guanidine and its analogues can be used in place of urea or thiourea.

Formation of N-acyliminium intermediate

Ar
O H
Aryl aldehyde
NH$_2$
H$_2$N X
Urea (X=O) / Thiourea (X=S)
Ar H
O$^-$ N$^+$-H
H$_2$N X
Ar
HO N-H
H$_2$N X
Hemiaminal
H^+
-H_2O
Ar
H_2O^+ N-H
H$_2$N X
Ar
N$^+$-H
H$_2$N X
N-Acyliminium (intermediate)

Formation of 3,4-dihydropyrimidinone/thione precursor

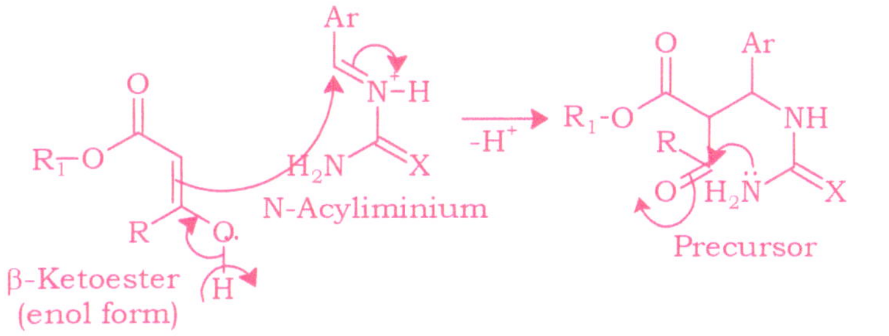

β-Ketoester (enol form)

N-Acyliminium

$-H^+$

Precursor

Formation of 3,4-dihydropyrimidinone/thione

Precursor

H^+

$-H_2O$

3,4-Dihydropyrimidin-2-one/2-thione

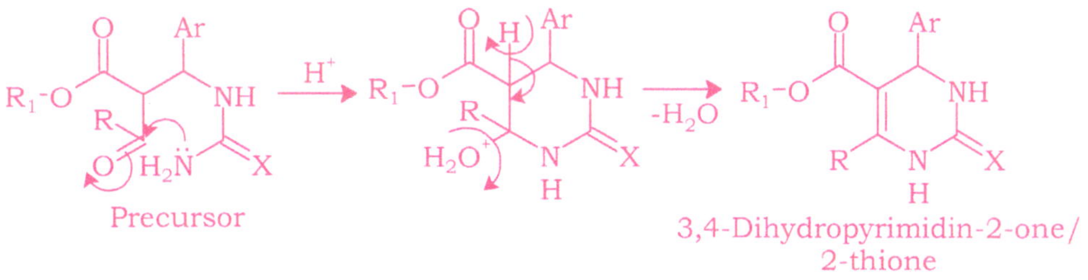

3,4-Dihydropyrimidines containing drugs

It is used to generate calcium channel blockers, mitotic kinesin Eg5 inhibitors, anti-viral and anti-bacterial compounds.

1) Antineoplastic drugs

Fluorastrol	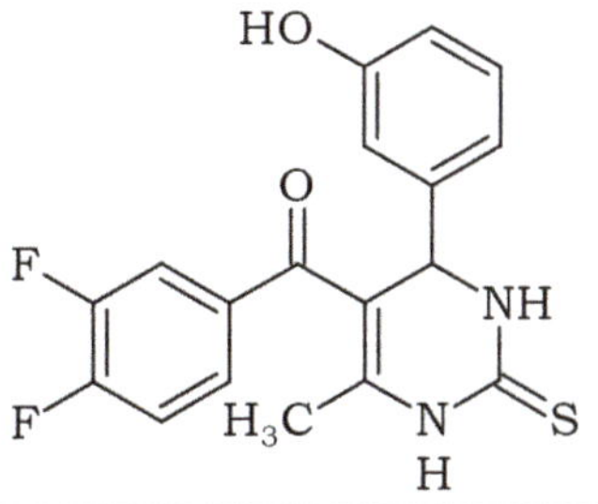
Monastrol	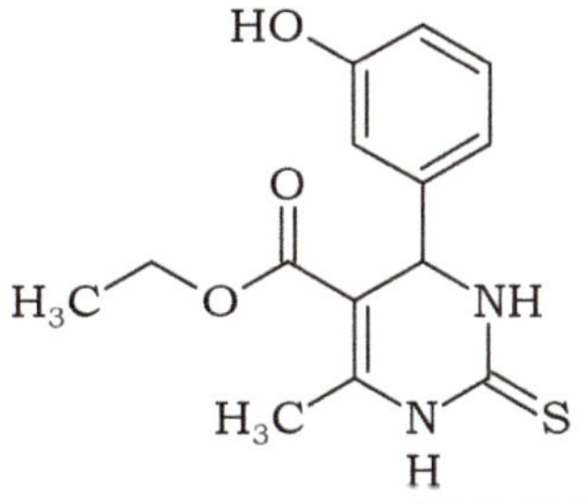

Table ***Contd...***

Enastron	[chemical structure]
Dimethylenastron	[chemical structure]

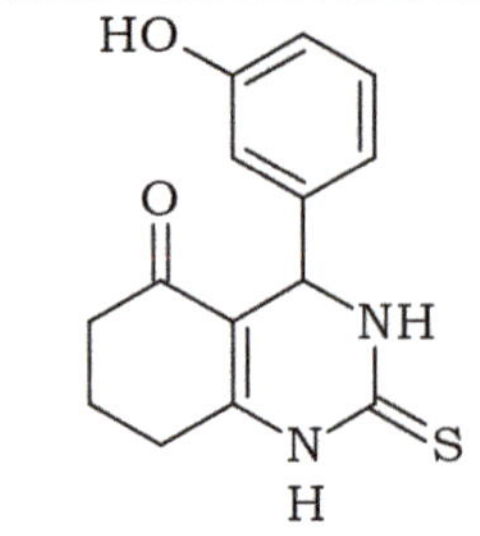

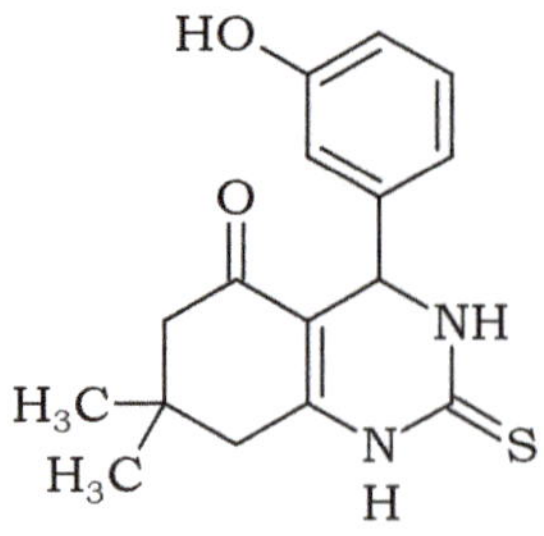

2) Antiviral drugs

Batzelladine B (anti-viral)
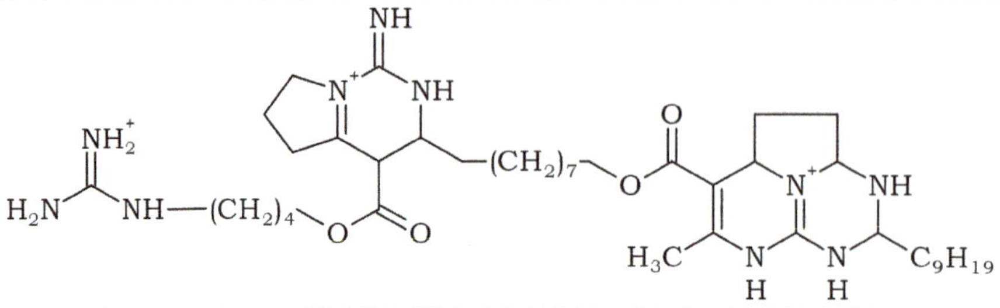 [chemical structure]
Ptilomycalin A (anti-HSV)
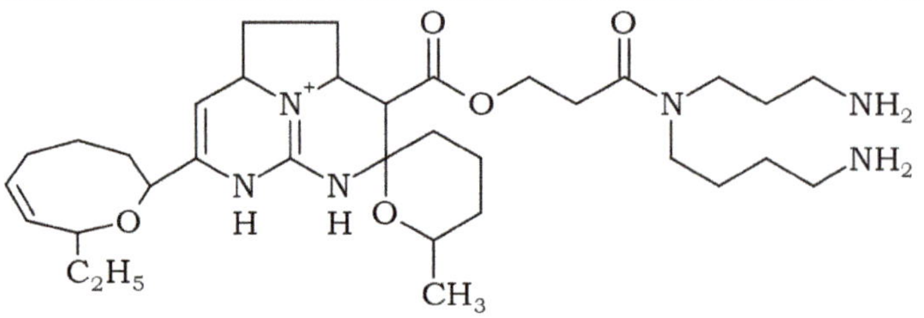 [chemical structure]
Crambescidin (anti-HSV)
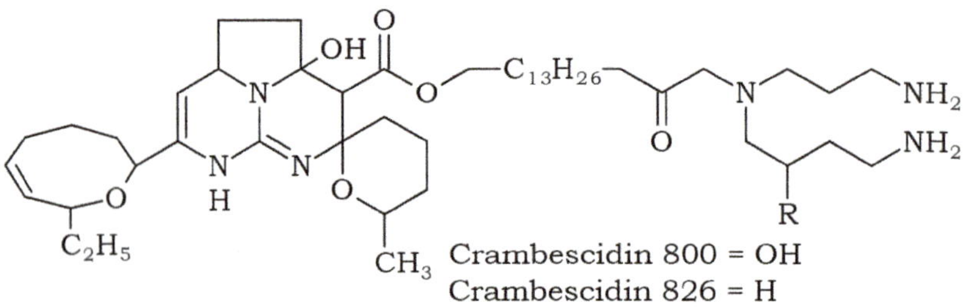 [chemical structure] Crambescidin 800 = OH Crambescidin 826 = H

Table *Contd...*

Dehydrocrambine
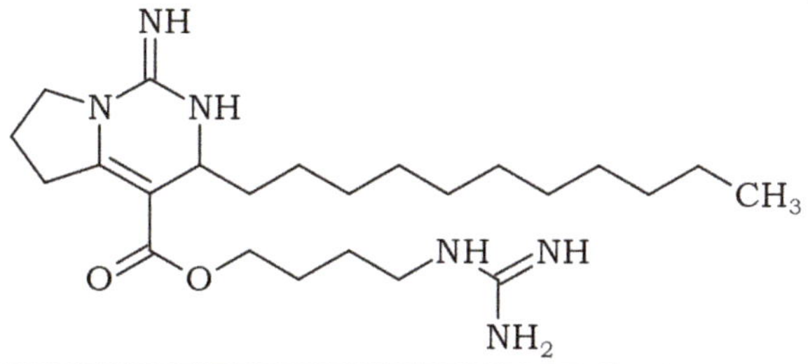 NH, N, NH, CH_3, O, O, NH, NH, NH_2

8.1 Preparation of 5-(Ethoxycarbonyl)-6-methyl-4-phenyl-3,4-dihydropyrimidin-2(1H)-one

Principle: Biginelli synthesis of 5-(ethoxycarbonyl)-4-phenyl-6-methyl-3,4-dihydropyrimidin-2(1*H*)-one involves the condensation of benzaldehyde, ethyl acetoacetate and urea in ethanol medium. The reaction can be catalyzed by calcium chloride ($CaCl_2$) or tetra-*n*-butylammonium bromide (TBAB).

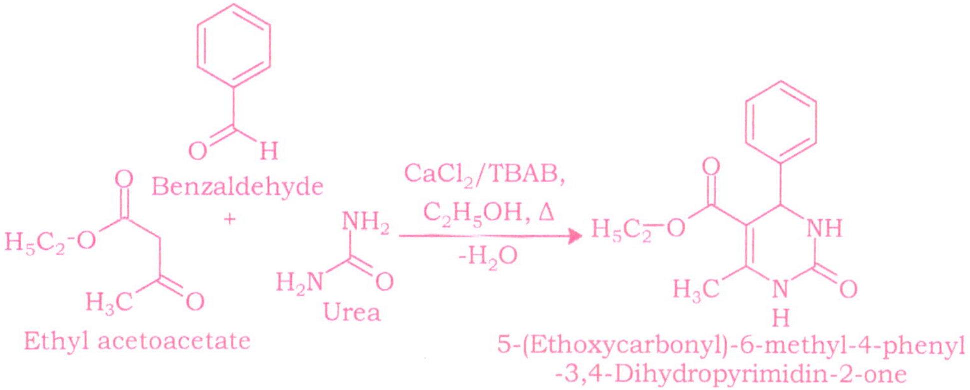

Benzaldehyde + Ethyl acetoacetate + Urea $\xrightarrow[-H_2O]{CaCl_2/TBAB,\ C_2H_5OH,\ \Delta}$ 5-(Ethoxycarbonyl)-6-methyl-4-phenyl-3,4-Dihydropyrimidin-2-one

Reaction Mechanism

Formation of N-acyliminium intermediate

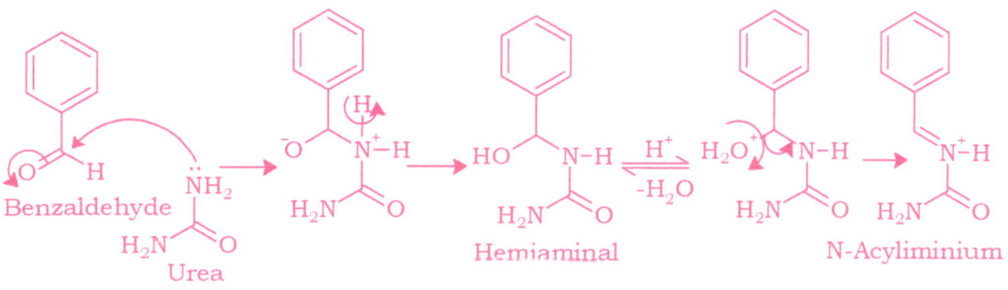

Benzaldehyde + Urea → → Hemiaminal $\underset{-H_2O}{\overset{H^+}{\rightleftharpoons}}$ → N-Acyliminium

Formation of 3,4-dihydropyrimidinone/thione precursor

Ethyl acetoacetate (enol form)

N-Acyliminium

$-H^+$

Precursor

Formation of 3,4-dihydropyrimidinone/thione

Precursor

H^+

$-H_2O$

5-(Ethoxycarbonyl)-4-phenyl-6-methyl-3,4-Dihydropyrimidin-2-one

Procedure:

Chemicals Required: Benzaldehyde, Ethyl acetoacetate, Ethanol/Glacial acetic acid, Calcium chloride/ Tetra-*n*-butylammonium bromide (TBAB).

1. Place ethyl acetoacetate (1.3 mL, 10 mmol), benzaldehyde (1 mL, 10 mmol) and urea (0.72 g, 12 mmol) in a round bottom flask containing ethanol / Glacial acetic acid (10 mL).
2. Add catalyst (calcium chloride = 0.16 g/ TBAB= 1.43 g) to the flask.
3. Attach reflux condenser to the flask and reflux the mixture for 2 h.
4. Pour the hot reaction mixture into the beaker containing crushed ice and stir well (~20 min).
5. Filter the product under vacuum and dry.
6. Purify the crude product by recrystallization with ethanol.
7. The melting range of pure 5-(ethoxy carbonyl)-4-phenyl-6-methyl-3,4-dihydro pyrimidin-2(*1H*)-one is 200 to 201 °C.

8.2 Preparation of Monastrol

Principle: Monastrol, a mitotic kinesin Eg5 inhibitor can be prepared through Biginelli synthesis. It involves the condensation of 3-hydroxybenzaldehyde, ethyl acetoacetate and thiourea in glacial acetic acid medium. The reaction can be catalyzed by benzyl-*n*-triethylammonium chloride (BTEAC).

3-Hydroxybenzaldehyde + Ethyl acetoacetate + Urea → (BTEAC, Gla CH_3COOH, Δ, $-H_2O$) → Monastrol

Reaction Mechanism

Formation of N-acyliminium intermediate

3-Hydroxybenzaldehyde + Thiourea → Hemiaminal ⇌ (H^+, $-H_2O$) → N-Acyliminium

Formation of 3,4-dihydropyrimidinthione precursor

Ethyl acetoacetate (enol form) + N-Acyliminium → ($-H^+$) → Precursor

Formation of dihydropyrimidinthione

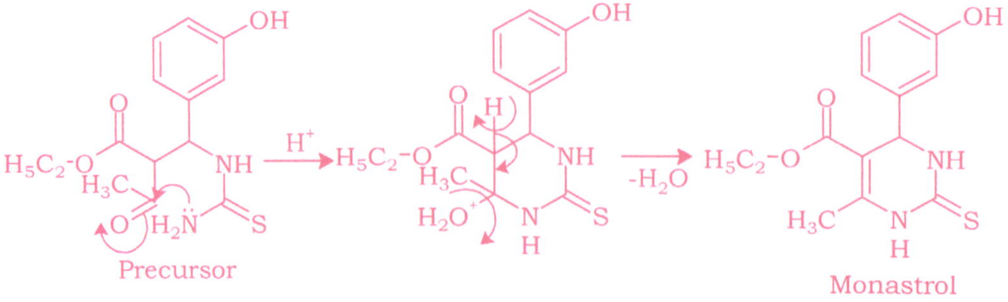

Precursor

$\xrightarrow{H^+}$ $\xrightarrow{-H_2O}$

Monastrol

Procedure:

Chemicals Required: 3-Hydroxybenzaldehyde, Ethyl acetoacetate, Thiourea, Benzyl-*n*-triethylammonium chloride (BTEAC), Ethanol.

1. Place ethyl acetoacetate (1.4 mL, 11 mmol), 3-hydroxy benzaldehyde (1.4 g, 11 mmol) and thiourea (0.72 g, 9.5 mmol) in a round bottom flask.
2. Add BTEAC (0.23 g, 10 mol%) to the flask and heat the mixture at 100 ºC for 60 min.
3. Pour the hot reaction mixture into the beaker containing crushed ice and stir well (~10 min).
4. Filter the product under vacuum, wash with ice-cold water (50 mL) and dry.
5. Purify the crude product by recrystallization with hot ethanol.
6. The melting range of pure monastrol is 185 to 187 °C.

KEY POINTS

- One pot condensation of an aryl aldehyde, β-ketoester and urea/thiourea produces dihydropyrimidinones and the reaction is known as Biginelli synthesis.
- Kappe mechanism, Folkers and Johnson mechanism, and Sweet and Fissekis mechanism are three plausible reactions mechanism for the Biginelli synthesis.
- Kappe mechanism explored the reaction mechanism using NMR spectroscopy, X-ray crystallographic analysis and trapping experiments.
- Fluorastrol (antineoplastic), monastrol (antineoplastic), Batzelladine (antiviral), and Ptilomycalin A (anti-HSV) contains Biginelli structure.

9

Biltz Synthesis

Heinrich Biltz first synthesized the diphenyl hydantoin in 1908. The condensation of benzil and urea produced phenytoin (diphenyl hydantoin). Phenytoin, an anti-convulsant agent belongs to the imidazolidine-2,4-dione (hydantoin) scaffold. Synthesis of phenytoin by base catalyzed condensation of benzil with urea is known as Biltz synthesis. This reaction is catalyzed by sodium ethoxide. This reaction occurs through Benzilic acid rearrangement.

Benzil + Urea $\xrightarrow[H^+]{NaOH,\ C_2H_5OH}$ Phenytoin

Pharmaceutical applications

1) Anticonvulsant drug: It is used in the treatment of grandmal epilepsy and psychomotor epilepsy.
2) Anti-ulcer drug: It is effective in treating epidermolysis bullosa, pressure ulcer, diabetic ulcers, venous stasis ulcers, traumatic wounds and burns.
3) Cutaneous drug: It is useful in linear scleroderma conditions in children's.
4) Anti-allergic drug: It is an effective immunomodulator. It suppresses the cytotoxic activities of natural killer (NK) cells and cytotoxic T-lymphocytes (CTL).
5) Neuroprotective drug: It is used in treating the neuropathic pain. It is effective in diabetic neuropathy and trigeminal neuralgia.
6) Cardioprotective Drug: It is drug for cardiac arrhythmias (class 1b antiarrythmic agent).

9.1 Preparation of Phenytoin

Traditional Name: Diphenyl hydantoin, Dihydantoin, Dilantin

***IUPAC Name*:** 5,5-Diphenylimidazolidine-2,4-dione **Mol wt**: 252.27 g/mol

History of phenytoin: In 1908, Heinrich Biltz synthesized the diphenyl hydantoin for the first time. In 1920s, Arthur Dox at parke –Davis prepared the same molecule for hypnotic property, but noticed inactive. Tracy. J. Putnam (1936) was attracted by the fact that the phenobarbitone is more active (hypnotic). Hence, stimulated to study on phenyl derivatives.

Principle: Base (sodium ethoxide) catalyzed condensation of benzil and urea forms phenytoin and the reaction is known as Biltz synthesis.

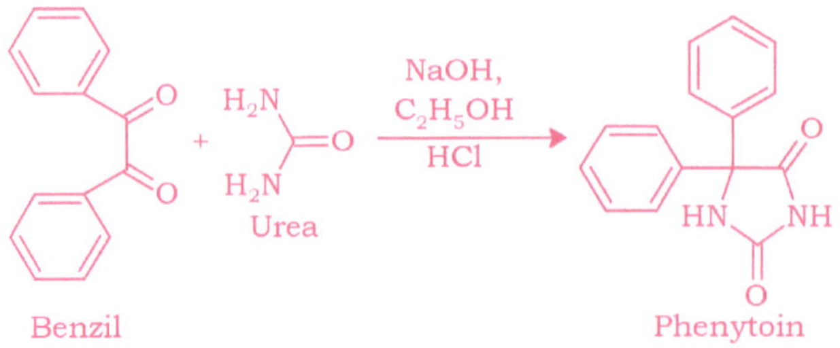

Benzil + Urea $\xrightarrow[\text{HCl}]{\text{NaOH, } C_2H_5OH}$ Phenytoin

This phenytoin preparation from benzil undergoes the Benzilic acid rearrangement reaction. The reaction also progresses through the Pinacol-Pinacolone rearrangement.

Benzilic acid rearrangement: Sodium ethoxide base (C_2H_5ONa) mediates the rearrangement of benzil into benzilic acid ester *via* phenyl group migration (1,2-rearrangement). This rearrangement reaction is known as Benzilic acid rearrangement. The ethoxide anion attacks one of the carbonyl carbon (polarization) of benzil. This prompts the phenyl group migration into the next carbon (1,2-aryl shift) and generates benzilic acid ester. The lone pair electrons of the urea nitrogen attack the ester carbonyl carbon and eliminates the ethanol. The acid protonates the hydroxyl group and promotes water elimination. The formed carbocation intermediate undergo cyclization by the attack of lone pair of electrons of urea nitrogen to generate phenytoin.

Generation of nucleophile

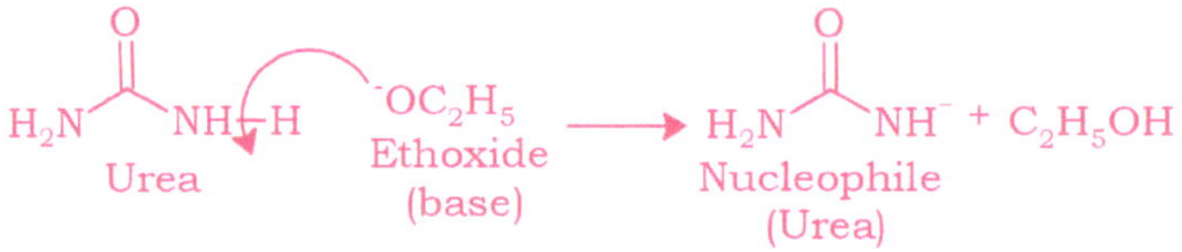

Urea + $^-OC_2H_5$ Ethoxide (base) ⟶ $H_2N\text{–CO–}NH^-$ Nucleophile (Urea) + C_2H_5OH

Benzilic acid rearrangement

Benzil + $^-OC_2H_5$ Ethoxide (base) ⟶ ⟶ Benzilic acid ester + Nucleophile (Urea) ⟶

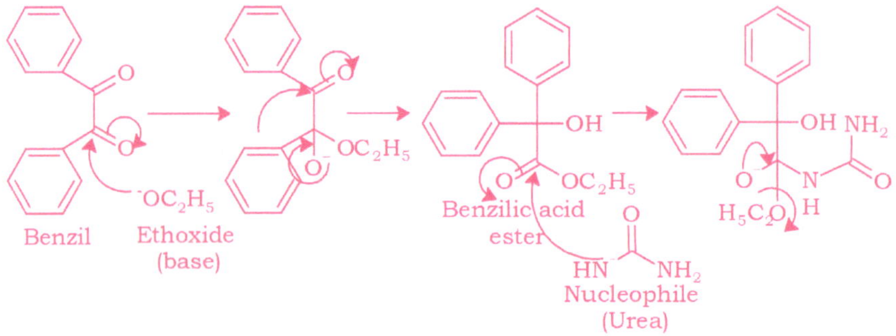

Cyclization and phenytoin formation

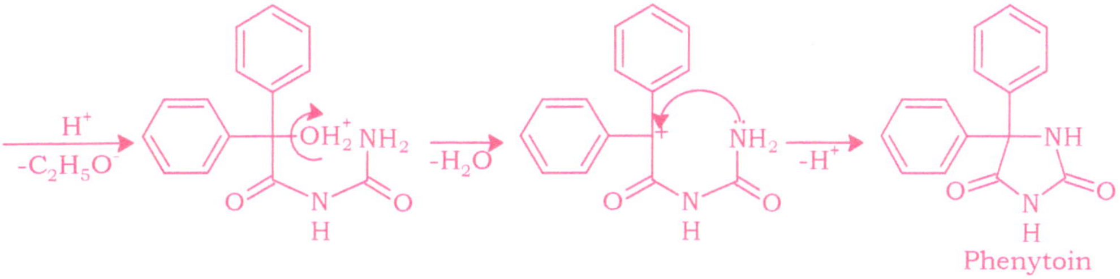

Phenytoin

Pinacol-Pinacolone rearrangement : Phenyl group shift and carbonyl group generation is characteristic of Pinacol-Pinacolone rearrangement reaction. Completely substituted 1,2-diols are known as pinacols. Base (sodium ethoxide) abstracts proton (H^+) from the urea and generates urea nucleophile. The nucleophile attacks the electrophilic center of carbonyl carbon of benzil and forms 1,2-diol (1,2-glycol/pinacol) through cyclization. Acid protonation of one of the hydroxyl group prompts the elimination of water molecule and generates electron deficient carbon atom. Phenyl group shift (1,2-shift) to electron deficient carbon and oxidation of another hydroxyl group generates carbonyl group (pinacolone).

Generation of nucleophile

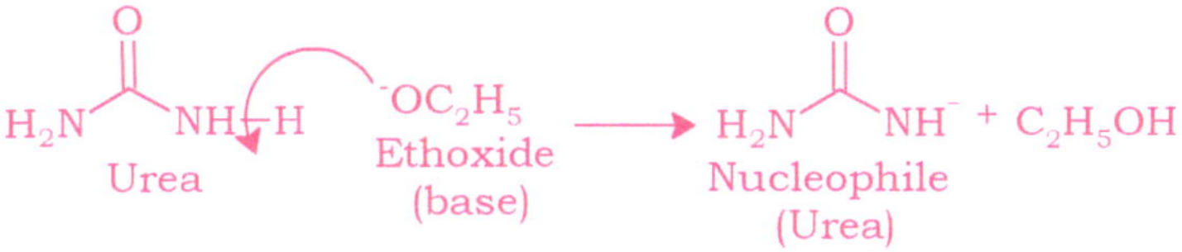

Urea Ethoxide (base) Nucleophile (Urea) + C_2H_5OH

Nucleophilic attack and pinacol formation

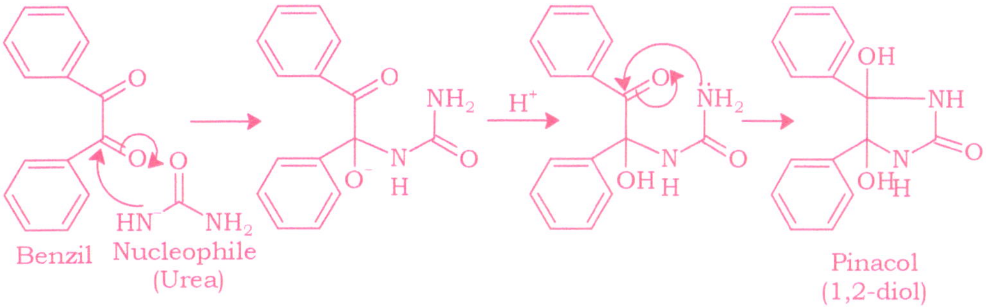

Benzil Nucleophile (Urea)

Pinacol (1,2-diol)

Rearrangement and pinacolone formation

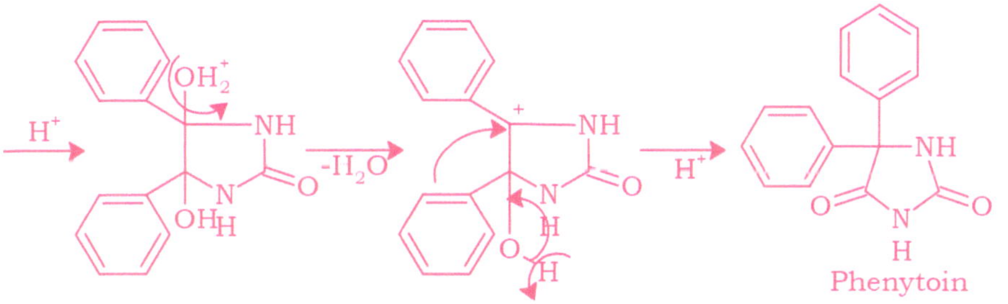

Phenytoin

Procedure:

Chemicals Required: Benzil, Urea, Ethanol, Sodium hydroxide (30%), Hydrochloric acid (dilute), Rectified Spirit.

1. Place benzil (1.1 g, 5 mmol), urea (0.6 g, 10 mmol), sodium hydroxide (3 mL, 30%) and ethanol (15 mL) in a round bottom flask.
2. Attach reflux condenser to the flask and reflux the mixture for 2 h.
3. Cool the reaction mixture to room temperature and pour into the beaker containing water (25 mL).
4. Stir thoroughly, allow it to stand for 15 min and filter (to remove any insoluble by product).
5. Acidify the filtrate with hydrochloric acid and cool in an ice bath.
6. Filter the precipitate immediately under vacuum and dry.
7. Purify the crude phenytoin by recrystallization with rectified sprit.
8. The melting range of pure phenytoin is 297 to 298 °C.

Note: Refer oxidation experiments 22 (Refer Page 179) for the preparation of benzil from benzoin

KEY POINTS

- Base catalyzed condensation of benzil and urea produces phenytoin, this reaction is known as Biltz synthesis.
- Phenytoin belongs to hydantoin scaffold and is well known anti-convulsant drug.
- Benzilic acid rearrangement mechanism and Pinacol-Pinacolone rearrangement are the two plausible reactions mechanism for the Biltz synthesis.

10

Borsche-Drechsel Cyclization

Two step conversion of arylhydrazine and cyclohexanone derivatives into corresponding carabazoles is known as Borsche-Drechsel cyclization. The first step involves the condensation of arylhydrazine and cyclohexanone, acid catalyzed sigmotropic rearrangement and ring closure leads to the formation of tetrahydrocarbazole. In the second step, the oxidation of tetrahydrocarbazole (aromatization) generates carbazole.

The reaction yields carbazole and its derivatives, hence the reaction refers to Borsche-Carbazole synthesis. The condensation step is very similar to that of Fisher Indole synthesis. Hence this reaction is also known as Fischer-Borsche synthesis.

Arylhydrazine + Cyclohexanone derivative $\xrightarrow{H^+}$ Tetrahydrocarbazole $\xrightarrow{(O)}$ Carbazole

Mineral acids (e.g., sulphuric acid), polyphosphoric acid, ceric ammonium nitrate and acidic ionic liquids (e.g., chloroaluminate) can be used as acid catalyst for the formation of tetrahydrocarbazole. The catalysts namely, palladium on carbon in acetonotrile, activated carbon in xylene, sulphur in boilng quinoline, raney nickel in refluxing xylene, chloranil in boiling xylene, pyridinium hydrochloride, mercurous acetate in glacial acetic acid, iodine in dimethylsulphoxide (DMSO) and 2,3-dichloro-5,6-dicyanobenzoquinone (DDQ) are useful for the chemical conversion of tetrahydrocarbazole into carbazole.

Reaction Mechanism

Step 1: Formation of tetrahydrocarbazole

Arylhydrazine + Cyclohexanone derivative → → Carbinolamine $\xrightarrow{-H_2O}$

Sigmotropic rearrangement
Tautomerization
Imine intermediate (schiff base)
Ene hydrazine
Double imine
Double imine
$-NH_3$
-H
Tetrahydrocarbazole

Step 2: Formation of carbazole

Oxidation
Tetrahydrocarbazole
Carbazole

Pharmaceutical Applications

1. Total synthesis of natural carbazole alkaloids

(a) Antibacterial Murrayafoline A can be constructed through Borsche-Carbazole synthesis.

Phenylhydrazine
4-Methyl cyclohexanone
Tetrahydrocarbazole
Murrayafoline A

(b) Total synthesis of antifungal carbazomycin G was reported through Borsche-Carbazole synthesis.

2-Methyl-tetrahydro carbazole
Carbazomycin G

2. Synthesis of pharmaceuticals

(a) Borsche-Carbazole synthesis is useful in the chemical synthesis of carvedilol (antihypertensive).

Phenylhydrazine + 1,3-Cyclohexane dione → Tetrahydrocarbazole-1-one → Carvedilol

(b) Synthesis of ciclindole and flucindole (antipsychotic) can be conducted through Borsche-Carbazole synthesis.

Substituted Phenylhydrazine + N,N-Dimethylcyclohexanone → Carbazole drugs
Ciclindole; R = H
Flucindole; R = F

10.1 Preparation of Carbazole

Traditional Name: Dibenzopyrrole, 9-Azafluorene, Diphenyleneimide

IUPAC Name: *9H*-Carbazole **Mol wt**: 167.21 g/mol

Principle: The reaction involved in the preparation of carbazole is known as Borsche-Drechsel cyclization. It involves a two step reaction. The condensation of phenylhydrazine and cyclohexanone followed by the acid catalyzed sigmotropic rearrangement leads to the formation of tetrahydrocarbazole. Phenyl hydrazine condenses with cyclohexanone and forms imine intermediate. This intermediate through sigmotropic rearrangement and ring closure produces 1,2,3,4-tetrahydrocarbazole (first step). The oxidation of tetrahydrocarbazole (aromatization) generates carbazole (second step).

Phenylhydrazine + Cyclohexanone $\xrightarrow{H^+}$ Tetrahydrocarbazole $\xrightarrow{\text{Oxidation}}$ Carbazole

Reaction mechanism

Step 1: Formation of tetrahydrocarbazole

Cyclohexanone

Phenylhydrazine

Carbinolamine

$-H_2O$

Sigmotropic rearrangement

H^+

Imine intermediate (schiff base)

Tautomerization

Ene hydrazine

Double imine

Double imine

$-NH_3$ -H

Tetrahydrocarbazole

Step 2: Formation of carbazole

Chloranil

Oxidation

Tetrahydrocarbazole

Carbazole

Procedure:

Step 1: Preparation of 1,2,3,4-tetrahydrocarbazole

Chemicals Required: Cyclohexanone, Phenylhydrazine, Glacial acetic acid, Charcoal, Ethanol (75%) , Methanol.

1. Place cyclohexanone (1 mL, 10 mmol), glacial acetic acid (3.5 mL) in a round bottom flask.
2. Attach reflux condenser and reflux the contents for 1 h with stirring.
3. Add phenylhydrazine (1 mL, 10 mmol) and continue stirring for 1 h.
4. Pour the mixture into beaker containing water (25 mL) and stir vigorously until the oily substance gets solidified.

5. Cool the mixture to 5 °C and filter the solid.
6. Wash it with water (5 mL) followed by ethanol (5 mL, 75%) and dry. *(Remove the coloured impurities, if any by charcoal treatment)*
7. Purify the crude product by recrystallization with methanol.
8. The melting range of pure 1,2,3,4-tetrahydrocarbazole is 116 to 117 °C.

Step 2: Preparation of carbazole

Chemicals Required: 1,2,3,4-tetrahydrocarbazole, Chloranil, Xylene, Diethyl ether, Sodium sulphate, Sodium hydroxide solution, Methanol.

1. Place tetrahydrocarbazole (2 g, 11 mmol), chloranil (5.66 g, 23 mmol) and sulphur free xylene (quantity sufficient to dissolve) into a round bottom flask.
2. Attach reflux condenser and reflux the contents until a few drops of solution produces no red colour with sodium hydroxide (~24 h).
3. Cool the hot reaction mixture to 5 °C and remove the solid.
4. Dilute the solution with diethyl ether, shake it with sodium hydroxide and with water.
5. Dry the solution by passing through sodium sulphate.
6. Evaporate the solvent and purify the crude solid carbazole by recrystallization with methanol and xylene.
7. The melting point of pure carbazole is 245 °C.

KEY POINTS

- The cylization of arylhydrazine and cyclohexanones forms carabazoles, and this reaction is known as Borsche-Drechsel cyclization.
- The reaction involves acid catalyzed sigmotropic rearrangement and aromatization to generate carbazole.
- This condensation reaction is also known as Fischer-Borsche synthesis. Murrayafoline A (antibacterial), carbazomycin G (antifungal), carvedilol (antihypertensive), ciclindole and flucindole (antipsychotic) can be synthesised by Borsche-Drechsel cyclization.

11

Claisen Isoxazole Synthesis

Oxazoles and Isoxazole based heterocycles are potential bioactive molecules. A five membered cyclic diene ring containing the two hetero atoms namely O and N adjacent to each other is known as isoxazole. If the hetero atoms are separated by carbon atom (1,3 position), the cyclic structure is named as oxazole.

Isoxazole Oxazole

The isoxazole is present in numerous therapeutic agents, such as sitaxentan (anti-hypertensive), valdecoxib (anti-inflammatory), leflunomide (anti-arthritic), glisoxepide (anti-diabetic) and isocarboxazid (anti-depressant).

Isoxazoles can be prepared by:

1. ***Claisen Isoxazole synthesis***: Active methylene compounds upon condensation with amino compounds produces cycloaddition products. The reaction between β-ketoester (1,3-diketones) and hydroxylamines generate isoxazole.

Ethyl acetoacetate $\xrightarrow[-H_2O]{NH_2OH,\ \Delta}$ 5-Methyl-isoxazol-3-ol

2. ***1,3-Dipolar cycloaddition***: The cycloaddition followed by electrophilic cyclization of nitrile oxides with alkynes produce isoxazole.

Aldehyde $\xrightarrow[-H_2O]{NH_2OH,\ \Delta}$ Nitrile oxide (in situ) $\xrightarrow{R_1-C\equiv CH}$ 3,5-Disubstituted isoxazole

Claisen Isoxazole Synthesis

Claisen described the formation of isoxazoles. The condensation of β-keto esters with hydroxylamine and further cyclization generates two isoxazole molecules (3-isoxazolol and 5-isoxazolone).

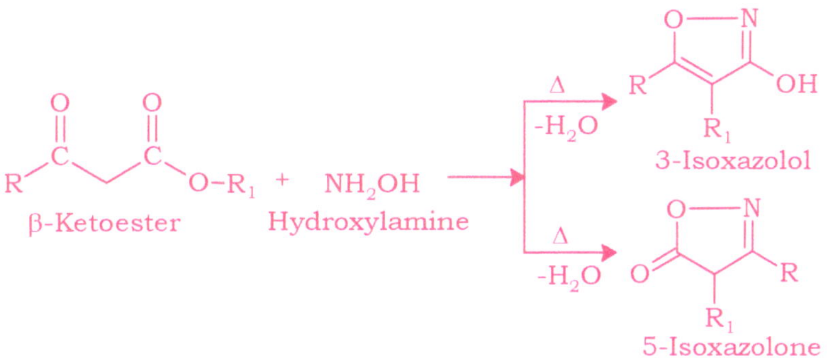

Reaction Mechanism

The substitution at α and β carbons (R_1 and R) generates differently substituted isoxazole (e.g., 4,5-disubstituted isoxazole).

- ***Formation of 5-isoxazololone***

  2-Substituted β-ketoester produces 5-isoxazololone

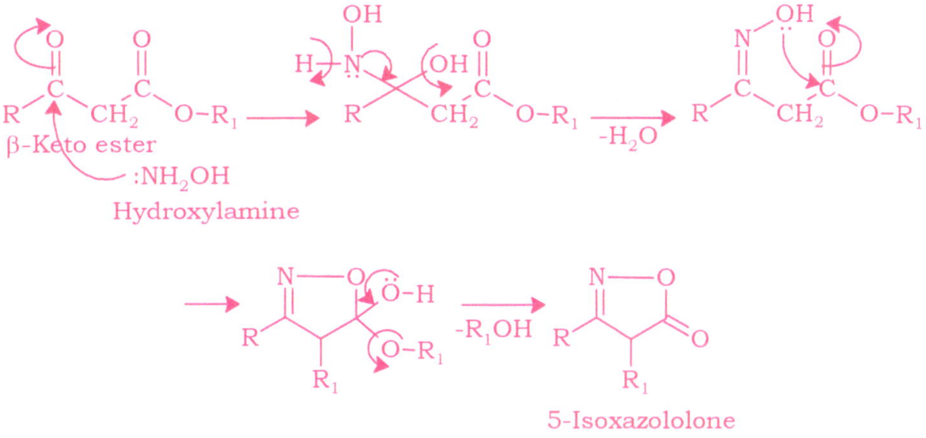

- ***Formation of 3-isoxazolol***

  2-Unsubstituted β-ketoester produce 3-isoxazolone.

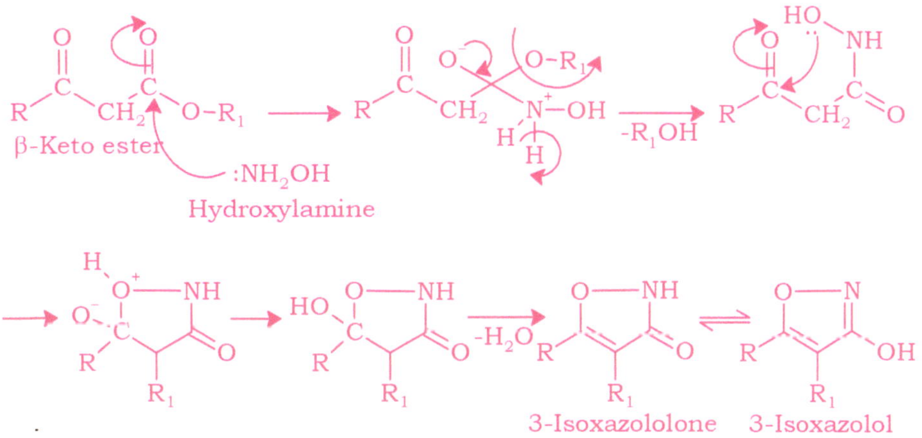

11.1 Preparation of 3,5-Dimethylisoxazole

IUPAC Name*:* 3,5-Dimethyl-1,2-oxazole **Mol wt**: 97.12 g/mol

Principle:. The cycloaddition reaction between β-ketoester (1,3-diketones) and hydroxylamine generates isoxazole. Acetyl acetone (1,3-diketones) condenses with hydroxylamine followed by the cyclization to produce 3,5-dimethylisoxazole.

$$H_3C-CO-CH_2-CO-CH_3 + NH_2OH \xrightarrow[-H_2O]{\Delta} \text{3,5-Dimethylisoxazole}$$

Acetyl acetone Hydroxylamine 3,5-Dimethylisoxazole

Reaction mechanism

Acetyl acetone + :NH_2OH (Hydroxylamine) → $\xrightarrow{-H_2O}$ → $\xrightarrow{-H_2O}$ 3,5-Dimethylisoxazole

Procedure:

Chemicals Required: Acetyl acetone, Hydroxylamine, Diethyl ether, Ferric chloride, Ethanol.

Experimental steps

1. Place hydroxylamine (7 g, 100 mmol) in a round bottom flask containing water (15 mL) and ethanol (10 mL).
2. Add acetyl acetone (10.2 mL, 100 mmol) in ethanol (10 mL) to the flask and attach the reflux condenser to the flask.
3. Reflux the contents until the negative ferric chloride test is obtained.
4. Pour the hot reaction mixture into beaker containing cold water (60 mL).
5. Extract the aqueous mixture with diethyl ether (5 mL, three times).
6. Combine the three ether extracts (in RBF) and evaporate the ether layer.
7. Brown oil residue remains in the flask and distill the oil (purification) to get colourless oil.
8. The boiling range of pure 3,5-dimethylisoxazole is 140 to 142 ºC.

Ferric chloride test: Test for detecting the presence of hydroxylamine.

KEY POINTS

- The condensation between β-ketoester (1,3-diketone) and hydroxylamine generates isoxazole, this reaction is known as Claisen isoxazole synthesis.
- Sitaxentan (anti-hypertensive), valdecoxib (anti-inflammatory), leflunomide (anti-arthritic), glisoxepide (anti-diabetic) and isocarboxazid (anti-depressant) contains isoxazole in the structure.
- Ferric chloride test is useful in the detection of unreacted hydroxylamine. Hydroxylamine produces blue colour with ferric chloride

12

Claisen-Schmidt Reaction

The condensation of two carbonyl compounds (aldehydes and or ketones) containing at least one α-hydrogen atom generates β-hydroxylcarbonyl compound (condensation product). The reaction can be catalyzed by base (e.g., NaOH) and acid (e.g., HCl). This condensation is applicable for aromatic and aliphatic carbonyl compounds.

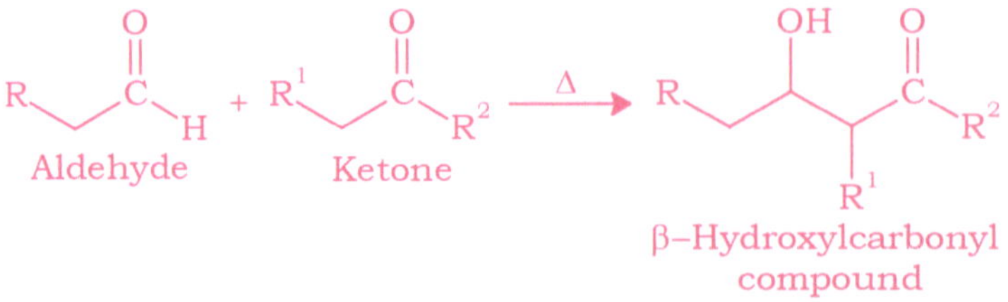

Aldehyde + Ketone →(Δ) β–Hydroxylcarbonyl compound

The condensation product upon base mediated reaction eliminates water molecule and forms α,β-unsaturated compound (conjucated double bond, C=C).

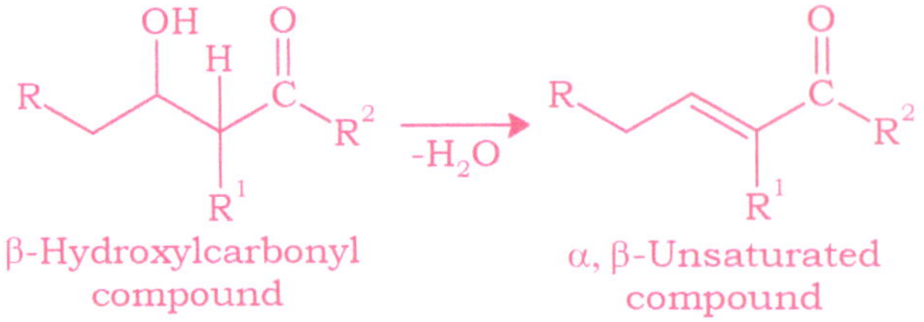

β-Hydroxylcarbonyl compound →($-H_2O$) α, β-Unsaturated compound

Cross aldol condensation reaction is known as Claisen-Schmidt condensation (also known as Claisen reaction). The condensation of benzaldehyde (contains no α-hydrogen and acetophenone (contains α-hydrogen) is typical example for this reaction. This reaction produces benzylidene acetophenone. Benzylidene acetophenone is the parent member of chalcone.

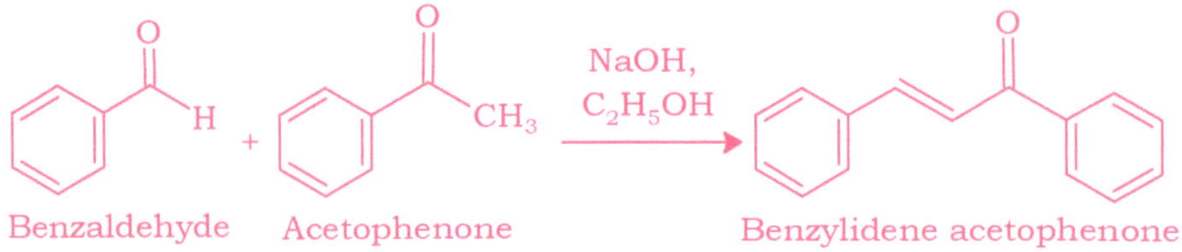

Benzaldehyde + Acetophenone →(NaOH, C_2H_5OH) Benzylidene acetophenone

The condensation of esters (e.g., β-keto ester) is known as Claisen condensation.

This condensation occurs as follows:

(a) Condensation between two aldehydes (identical/different). At least one α-hydrogen atom is required.

$$\underset{\text{Aldehyde}}{RCH_2CHO} + \underset{\text{Aldehyde}}{RCH_2CHO} \xrightarrow{\Delta} \underset{\beta\text{-Hydroxycarbonyl compound}}{RCH_2CH(OH)CH(R)CHO}$$

$$\underset{\text{Aldehyde}}{RCH_2CHO} + \underset{\text{Aldehyde}}{R^1CH_2CHO} \xrightarrow{\Delta} \underset{\beta\text{-Hydroxycarbonyl compound}}{RCH_2CH(OH)CH(R^1)CHO}$$

This condensation product (α-hydroxylcarbonyl compound) contains an aldehyde (*ald*) and a hydroxyl (*ol*) group, and is known as *aldol* (aldehyde +alcohol). Hence this reaction is named as aldol condensation. The consdensatin between different aldehydes are known as mixed aldol condensation.

In general two different aldehydes can generate four possible condensation products. It includes self condensation products (2) and condensation products of two different carbonyl compounds (2).

(b) Condensation between an aldehyde and ketone. At least one α-hydrogen atom is required. This reaction occurs between two different carbonyl members (aldehydes and ketones), hence known as Cross-aldol condensation.

$$\underset{\text{Aldehyde}}{RCH_2CHO} + \underset{\text{Ketone}}{R^1CH_2COR^2} \xrightarrow{\Delta} \underset{\beta\text{-Hydroxycarbonyl compound}}{RCH_2CH(OH)CH(R^1)COR^2}$$

(c) Condensation between two ketones (identical/different). At least one α-hydrogen atom is required.

Ketone + Ketone $\xrightarrow{\Delta}$ β-Hydroxycarbonyl compound

Ketone + Ketone $\xrightarrow{\Delta}$ β-Hydroxycarbonyl compound

Reaction Mechanism

Base-catalyzed condensation is classical method for the preparation of chalcones. The aldehyde is more reactive towards nucleophiles of ketone (ketone enolate) and avoids the self condensation of ketone enolate. This can be achieved by the addition of ketone to mixture of aldehyde and base. Piperidine mediated chalcone synthesis avoids multiple condensation, polymerization and rearrangement reactions.

Step 1: Base abstracts α-hydrogen and generates nucleophile (enolate ion)

Ketone + ^-OH $\underset{-H_2O}{\rightleftharpoons}$ Nucleophile (enolate ion)

Step 2: Nucleophilic attack of enolate ion on carbonyl group of aldehyde

Aldehyde + Nucleophile (enolate ion) $\rightleftharpoons$ … $\underset{H_2O}{\rightleftharpoons}$ …

Step 3: Generation of α, β- unsaturated compound

… $\xrightarrow{H^+}$ … $\xrightarrow{-H_2O}$ α, β-Unsaturated compound

Pharmaceutical Applications

1) Flavanone is the core structure of several natural flavanoids such as naringenin and hesperidin. Flavanone can be synthesized by Claisen-Schmidt reaction.

2-Hydroxy acetophenone + Benzaldehyde —Base→ Flavanone

2) Raspberry ketone, also known and rheosmin is an important flavouring agent in the perfume and food industry. It can be synthesized through Claisen-Schmidt reaction.

4-Hydroxy benzaldehyde + Acetone —Base→ 4-Hydroxybenzalacetone (PHBA) → Raspberry ketone (Rheosmin)

12.1 Preparation of Benzylidene Acetophenone

Traditional Name: Chalcone, Benzalacetophenone

IUPAC Name: 1,3-Diphenylprop-2-en-1-one **Mol wt**: 208.26 g/mol

Principle: Benzylidene acetophenone (chalcone) can be prepared through the Claisen-Schmidt reaction. Acetophenone condenses with benzaldehyde under alkaline condition (sodium hydroxide) in ethanol medium produces benzylidene acetophenone.

Benzaldehyde + Acetophenone —NaOH, C_2H_5OH→ Benzylidene acetophenone

Reaction Mechanism

Step 1: Sodium hydroxide abstracts α-hydrogen from acetophenone and generates nucleophile (enolate ion).

Acetophenone

$-H_2O$

Nucleophile (enolate ion)

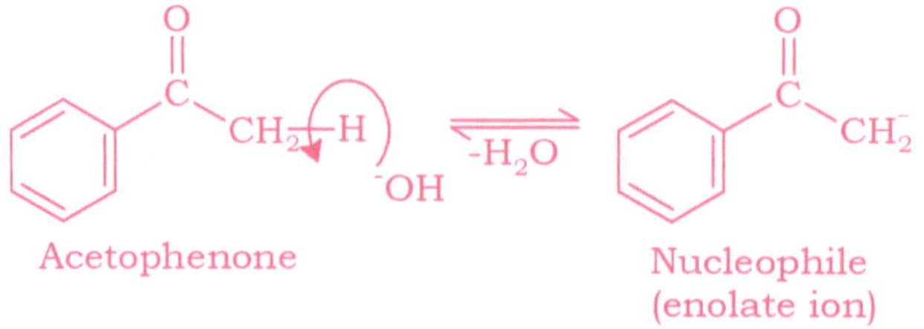

Step 2: Nucleophilic attack of enolate on carbonyl group of benzaldehyde.

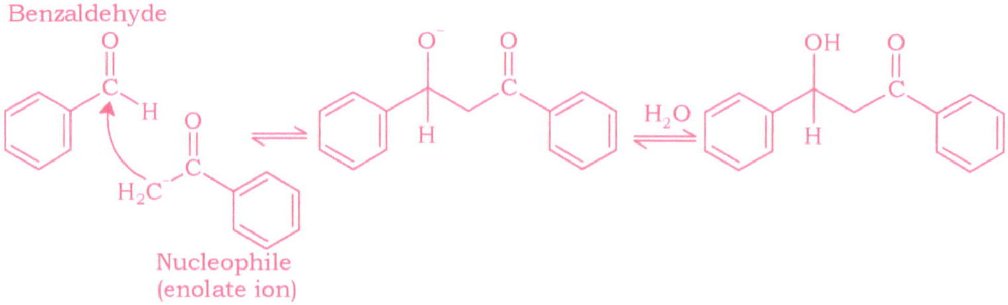

Benzaldehyde

Nucleophile (enolate ion)

Step 3: Generation of benzylidene acetophenone (α, β- unsaturated compound).

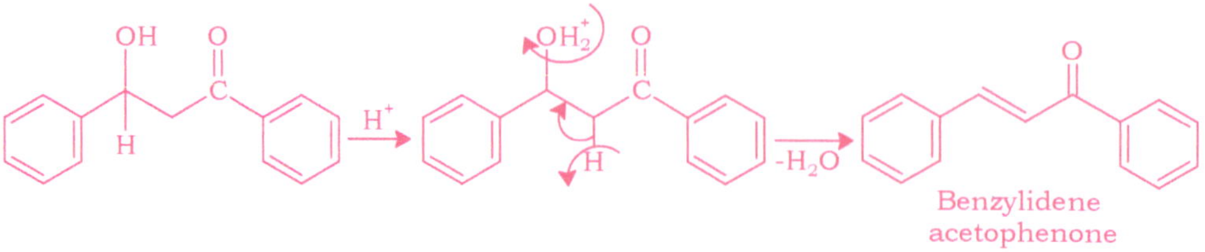

Benzylidene acetophenone

Procedure:

Chemicals Required: Acetophenone, Benzaldehyde, Sodium hydroxide, Ethanol

Experimental steps

1. Place a solution of sodium hydroxide (2.2 g, 55 mmol) in water (20 mL) and ethanol (15 mL) in a flask.
2. Immerse the flask on an ice-bath to maintain the temperature between 20-30 °C (optimum temperature is 25 °C).

   Higher temperature (>30 °C) promotes secondary reactions. It reduces the purity and yield.
3. Pour freshly distilled acetophenone (5 mL, 43 mmol) and add benzaldehyde (4.4 mL, 43 mmol).
4. Stir the mixture vigorously until it becomes thick (~ 3 h).

5. Keep the reaction mixture in refrigerator for overnight.

   The product separates as an oil, if the temperature is low and high, and/srtirring is slow (which forms lumps).
6. Filter the solid separated through vacuum filtration, wash with cold water (until the washings are neutral to litmus) and with 20 mL of cold ethanol.
7. Recrystallize the product from ethanol.
8. The melting range of the pure benzylidene acetophenone is 56 to 57 °C.

Caution: Benzylidene acetophenone is skin irritant, hence handle with gloves.

KEY POINTS

- Condensation of two carbonyl compounds (aldehydes and or ketones) containing at least one α-hydrogen atom generates β-hydroxylcarbonyl compound (aldol).
- Cross aldol condensation (between an aldehyde and ketone) is known as Claisen-Schmidt condensation (also known as Claisen reaction).
- Piperidine mediated chalcone synthesis avoids multiple condensation, polymerization and rearrangement reactions.
- Naringenin and hesperidin (flavanoids), and Raspberry ketone (rheosmin), can be synthesized by Claisen-Schmidt reaction.

13

Diazotization Reaction

Diazotization is an important chemical reaction in the synthesis of pharmaceuticals. It involves the reaction between aromatic primary amine and nitrous acid under ice-cold condition (0 to 5 °C) to form diazonium salt. Sodium nitrite reacts with hydrochloric acid and generates nitrous acid (HONO) *in situ*. In place of hydrochloric acid, any other mineral acids and inorganic acids can be used. The use of glacial acetic acid also reported.

$$\underset{\text{Arylamine}}{Ar{-}NH_2} + \underset{\text{Sodium nitrite}}{NaNO_2} \xrightarrow[0 \text{ to } 5\ ^\circ C]{HCl} \underset{\text{Aryldiazonium salt}}{Ar{-}N_2^{+}Cl^{-}} + H_2O$$

Aliphatic primary amines do not produce diazonium salt. Instead, it forms alcohol and evolves nitrogen.

$$\underset{\text{Arylamine}}{R{-}NH_2} + \underset{\text{Sodium nitrite}}{NaNO_2} \xrightarrow[0 \text{ to } 5\ ^\circ C]{HCl} \underset{\text{Alcohol}}{R{-}OH} + N_2 + H_2O$$

General method

1) Dissolve the amine in excess of aqueous mineral acid (2.5 to 3 equivalents of water).
   Heat if necessary to effect the dissolution.
2) Cool the solution in an ice-bath to bring the temperature in the range of 0 to 5 °C.
3) Add cold aqueous solution of sodium nitrite, slowly with stirring.
4) The completion of the reaction can be assessed by potassium iodide-starch paper (external indicator) test. The appearance of blue colour, when a drop of reaction mixture placed on the starch paper confirms the excess of nitrous acid (completion of the reaction).

Reaction temperature: The reaction is exothermic, hence should be conducted in the ice-bath (0 to 5 °C). If the temperature is high (> 5 °C), it hydrolyses the diazonium compound into corresponding phenol.

Reaction Mechanism

***Step 1*: Generation of nitrosonium ion (electrophile):** Sodium nitrite reacts with mineral/inorganic acid under ice cold condition (0 to 5 °C) and gives nitrous acid, *in situ*. Nitrous acid upon protonation by mineral acid forms nitrosonium ion (electrophile).

$$NaNO_2 + HCl \xrightarrow[-NaCl]{0\text{ to }5\,°C} HONO \xrightarrow{HCl} O{=}N{-}\overset{+}{O}H_2 \underset{H_2O}{\overset{-H_2O}{\rightleftharpoons}} O{=}N^+ \longrightarrow O\overset{+}{\equiv}N$$

Sodium nitrite; Nitrous acid; Nitrosonium ion (Electrophile)

***Step 2*: Nucleophilic attack on nitrosonium ion:** The electrons of amino group (aromatic primary amine) attacks nitrosonium ion (electrophile) and forms diazonium salt.

$$Ar{-}\ddot{N}H_2 + O{=}N^+ \xrightarrow[0\text{ to }5\,°C]{} Ar{-}\overset{H}{\overset{|}{N^+}}(H){-}N{=}O \xrightarrow[-H^+]{} Ar{-}N(H){-}N{=}O \overset{H^+}{\rightleftharpoons}$$

Arylamine; Nitrosonium ion (Electrophile)

$$\overset{H^+}{\rightleftharpoons} Ar{-}N(H){-}N{=}\overset{+}{O}{-}H \longrightarrow Ar{-}N{=}N{-}O{-}H \xrightarrow{H^+} Ar{-}N{=}N{-}\overset{+}{O}H_2 \underset{-H_2O}{\rightleftharpoons} Ar{-}\overset{+}{N}{\equiv}N$$

Hydroxy diazo intermediate; Aryldiazonium compound

Pharmaceutical Applications

Diazonium salts are important synthetic reagents for the preparation of drugs.

1. Pentetrazol (respiratory stimulant) can be synthesized through diazotization followed by cyclization.

Hydrazinyl caprolactum + $NaNO_2$ (Sodium nitrite) $\xrightarrow{\text{Gla } CH_3COOH}$ Pentetrazol

2. Riboflavin (Vitamin B_2) preparation requires the phenyldiazonium salt (reactant).

N-(3,4-dimethylphenyl)-D-1'-ribamine + Benzenediazonium chloride → Riboflavin

3. Japp-Klingemann hydrazone synthesis: The tranquilizer drug diazepam can be synthesized from 4-chlorolaniline through diazotization step.

4-Chloroaniline + $NaNO_2$ Sodium nitrite —HCl, 5 to 10 °C→ Diazonium salt → Diazepam

4. Japp-Klingemann Fisher indole synthesis: The condensation of aryldiazonium salt and an active methylene compound under acidic (or basic) conditions forms a hydrazone. The hydrazone upon cyclization produces a substituted phenylindole.

Diazonium salt Active methylene compound Phenylindole derivative

5. Drug estimation: Coupling of diazonium ion with drug molecules in acidic or basic medium forms azodyes. It has been used for the estimation of drugs.
   - Diazonium salt condenses with aromatic amine in weak acidic medium to form highly coloured azo compound.
   - Diazonium salt condenses with hydroxyl group of aromatic compounds in weak alkaline condition to form highly coloured azodye.

13.1 Preparation of Benzotriazole

Traditional Name: Aziminobenzene, Benzene azimide

IUPAC Name: 2H-Benzotriazole **Mol wt**: 119.13 g/mol

Principle: Benzotriazole can be prepared by diazotization followed by cyclization. The reaction between sodium nitrite and glacial acetic acid generates nitrous acid, *in situ*. Nitrous acid diazotizes the amino group of *ortho*-phenylenediamine and forms diazonium salt. The formed diazonium group couples with adjacent amino group (of *ortho*-phenylenediamine) and produces benzotriazole.

ortho-Phenylene diamine Benzotriazole

Reaction Mechanism

Step 1: Generation of nitrosonium ion (electrophile)

$$NaNO_2 + HCl \xrightarrow[-NaCl]{0\text{ to }5\ °C} HONO \xrightarrow{HCl} O{=}N{-}\overset{+}{O}H_2 \underset{H_2O}{\overset{-H_2O}{\rightleftharpoons}} O{=}N^+ \longleftrightarrow \overset{+}{O}{\equiv}N$$

Sodium nitrite Nitrous acid Nitrosonium ion (Electrophile)

***Step 2*:** Nucleophilic attack on nitrosonium ion

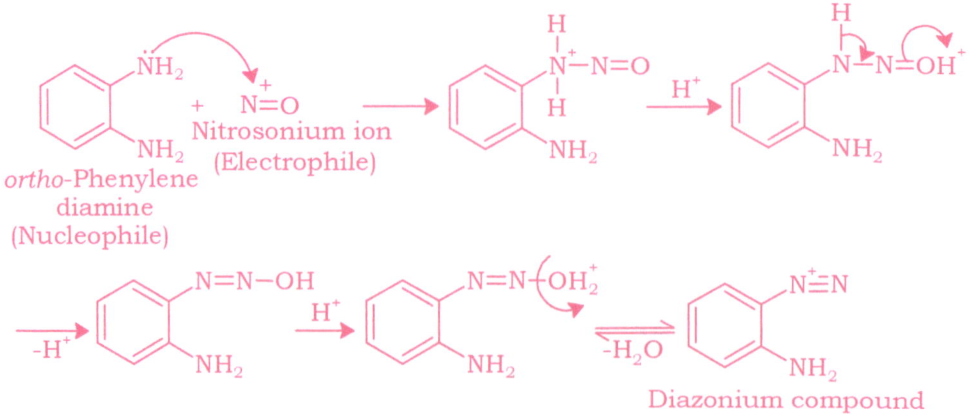

ortho-Phenylene diamine (Nucleophile) + $\overset{+}{N}=O$ Nitrosonium ion (Electrophile) → H^+ → $-H^+$ → H^+ → $-H_2O$ → Diazonium compound

***Step 3*:** Cyclization of diazonium compound into benzotriazole

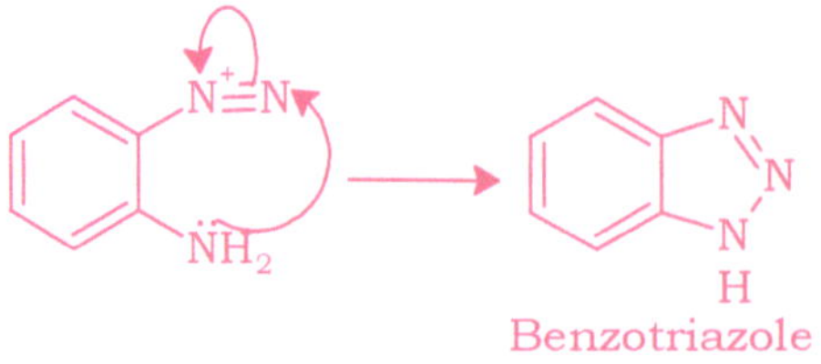

→ Benzotriazole

Procedure:

Chemicals Required: *ortho*-Phenylenediamine, Sodium nitrite, Glacial acetic acid, Charcoal.

Experimental steps

1. Transfer *ortho*-phenylenediamine (1 g, 9 mmol) into a beaker (25 mL) and dissolve with aqueous acetic acid (1 mL in 3 mL of water).
   (warm if necessary to effect the solution)
2. Cool the clear solution by placing in an ice bath to bring the temperature below 5 °C with stirring (magnetic stirring).
3. Add cold aqueous solution of sodium nitrite (0.7 g, 10 mmol) in water (2 mL) to the beaker.
4. The reaction is exothermic (evolves heat). It decomposes the product into corresponding phenol. Hence place the flask in an ice bath to maintain the temperature below 5 ºC (*add crushed ice to the solution, if necessary*).
5. Continue stirring for 15 min and place it in an ice bath for 30 min.
6. Collect the pale brown solid by vacuum filtration and wash with ice-cold water.
7. Dissolve the solid in boiling water (15 mL) and add charcoal for decolourization.
8. Filter and allow the filtrate to cool by placing in an ice bath.
9. Collect the pale straw-coloured needles of crude benzotriazole.

10. Dry the product and purify the crude benzotriazole by recrystallization with benzene.
11. The melting range of pure benzotriazole is 90 to 95 °C.

13.2 Preparation of p-Iodotoluene

Traditional Name: 4-Iodotoluene, *p*-Tolyl iodide

IUPAC Name: 1-Iodo-4-methylbenzene **Mol wt**: 218.04 g/mol

Principle: The preparation of *p*-iodotoluene involves diazotization followed by iodination with potassium iodide. The reaction between sodium nitrite and glacial acetic acid generates nitrous acid, *in situ*. Diazotization of *p*-toluidine with nitrous acid forms diazonium salt. The diazonium salt upon iodination by potassium iodide generates *p*-iodotoluene.

NH_2 / CH_3 — $\xrightarrow[\text{0 to 5 °C}]{NaNO_2,\ HCl}$ — N_2Cl / CH_3 — $\xrightarrow{KI}$ — I / CH_3 + N_2 + KCl

p-Toluidine Diazonium salt *p*-Iodotoluene

Reaction Mechanism

***Step 1*:** Generation of nitrosonium ion (electrophile)

$NaNO_2$ + HCl $\xrightarrow[\text{-NaCl}]{\text{0 to 5 °C}}$ HONO $\xrightarrow{HCl}$ $O{=}N{-}\overset{+}{O}H_2$ $\underset{H_2O}{\overset{-H_2O}{\rightleftharpoons}}$ $O{=}N^+$ ⟷ $\overset{+}{O}{\equiv}N$

Sodium nitrite Nitrous acid Nitrosonium ion (Electrophile)

***Step 2*:** Electrophilic attack on nitrosonium ion

$\ddot{N}H_2$ / CH_3 + $\overset{+}{N}{=}O$ ⟶ $H{-}\overset{+}{N}(H){-}N{=}O$ / CH_3 $\xrightarrow{-H^+}$ $H{-}N{-}N{=}O$ / CH_3 $\xrightarrow{H^+}$ $H{-}N{-}N{=}OH^+$ / CH_3 ⟶

p-Toluidine (Nucleophile) Nitrosonium ion (Electrophile)

$\xrightarrow{-H^+}$ $N{=}N{-}OH$ / CH_3 $\xrightarrow{H^+}$ $N{=}N{-}\overset{+}{O}H_2$ / CH_3 $\xrightarrow{-H_2O}$ $\overset{+}{N}{\equiv}N$ / CH_3 ⟶ N_2Cl / CH_3

Diazonium salt

***Step 3*:** Conversion of diazonium salt into *p*-iodotoluene

N_2Cl (Diazonium salt, CH_3) $\xrightarrow{KI}$ I (CH_3) (p-Iodotoluene) + N_2 + KCl

Diazonium salt *p*-Iodotoluene

Procedure

***Chemical Required*:** *p*-Toluidine, Sodium nitrite, Dilute hydrochloric acid, Potassium iodide, Sodium hydroxide (10%), Sodium metabisulphite.

Experimental steps

1. Transfer *p*-toluidine (2.7 g, 250 mmol) into a reaction flask and dissolve with dilute hydrochloric acid (6. 3 mL in 6.3 mL of water) (*warm if necessary, to effect the solution*)
2. Cool the clear solution to 0 to 5 °C by placing in a salt water bath / ice bath. (add crushed ice to the solution, if necessary)
3. Add cold aqueous solution of sodium nitrite (1.9 g, 270 mmol) in water (4 mL) slowly to the reaction flask with vigorous stirring.
4. Maintain the temperature at 0 to 5 °C, ensure that it is not above 10 °C.
5. Add potassium iodide solution (4.4 g, 265 mmol) in water (4. 4 mL) slowly to the reaction flask with stirring.
6. Allow to the reaction mixture to stand for 1 h at room temperature.
7. Heat cautiously on a water bath, until the evolution of nitrogen gas ceases.
8. Allow it to cool, a dark coloured oil settles to the bottom and solidifies.
9. Decant the aqueous layer, add sodium metabisulphite (0.2 g) to remove dark colour.
10. Alkalize the solution with sodium hydroxide solution (10%) to retain cresol (byproduct, if any formed).
11. Steam distil the mixture (turn off to melt the condensed solid or the condenser, if required).
12. Purify the crude *p*-iodotoluene by recrystallization with ether.
13. The melting point of the pure *p*-iodotoluene is 35 °C.

13.3 Preparation of 1-Phenylazo-2-naphthol (Sudan-1)

Traditional Name: Sudan-1, Solvent yellow, Spirit orange

IUPAC Name*:* (1-Phenylhydrazinylidene)naphthalene-2-one

Mol wt: 248.29 g/mol

Principle: Azodyes are synthetic dyes and are made from primary arylamines. These dyes are useful in biological testing, titrations as indicators, cosmetics and other chemical processes. 1-Phenylazo-2-naphthol (Sudan-1) is a typical example for azo dye. It can be prepared by two-pot reaction. First aniline (primary aryl amine) gets converted into phenyl diazonium salt under diazotization condition (0 to 5 °C). Nitrous acid formed *in situ* by the reaction between sodium nitrite and hydrochloric acid converts the aniline into diazonium salt. In the next step, the phenyl diazonium salt couples with 2-naphthol and produces 1-phenylazo-2-naphthol (Sudan-1). Chromophoric groups of Sudan-1 (azo, -N=N-) gives bright red colour. It absorbs the light in the range of 480 to 516 nm.

Aniline (NH_2) --[$NaNO_2$, HCl; 0 to 5 °C]--> Phenyl diazonium salt (N_2Cl) --[β-Naphthol (OH); NaOH]--> 1-Phenylazo-2-naphthol (Sudan-1)

Reaction Mechanism

***Step 1*:** Generation of nitrosonium ion (electrophile)

$$NaNO_2 + HCl \xrightarrow[-NaCl]{0\ to\ 5\ °C} HONO \xrightarrow{HCl} O{=}N{-}\overset{+}{O}H_2 \underset{H_2O}{\overset{-H_2O}{\rightleftharpoons}} O{=}N^+ \longleftrightarrow O{\equiv}\overset{+}{N}$$

Sodium nitrite; Nitrous acid; Nitrosonium ion (Electrophile)

***Step 2*:** Nucleophilic attack on nitrosonium ion

Aniline (Nucleophile) ($\ddot{N}H_2$) + $\overset{+}{N}{=}O$ Nitrosonium ion (Electrophile) → $H{-}\overset{+}{N}(H){-}N{=}O$ (Ph) $\xrightarrow{-H^+}$ $H{-}N{-}N{=}O$ (Ph) $\xrightarrow{H^+}$ $H{-}N{-}N{=}OH^+$ (Ph) →

$\xrightarrow{-H^+}$ $N{=}N{-}OH$ (Ph) $\xrightarrow{H^+}$ $N{=}N{-}\overset{+}{O}H_2$ (Ph) $\xrightarrow{-H_2O}$ $\overset{+}{N}{\equiv}N$ (Ph) → N_2Cl (Ph)

Diazonium salt

***Step 3*:** Coupling between phenyl diazonium salt and 2-naphthol

Procedure:

***Step 1:* Preparation of phenyldiazonium salt**

***Chemical Required*:** Aniline, Sodium nitrite, Dilute hydrochloric acid.

Experimental steps

1. Transfer aniline (2.5 mL, 27 mmol) into the round bottom flask and dissolve with the aid of dilute hydrochloric acid (8 mL).
   (*warm if necessary, to effect the solution*)
2. Immerse the flask in an ice-bath (to reduce the temperature below 5 ºC).
3. Add aqueous sodium nitrite solution (2 g in 10 mL of water) in small portions (1 mL at a time) to the flask with stirring and maintain the temperature below 5 ºC.
4. The reaction is exothermic (evolves heat). It decomposes the product into corresponding phenol. Hence place the flask in an ice bath to maintain the temperature below 5 ºC (*add crushed ice to the solution, if necessary*).
5. Add the last 5% of sodium nitrite solution very slowly (0.5 mL at a time), stir (3-4 min) and test the solution with potassium iodide starch paper (external indicator).
6. The appearance of blue colour indicates the completion of reaction (excess of nitrous acid).

***Step 2:* Preparation of anilinediazonium salt**

***Chemical Required*:** Phenyl diazonium compound, 2-Naphthol, Sodium hydroxide, Glacial acetic acid, Ethanol.

Experimental steps

1) Transfer 2-naphthol (3.9 g, 27 mmol) into a beaker and dissolve with aqueous sodium hydroxide solution (22.5 mL, 10%).
2) Cool the solution by placing in an ice-bath to reduce the temperature below 5 ºC (*add crushed ice to the solution, if necessary*).
3) Add the cold diazonium salt solution very slowly with vigorous stirring.

4) Red colour develops and red crystals of 1-phenylazo-2-naphthol separate out.
5) Allow to stand the reaction mixture in an ice-bath for 10 min with occasional stirring.
6) Filter through Buchner funnel and wash the solid with water.
7) Purify the crude product by recrystallization with glacial acetic acid (~35 mL).
8) Wash the recrystallized product with ethanol to remove glacial acetic acid.
9) The melting point of the pure 1-phenylazo-2-naphthol is 131 °C.

KEY POINTS

- The reaction between aromatic primary amine and nitrous acid under ice-cold condition (0 to 5 °C) forms diazonium salt (orange colour dye), and the reaction is known as diazotization.
- The appearance of blue colour, when a drop of reaction mixture placed on the starch paper confirms the excess of nitrous acid (indicates the reaction completion).
- Diazotization reaction is exothermic, hence should be conducted in the ice-bath (0 to 5 °C).
- Synthesis of pentetrazol (respiratory stimulant), diazepam (tranquilizer) and riboflavin (Vitamin B_2) involves diazotization.

14

Erlenmeyer-Plochl Azlactone Synthesis

The acylation of glycine (amino acid) with acetic anhydride (or benzoyl chloride) forms N-acylated glycine derivatives (acetyl/benzoyl glycine). Intramolecular cyclization of acylglycines (dehydration) in the presence of acetic anhydride and sodium acetate forms azlactone (five membered heterocycle). Knoevenagel condensation of azlactone with aromatic aldehydes (or ketones) produces 4-arylideneazalactone. This occurs under base catalyzed reaction. The condesation with benzaldehyde offers 4-benzylidene-2-substituted azlactone. Erlenmeyer and Plochl reported this reaction, hence the name Erlenmeyer-Plochl azlactone synthesis is given.

The benzylidene azlactone upon hydrolysis yields unsaturated α-acetylamino acids. This α-acetylamino acid upon reduction and hydrolysis forms amino acid. The conversion of glycine into phenylalanine (or any other) is known as Erlenmeyer-Plochl synthesis.

Formation of acyl glycine

HOOC–CH_2–NH_2 (Glycine) → with H_3C–CO–CH_2–CO–CH_3 (Acetyl acetone) → HOOC–CH_2–NH–CO–CH_3 (Acetyl glycine)

HOOC–CH_2–NH_2 (Glycine) → with C_6H_5COCl (Benzoyl chloride) → HOOC–CH_2–NH–CO–C_6H_5 (Benzoyl glycine)

Formation of azlactone

$$\text{HN(CO–R)–CH}_2\text{–COOH} \xrightarrow[\text{Cyclization}]{\text{Acetic anhydride}} \text{Azlactone}$$

Acyl glycine
R= CH_3; C_6H_5

Azlactone

Formation of arylidene azlactone

2-Substituted azlactone + Benzaldehyde → 4-Benzylidene 2-subtituted azlactone

Formation of amino acid

4-Benzylidene 2-subtituted azlactone $\xrightarrow{H_2O}$ $\xrightarrow{[H]}$ $\xrightarrow{H_2O}$ Phenylalanine

Heating azlactone in acetic anhydride solution with red phosphorous and hydroiodic acid also yields acylamino acrylic acid in single step.

14.1 Preparation of 4-Benzylidene-2-methylazlactone

IUPAC Name: 4-Benzylidene-2-methyl-1,3-oxazol-5-one

Mol wt: 187.20 g/mol

Principle: Preparation of 4-benzylidene-2-methylazlactone (intermediate in the Erlenmeyer Plochl reaction) can be prepared by the condensation of acetyl glycines in one pot. Acetyl glycine undergoes dehydration in the presence of acetic anhydride and sodium acetate to produce 2-methylazlactone (2-methyloxazolone). This follows the Knoevenagel condensation of benzaldehyde with azlactone. The reactive methylene group of the azlactone under the influence of sodium acetate promotes this reaction.

Acetyl glycine $\xrightarrow[\text{Cyclization}]{\text{Acetic anhydride}}$ 2-Methyl azlactone → 4-Benzylidene 2-methylazlactone

Reaction Mechanism

***Step 1*: Formation of azlactone**

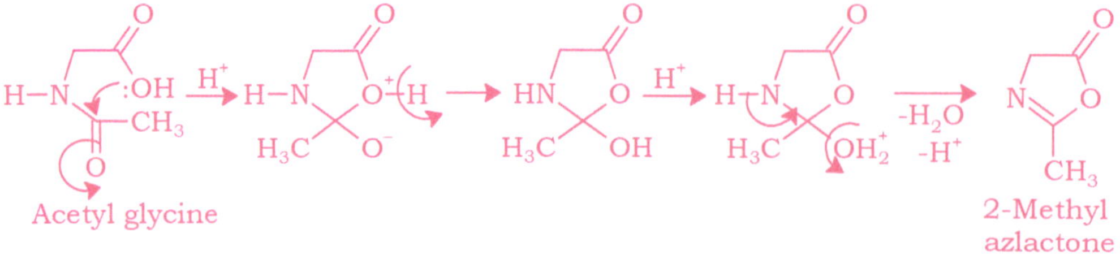

Acetyl glycine

2-Methyl azlactone

***Step 2:* Formation of 4-benzylidene-2-methyloxazol-5-one**

Generation of nucleophile

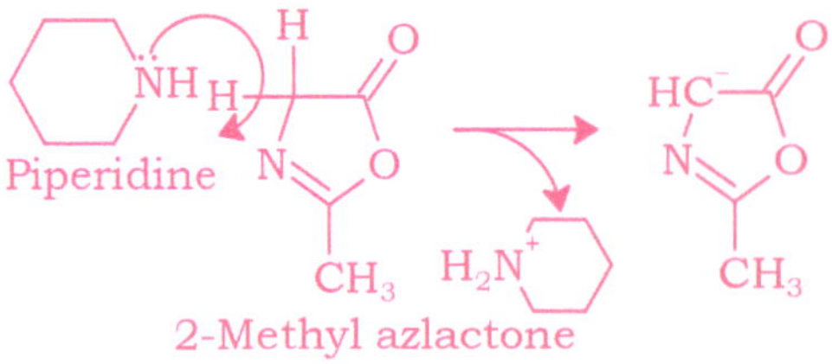

Piperidine

2-Methyl azlactone

Generation of 4-benzylidene-2-methyloxazol-5-one

Benzaldehyde

4-Benzylidene 2-methylazlactone

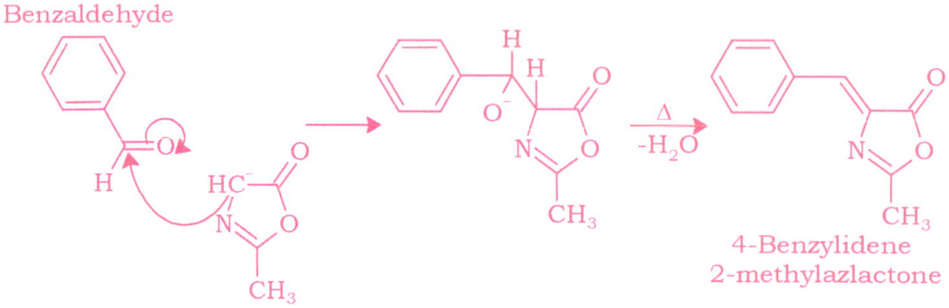

Procedure:

Chemicals Required: *N*-Acetylglycine, Acetic anhydride, Benzaldehyde, Sodium acetate, Carbon tetrachloride

1. Place acetylglycine (1 g, 8.6 mmol), distilled benzaldehyde (1.3 mL, 13 mmol), anhydrous sodium acetate (0.517 g, 6.3 mmol) and acetic anhydride (2 mL, 21 mmol) into the round bottom flask.
2. Stir the mixture to effect the solution (*warm if necessary*).
3. Attach reflux condenser to the flask and boil the reaction mixture for 1 h (water bath).
4. Cool the reaction mixture to room temperature and place the flask in a refrigerator overnight.
5. Stir the resulting yellow crystalline solid with cold water (5 mL).

6. Isolate the yellow solid product by filtration and wash with cold water.
7. Purify the crude product by recrystallization with carbon tetrachloride. (*ethyl acetate-light petroleum mixture also useful*).
8. The melting point of pure 4-benzylidene-2-methylazlactone is 150 °C.

Note: *Refer 3.4 (page 54) for the preparation of acetyl glycine.

KEY POINTS

- The chemical conversion of glycine into phenylalanine (or any other) through number of chemical reactions is a typical example for Erlenmeyer-Plochl synthesis.
- The reaction involves-alkylation, intramolecular cyclization, Knoevenagel condensation and hydrolysis.
- Sodium acetate acts as a base and provides azeotropic condition for the reaction.

15

Fischer Indole Synthesis

Adolph Baeyer (1866) discovered indole in the investigations of indigo. The reduction of isatin (indigo derivative) formed oxindole and dioxindole. Further, he successfully reduced oxindole into indole by zinc distillation.

Emil Fischer and V.F Hess (1884) reported the chemical synthesis of indole. This reaction is named as Fischer-Indole synthesis. Fischer discovered the phenylhydrazine derivatives (salt form), a condensation product of phenyl hydrazine and aldehydes (aromatic and aliphatic). The methylphenylhydrazone and pyruvic acid generated corresponding phenylhydrazones. Fischer warmed this methylhydrazones with dilute hydrochloric acid and recognized the formation of indole carboxylic acid.

Formation of indoles on heating arylhydrazones of aldehydes/ketones in the presence of acid catalysts (lewis/proton acids) is known as Fischer Indole synthesis.

NH_2 + O OH → N N OH

CH_3 CH_3 CH_3 CH_3

1-Methylphenyl hydrazine Pyruvic acid Pyruvic acid 2-methylphenylhydrazone

HCl | $-NH_3$

COOH N CH_3

1-Methylphenylindole 2-carboxylic acid

Reaction Mechanism

G. M. Robinson and R. Robinson (1918) explained the most acceptable reaction mechanism for Fischer Indole synthesis. They explained the enolization of imine nitrogen (similar to carbonyl compounds). Tautomeric shift of hydrogen from the methyl group (α-carbon) to nitrogen makes it more basic. Protonation of imine nitrogen initiates the attack of α-carbon on the aromatic ring and cleaves N-N bond.

Polyphosphoric acid is the source of proton and serves as a solvent and drying agent (water hydrolyses imine). Polyphosphoric acid forms ammonium phosphate with the liberated ammonia and drives the reaction to completion. Elimination of β-hydrogen restores the aromaticity and generates nucleophilic center on the nitrogen bound ring. Nucleophilic center attacks imine carbon and forms 5-membered ring. Loss of nitrogen as amine group generates 2-phenylindole.

Fischer indole synthesis involves the following two steps:

***Step 1*: Formation of arylhydrazone:** Condensation of aromatic carbonyl compounds (e.g., acetophenone) with phenylhydrazine (and its derivatives) forms corresponding arylhydrazones.

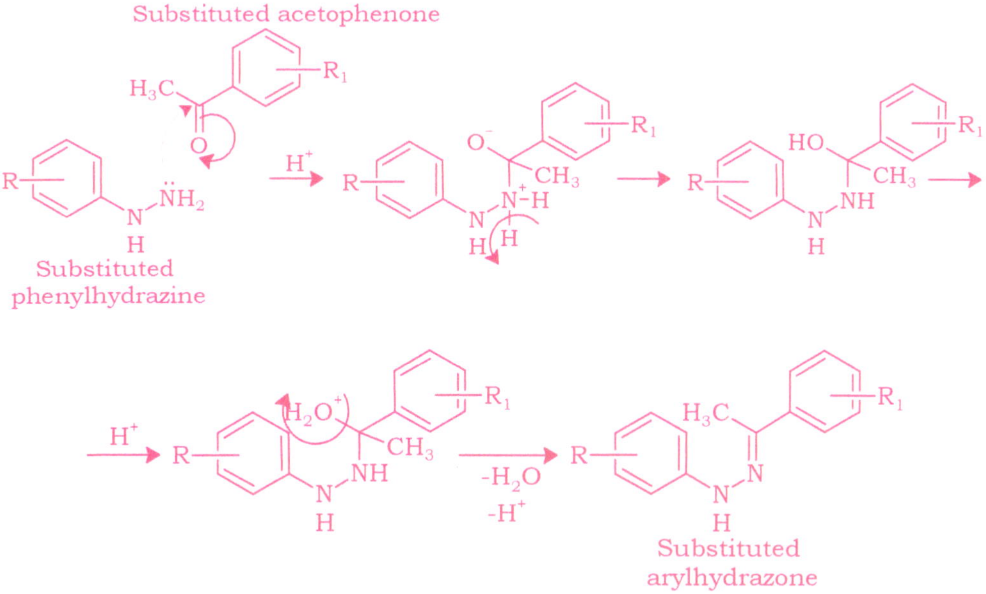

Substituted acetophenone

Substituted phenylhydrazine

Substituted arylhydrazone

***Step 2*: Cyclization of arylhydrazone into 2-phenylindole:** Hydrazone undergoes cyclization in presence of acid catalysts to yield 2-phenylindole derivatives. One of the nitrogen present in the hydrazine will be eliminated as ammonia.

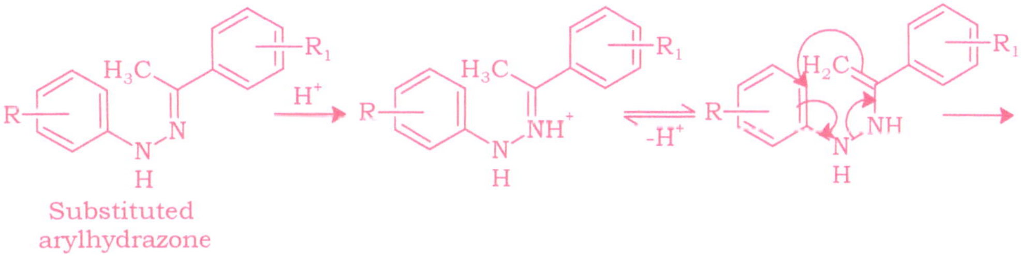

Substituted arylhydrazone

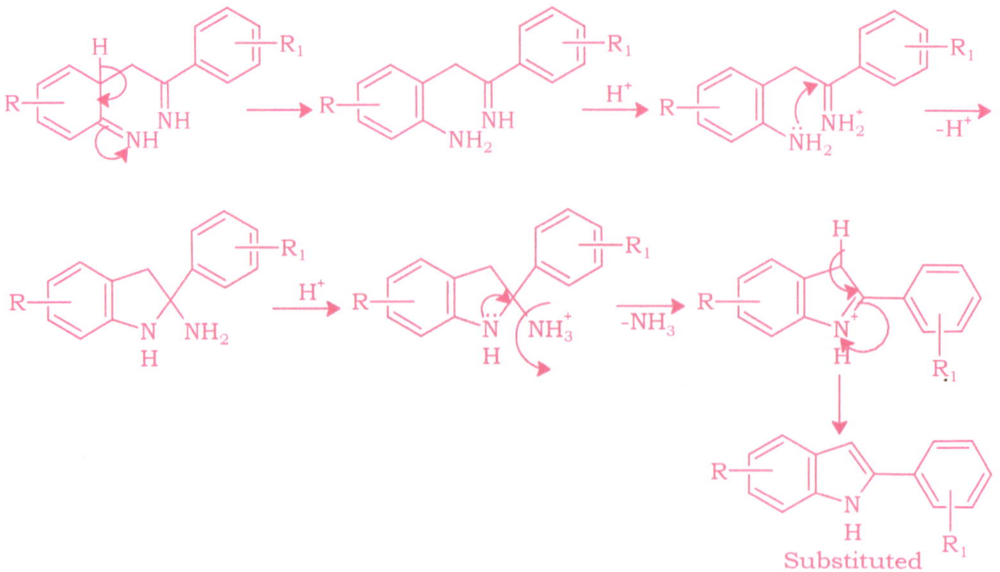

Substituted 2-phenylindole

N,N-Disubstituted phenylhydrazones readily transform (cyclizes) into phenylindoles, when compared with unsubstituted phenylhydrazones. The ring substitution of phenylhydrazones has no influence on the reaction.

Catalysts: The yield of first Fischer-Indole synthesis product (1-methyl-indole-2-carboxylic acid) was very low (%). In an attempt to improve the yield, Fischer identified zinc chloride (anhydrous) as an effective catalyst. It improved the yield (~50%). Sulphuric acid, cuprous chloride, cobaltous chloride, nickel chloride, stannous chloride, boron trifluoride, methane sulphonic acid, polyphosphoric acid and Grignard reagent are identified as an effective catalyst.

Pharmaceutical Applications

1. Anti-inflammatory drug, indomethacin can be synthesized through Fischer Indole synthesis.

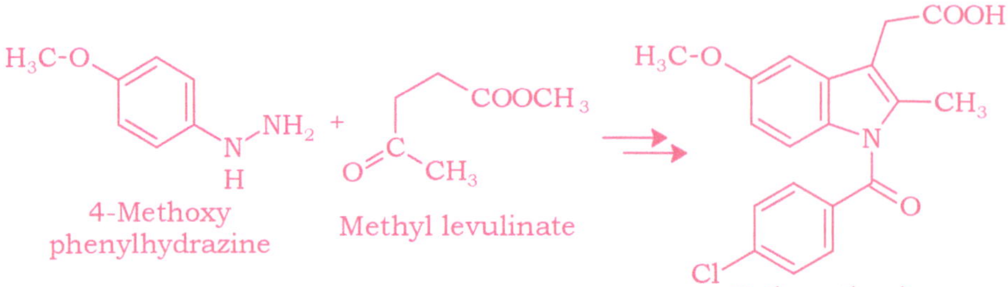

4-Methoxy phenylhydrazine + Methyl levulinate → Indomethacin

2. Anti-emetic drug, ondansetron can be synthesized through Fischer Indole synthesis.

1-Methyl-1-phenylhydrazine + Imidazolo cyclohexanone → Ondansetron

15.1 Preparation of 2-Phenylindole

Traditional Name: Phenylindole

IUPAC Name: 2-Phenyl-1*H*-indole **Mol wt**: 193.25 g/mol

Principle: Polarization of acetophenone carbonyl group generates electron deficient carbonyl carbon. Lone pair of electrons present in nitrogen of phenyl hydrazine attacks (nucleophilic attack) electron deficient carbon and forms an intermediate. Protonation followed by dehydration produces aryl hydrazone. Polyphosphoric acid is the source of proton and serves as a solvent and drying agent. Imine nitrogen of aryl hydrazone undergoes enolization and tautomeric shift of the hydrogen of α-carbon to the imine nitrogen makes it more basic. Protonation of this nitrogen allows the attack of the α-carbon on the aromatic ring and breaks N-N bond of phenylhydrazine.

Elimination of β-hydrogen restores the aromaticity and forms nucleophilic center on the nitrogen bound ring. Nucleophilic center attacks imine carbon and forms 5-membered ring. Loss of nitrogen as amine group generates 2-phenylindole. Polyphosphoric acid forms ammonium phosphate with the liberated ammonia and drives the reaction to completion.

Phenylhydrazine + Acetophenone $\xrightarrow[-H_2O]{C_2H_5OH}$ Phenylhydrazone $\xrightarrow{\text{PPA, 90 to 100 °C}}$ 2-Phenylindole

***Step 1*: Formation of phenylhydrazone**

Acetophenone

H_3C O $\ddot{N}H_2$ N H

Phenylhydrazine

H^+ O^- CH_3 N $\overset{+}{N}$–H H H

HO CH_3 NH N H

H^+ $H_2\overset{+}{O}$ CH_3 NH N H

$-H_2O$ $-H^+$

H_3C N N H

Phenylhydrazone

***Step 2*: Cyclization of phenylhydrazone into 2-phenylindole**

H_3C N N H

Phenylhydrazone

H^+ H_3C NH^+ N H

H_2C NH N H

H NH NH

NH NH_2

H^+ NH_2^+ $\ddot{N}H_2$ $-H^+$

N H NH_2

H^+ $\ddot{N}$ H NH_3^+

$-NH_3$

H N^+ H

N H

2-Phenylindole

Procedure

Step 1: Preparation of acetophenone phenylhydrazone

Chemicals Required: Acetophenone, Phenylhydrazine, Ethanol, Glacial acetic acid, Hydrochloric acid.

1. Mix acetophenone (5 mL, 43 mmol) and phenylhydrazine (4.1 mL, 42 mmol) with ethanol (15 mL) and few drops of glacial acetic acid.
2. Warm the mixture and cool to room temperature.
3. Filter the reaction mixture, wash the solid with dilute hydrochloric acid and cold ethanol (4 mL).
4. Purify the product by recrystallization with ethanol.
5. The melting point of pure acetophenone phenylhydrazone is 106 °C.

Step 2: Preparation of 2-phenylindole

Chemicals Required: Acetophenone phenylhydrazone, Ethanol, Polyphosphoric acid, Charcoal.

1. Place acetophenone phenylhydrazone (1 g) in a beaker containing polyphosphoric acid (6.4 g).
2. Heat the mixture by placing on a water bath, stir and maintain the temperature between 100-120 °C for about 10 min (exothermic reaction).
3. Add cold water (16 mL) to the reaction mixture, stir well, filter and wash the residue with water.
4. Add ethanol (11 mL) to the solid and reflux the mixture for 30 min.
5. Add charcoal to the reaction mixture and filter through preheated Buchner funnel.
6. Wash the residue with of hot ethanol (2 mL).
7. Cool the filtrate to room temperature and filter 2-phenylindole separated.
8. Wash the isolated 2-phenylindole with 1 mL portions of cold alcohol (three times) and dry in vacuum desiccator.
9. The melting range of pure 2-phenylindole is 188 to 189 °C.

Precaution:

- Phenylhydrazine is highly poisonous (carcinogen) and produces burns when it comes in contact with skin.
- If any liquid does come in contact with the skin, wash off immediately with 2% acetic acid then with soap and water.

KEY POINTS

- Condensation of hydrazines with carbonyl compounds in the presence of acid catalysts produces indole and the reaction is known as Fischer Indole synthesis.

- Indomethacin (anti-inflammatory) and ondansetron (anti-emetic) can be synthesized through Fischer Indole synthesis.
- Polyphosphoric acid is the widely useful acid catalyst serves as a source of proton, solvent and drying agent.
- Skin contact of phenylhydrazine (carcinogen) produces burns; washing with 2% acetic acid followed by soap water is the first aid.

16

Fischer-Speier Esterification

The chemical interaction between a carboxylic acid and an alcohol forms an ester. The reaction is called as an esterification, which is very slow and reversible in nature.

Fisher-Speier Esterification

The chemical equilibrium for the ester formation occurs after several days of reflux. But the use of mineral acids namely concentrated sulphuric acid or dry hydrochloride with alcohol (3%) helps attaining the equilibrium within few hours. This method is known as Fisher-Speier esterification (acid catalysed esterification). The use of excess of one reactants (in particular acid) favors the ester formation. Primary alcohols produce best yields of an ester and secondary alcohols offer good yields. But, the tertiary alcohols through acid catalyzed dehydration promote the formation of an alkene. Dean-Stark apparatus is useful in the removal of water (azeotropic condition) and promotes the ester formation. Varieties of other catalysts such as cation exchange resin, toluene-*p*-sulphonic acid are best catalysts.

$$\underset{\text{Carboxylic acid}}{R-\overset{O}{\overset{\|}{C}}-OH} + \underset{\text{Alcohol}}{R_1\text{-}OH} \xrightarrow{H^+} \underset{\text{Ester}}{R-\overset{O}{\overset{\|}{C}}-O-R_1}$$

General reaction mechanism

***Step 1* Protonation of carbonyl oxygen**: The carbonyl oxygen abstracts proton from the mineral acid. This generates positive charge on oxygen. The electrons between carbon and oxygen (of carbonyl group) stabilize the positive charge. This cause the electron loss at carbon level and forms positive charge (electron deficient).

***Step 2* Nucleophilic attack on carbonyl carbon**: The oxygen with lone pair of electrons (nucleophile) attacks positively charged carbonyl carbon (electrophile).

Step 3 **Proton transfer**: Transfer of proton attached to the alcohol to the hydroxyl group of carboxylic acid.

Step 4 **Dehydration**: Loss of water molecule.

Step 5 **Deprotonation**: Hydrogen sulphate abstracts hydrogen.

$$R{-}C(=O){-}OH \underset{-HSO_4^-}{\overset{\text{Step 1},\ H_2SO_4}{\rightleftharpoons}} R{-}C(=\overset{+}{O}H){-}OH \xrightarrow{R_1{-}\ddot{O}H} \overset{\text{Step 2}}{\rightleftharpoons} R{-}C(OH)(OH){-}\overset{+}{O}(H)R_1 \overset{\text{Step 3}}{\rightleftharpoons} R{-}C(\overset{+}{O}H_2)(OH){-}OR_1$$

Carboxylic acid; Alcohol

$$\overset{\text{Step 4}}{\rightleftharpoons} R{-}C(=\overset{+}{O}H){-}OR_1 \underset{-H_2SO_4}{\overset{\text{Step 5},\ HSO_4^-}{\longrightarrow}} R{-}C(=O){-}O{-}R_1$$

Ester

The esterification reaction also can be performed using thionyl chloride, 1,8-diazabicyclo[5.4.0]undec-7-ene and N,N-dicyclohexylcarbodimide (DCC) with 4-methyl-diaminopyridine (DMAP).

Pharmaceutical applications

1. Preparation of local anaesthetic drug benzocaine.

$$H_2N{-}C_6H_4{-}C(=O){-}OH + C_2H_5OH \xrightarrow{H_2SO_4} H_2N{-}C_6H_4{-}C(=O){-}O{-}C_2H_5 + H_2O$$

4-Aminobenzoic acid; Ethanol; Benzocaine

2. Preparation of clofibrate (lipid lowering agent).

$$Cl{-}C_6H_4{-}O{-}C(CH_3)_2{-}C(=O){-}OH + C_2H_5OH \xrightarrow{H_2SO_4} Cl{-}C_6H_4{-}O{-}C(CH_3)_2{-}C(=O){-}O{-}C_2H_5$$

Clofibric acid; Ethanol; Clofibrate

3. Preparation of methyl benzoate (analgesic).

$$C_6H_5{-}C(=O){-}OH + CH_3OH \xrightarrow{H_2SO_4} C_6H_5{-}C(=O){-}O{-}CH_3 + H_2O$$

Benzoic acid; Methanol; Methyl benzoate

4. Preparation of methyl salicylate (analgesic).

$$o\text{-}HO{-}C_6H_4{-}C(=O){-}OH + CH_3OH \xrightarrow{H_2SO_4} o\text{-}HO{-}C_6H_4{-}C(=O){-}O{\cdot}CH_3 + H_2O$$

Salicylic acid; Methanol; Methyl salicylate

16.1 Preparation of *n*-Butyl Acetate

Traditional Name: Butyl ethanoate, Butylacetaten

***IUPAC Name*:** Butyl acetate **Mol wt**: 116.16 g/mol

Principle: The esterification of *n*-butanol with glacial acetic acid forms *n*-butyl acetate using concentrated sulphuric acid as a catalyst. Sulphuric acid also acts as a dehydrating agent.

$$\underset{\text{Glacial acetic acid}}{H_3C-\overset{O}{\overset{||}{C}}-OH} + \underset{n\text{-Butanol}}{H_9C_4\text{-}OH} \xrightarrow{H_2SO_4} \underset{n\text{-Butyl acetate}}{H_3C-\overset{O}{\overset{||}{C}}-O-C_4H_9}$$

The large excess of *n*-butanol promotes the reversible reaction, hence should be avoided.

Reaction Mechanism

$$\underset{\text{Glacial acetic acid}}{H_3C-\overset{O}{\overset{||}{C}}-OH} \underset{-HSO_4^-}{\overset{\text{Step 1}}{\overset{H_2SO_4}{\rightleftharpoons}}} H_3C-\overset{\overset{+}{O}-H}{\overset{||}{C}}-OH \;\; + \underset{n\text{-Butanol}}{H_9C_4\text{-}\ddot{O}H} \overset{\text{Step 2}}{\rightleftharpoons} H_3C-\overset{OH}{\overset{|}{C}}-OH \;(\text{with } H_9C_4\text{-}\overset{+}{O}H) \overset{\text{Step 3}}{\rightleftharpoons} H_3C-\overset{H-\overset{+}{O}-H}{\overset{|}{C}}-O-H \;(\text{with } H_9C_4\text{-}O)$$

$$\underset{-H_2O}{\overset{\text{Step 4}}{\rightleftharpoons}} H_3C-\underset{H_9C_4\text{-}O}{\underset{|}{C}}=\overset{+}{O}-H \underset{-H_2SO_4}{\overset{\text{Step 5}}{\overset{HSO_4^-}{\longrightarrow}}} \underset{n\text{-Butyl acetate}}{H_3C-\overset{O}{\overset{||}{C}}-O-C_4H_9}$$

Procedure:

Chemicals Required: *n*-Butanol, Glacial acetic acid, Concentrated sulphuric acid, Sodium bicarbonate and Magnesium sulphate (anhydrous).

1. Place *n*-butanol (10 mL, 109 mmol) and glacial acetic acid (13 mL, 229 mmol) into a round bottom flask.
2. Mix the contents of flask well and add three drops of sulphuric acid cautiously.
3. Attach reflux condenser to the flask and reflux gently for about 1.5 h.
4. Allow the hot reaction mixture to cool and transfer into separating funnel containing water (8 mL).
5. Rinse the flask with water and return to separating funnel containing water (50 mL).
6. Swirl the separatory funnel gently to remove the upper organic layer.

7. Wash the organic layer with water (20 mL), saturated sodium bicarbonate solution (5 mL) and water (10 mL).
8. Collect the organic layer and dry by passing through (filtration) magnesium sulphate (anhydrous, 1.3 g).
9. Distil the organic filtrate at 124-125 °C to collect *n*-butyl acetate.
10. The boiling point of the pure *n*-butyl acetate is 126 °C.

16.2 Preparation of Methyl Benzoate

Traditional Name: Niobe oil, Oniobe oil

IUPAC Name: Methyl benzoate **Mol wt**: 136.15 g/mol

Principle: The esterification of benzoic acid with methanol in the presence of sulphuric acid forms methyl benzoate. Concentrated sulphuric acid also acts as a dehydrating agent and removes water. The excess of methanol promotes the reversible reaction, hence should be avoided.

$$C_6H_5-COOH + CH_3OH \xrightarrow{H_2SO_4} C_6H_5-CO-O-CH_3 + H_2O$$

Benzoic acid Methanol Methyl benzoate

Reaction Mechanism

Step 1: Benzoic acid $\underset{-HSO_4^-}{\overset{H_2SO_4}{\rightleftharpoons}}$ $C_6H_5-C(=\overset{+}{O}-H)-OH$; attack by $H_3C-\ddot{O}H$ (Methanol)

Step 2: $\rightleftharpoons$ $C_6H_5-C(OH)(OH)-\overset{+}{O}(H)-CH_3$

Step 3: $\rightleftharpoons$ $C_6H_5-C(\overset{+}{O}H_2)(OH)-O-CH_3$

Step 4: $\underset{-H_2O}{\rightleftharpoons}$ $C_6H_5-C(=\overset{+}{O}-H)-O-CH_3$

Step 5: $\xrightarrow[-H_2SO_4]{HSO_4^-}$ $C_6H_5-CO-O-CH_3$ (Methyl benzoate)

Procedure:

Chemicals Required: Benzoic acid, Methanol, Concentrated sulphuric acid, Carbon tetrachloride, Magnesium sulphate (anhydrous) and Sodium bicarbonate.

1. Place benzoic acid (1 g, 8.2 mmol) and absolute methanol (4 mL) into a round bottom flask.
2. Mix the contents and add and three drops of sulphuric acid.
3. Add boiling chips to the flask, attach reflux condenser and boil gently for 4 h (*longer heating improves yield*).

4. Allow the hot reaction mixture to cool and transfer into separating funnel containing water (8 mL).
5. Rinse the flask with water and return to separating funnel.
6. Add carbon tetrachloride (1 mL) to the separating funnel (diethyl ether can be used) to enhance the separation of two distinct layers and shake vigorously.
7. Methyl benzoate gets into carbon tetrachloride and separates at the bottom (upon standing).
8. Collect the lower carbon tetrachloride layer and transfer back to separating funnel.
9. Shake the contents of separating funnel with sodium bicarbonate solution until effervescence ceases.
10. Wash the organic layer with excess of water and dry it by passing (flirtation) into magnesium sulphate (anhydrous, 0.17 g).
    (*anhydrous sodium sulphate also can be used*)
11. Stopper the flask containing filtrate and shake for 5 min.
12. Allow it to stand for 30 minutes with occasional shaking.
13. Distil the filtrate at 198-200 °C to collect the colourless liquid of methyl benzoate.
14. The boiling point of the pure methyl benzoate is 199 °C.

16.3 Preparation of Methyl Salicylate

Traditional Name: Wintergreen oil, Teaberry oil, Sweet birch oil, Spicewood oil

***IUPAC Name*:** Methyl-2-hydroxy benzoate **Mol wt**: 152.15 g/mol

Principle: The esterification of salicylic acid with methanol in the presence of sulphuric acid forms methyl salicylate. Concentrated sulphuric acid also acts as a dehydrating agent and removes water. The excess of methanol promotes the reversible reaction, hence should be avoided.

$$\text{Salicylic acid} + CH_3OH \xrightarrow{H_2SO_4} \text{Methyl salicylate} + H_2O$$

Salicylic acid Methanol Methyl salicylate

Reaction Mechanism

Procedure:

Chemicals Required: Salicylic acid, Methanol, Concentrated sulphuric acid, Ether, Sodium bicarbonate, Magnesium sulphate (anhydrous).

1. Place salicylic acid (0.2 g, 15 mmol) and absolute methanol (2 mL) into a round bottom flask.
2. Mix the contents and add five drops of concentrated sulphuric acid.
3. Add boiling chips to the flask, attach reflux condenser and boil gently for 4 h (*longer heating improves yield*).
4. Distil the excess methanol (unreacted).
5. Cool the hot reaction mixture under tap and transfer the residue into a separating funnel containing ether (7 mL).
6. Wash the ethereal layer with water (50 mL, two times).
   (*Removes the unreacted methanol and sulphuric acid*)
7. Add sodium bicarbonate solution (5 mL, 10%) to neutralize the traces of sulphuric acid.
   (*this step separates the methyl salicylate from unreacted salicylic acid*)
8. Wash the organic layer with excess of water and dry it by passing (flirtation) into anhydrous magnesium sulphate (0.17 g).
   (*anhydrous sodium sulphate also can be used*)
9. Distil the organic layer at 222 °C (air-condenser is preferable, water condenser leads to cracking).
10. Collect the colourless liquid of methyl saliylate.
11. The boiling point range of the pure methyl salicylate 222 to 224 °C.

16.4 Preparation of Benzocaine

Traditional Name: Americaine, Anaesthesin, Ethoform

***IUPAC Name*:** Ethyl-4-amino benzoate **Mol wt**: 165.19 g/mol

Principle: The local anesthetic agent benzocaine can be prepared by esterification reaction. The esterification of 4-amino benzoic acid (*para*-amino benzoic acid; PABA) with ethanol (absolute) in the presence of concentrated sulphuric acid forms benzocaine. Sulphuric acid also acts as a dehydrating agent and eliminates water. An excess of one reactant, usually the ethanol favours the benzocaine formation.

$$H_2N-C_6H_4-\overset{O}{\overset{\|}{C}}-OH + C_2H_5OH \xrightarrow{H_2SO_4} H_2N-C_6H_4-\overset{O}{\overset{\|}{C}}-O-C_2H_5 + H_2O$$

4-Aminobenzoic acid Ethanol Benzocaine

Reaction Mechanism

$$H_2N-C_6H_4-\overset{O}{\overset{\|}{C}}-OH \underset{-HSO_4^-}{\overset{H_2SO_4}{\rightleftharpoons}} H_2N-C_6H_4-\overset{\overset{+}{O}-H}{\overset{\|}{C}}-OH \rightleftharpoons H_2N-C_6H_4-\underset{H_5C_2-\overset{+}{O}-H}{\overset{OH}{C}}-OH$$

4-Aminobenzoic acid

$H_5C_2-\ddot{O}H$

Ethanol

$$\rightleftharpoons H_2N-C_6H_4-\underset{H_5C_2-O}{\overset{H-\overset{+}{O}-H}{C}}-O-H \xrightarrow[\substack{-H_2O \\ -H_2SO_4}]{HSO_4^-} H_2N-C_6H_4-\overset{O}{\overset{\|}{C}}-O-C_2H_5$$

Benzocaine

Procedure:

Chemicals Required: 4-Aminobenzoic acid, Absolute ethanol, Concentrated sulphuric acid and Sodium carbonate.

1. Place absolute ethanol (8 mL) and concentrated sulphuric acid (3 mL) into the round bottom flask.
2. Mix well the contents of flask and add 4-amino benzoic acid (1.2 g, 9 mmol) to the flask.

   Higher temperature is required, hence sand bath is preferable.
3. Add boiling chips, attach reflux condenser and reflux the mixture for 2 h.
4. Cool the reaction mixture to room temperature and transfer into beaker containing distilled water.
5. Neutralize the excess of acid with solid sodium carbonate (Litmus paper test)
6. Collect the white precipitate of benzocaine by vacuum filtration and wash the product with water (several times).
7. Purify the crude benzocaine by recrystallization with ethanol.
8. The melting point of pure benzocaine is 91 °C.

16.5 Preparation of Isoniazid

Traditional Name: Andrazide, Nydrazid, Pycazide

IUPAC Name: Pyridine-4-carbohydrazide **Mol wt**: 137.14 g/mol

Principle: The preparation of isoniazid involves esterification of nicotinic acid followed by hydrazide formation. Isonicotinic acid undergoes esterification catalyzed by sulphuric acid and forms ethyl isonicotinate. Ethyl isonicotinate reacts with hydrazine hydrate and gives isoniazid.

Isonicotinic acid + C_2H_5OH (Ethanol) $\xrightarrow{H_2SO_4}$ Ethyl isonicotinate $\xrightarrow[\text{Hydrazine hydrate}]{NH_2NH_2.H_2O}$ Isoniazid

Reaction Mechanism

Preparation of ethyl isonicotinate

Isonicotinic acid $\xrightarrow[-HSO_4^-]{H_2SO_4}$ … $\xrightarrow{\ddot{O}H\cdot C_2H_5 \text{ Ethanol}}$ … → … $\xrightarrow[-H_2O,\ -H_2SO_4]{HSO_4^-}$ Ethyl isonicotinate

Preparation of isoniazid

Ethyl isonicotinate + $:NH_2NH_2.H_2O$ (Hydrazine hydrate) → … $\xrightarrow{-C_2H_5OH}$ Isoniazid

Procedure:

Step 1: Preparation of ethyl isonicotinate

Chemicals Required: Isonicotinic acid, Ethanol, Concentrated sulphuric acid, Sodium bicarbonate, Ether.

1. Place isonicotinic acid (1.23 g, 10 mmol), ethanol (10 mL) and concentrated sulphuric acid (2 mL) into a round bottom flask.

2. Reflux the mixture for 3 h maintaining the temperature between 60-70 °C. (*the reaction produces irritating and toxic vapours, hence the reaction in fume hood is advisable*).
3. Pour the hot reaction mixture to a beaker containing ice-cold water (200 mL) and neutralize the excess of acid with sodium bicarbonate (Litmus paper test).
4. Extract the aqueous layer with diethyl ether in separating funnel.
5. Evaporate the ether layer to obtain the residue of ethyl isonicotinate.
6. The boiling point of pure ethyl isonicotinate is 220 °C

Step 2: Preparation of isoniazid

Chemicals Required: Ethyl isonicotinate, Ethanol, Hydrazine hydrate.

1. Place ethyl isonicotinate (1.6 mL, 10 mmol) into a round bottom flask.
2. Dissolve the ethyl isonicotinate in ethanol (10 mL).
3. Add hydrazine hydrate (0.6 mL, 12 mmol) to the flask and attach reflux condenser.
4. Reflux the reaction mixture for 2 h.
5. Cool to hot reaction mixture to room temperature.
6. Isolate the crude isoniazid and dry.
7. Purify the crude isoniazid by recrystallization with ethanol.
8. The melting range of pure isoniazid is 171 to 172 °C.

KEY POINTS

- The mineral acids catalyzed esterification reaction is known as Fisher-Speier esterification.
- Concentrated sulphuric acid or dry hydrochloride with alcohol (3%) helps attaining the equilibrium within few hours.
- Dean-Stark apparatus provides azeotropic condition and promotes the ester formation.
- Chemical synthesis of benzocaine (local anaesthetic), clofibrate (lipid lowering agent), methyl benozate (analgesic) and methyl salicylate (analgesic) involves Fisher-Speier esterification.

17

Haloform Reaction

The reaction between the methyl ketones (or secondary alcohols) and the hypohalites (OX^{-}) in the alkaline condition forms trihalomethane (haloform). This reaction is known as haloform reaction. The typical example for this reaction is the iodoform reaction. Acetone (methyl ketone) reacts with sodium hypoiodate and forms iodoform.

$$R{-}CO{-}CH_3 + OX^- \xrightarrow{OH^-} CHX_3 + R{-}CO{-}O^-$$

Methyl ketone + Hypohalite → Haloform + Carboxylate anion

Reaction Mechanism

$$OX^- + H_2O \rightleftharpoons X_2 + 2OH^-$$

Hypohalite ⇌ Dihalogen

$$R{-}CO{-}CH_2{-}H \xrightarrow[-H_2O]{^-OH} R{-}CO{-}CH_2^- \xrightarrow[-X]{X_2} R{-}CO{-}CH_2{-}X \xrightarrow[-X]{^-OH,\ X_2} R{-}CO{-}C{-}X_3$$

Methyl ketone → Nucleophile → ... → Trihalomethyl ketone

Step 1 — *Step 2* — *Step 3* (*Step 1 & 2*) *2 times*

$$\rightarrow R{-}CO{-}C{-}X_3 \xrightarrow{^-OH} R{-}C(O^-)(OH){-}C{-}X_3 \rightarrow CHX_3 + R{-}CO{-}O^-$$

Haloform + Carboxylate anion

Step 4 — *Step 5*

Pharmaceutical Applications

1. **Identification of methyl ketones:** The reaction between methyl ketone and iodine forms yellowish iodoform solid (indicative of the presence of methyl ketone). Bromine and chlorine also produces haloforms (bromoform and chloroform). But, they are liquid. Hence, iodoform test alone useful for identification of methyl ketones.

17.1 Preparation of Iodoform

Traditional Name: Tri-Iodomethane

IUPAC Name: Iodoform **Mol wt**: 393.73 g/mol

Principle: The reaction between the acetone and sodium hypochlorite-potassium iodide mixture forms iodoform (*tri*-iodomethane). This reaction is known as iodoform reaction (haloform reaction). Sodium hypochlorite (oxidizing agent) releases iodine from the potassium iodide. This liberated iodine is useful in iodination of acetone to form iodoform. This reaction is useful in the identification of methyl ketones, qualitatively.

$$\underset{\text{Acetone}}{H_3C-CO-CH_3} + \underset{\text{Sodium hypochlorite}}{NaOCl} \xrightarrow{KI} \underset{\text{Iodoform}}{CHI_3} + \underset{\text{Sodium acetate}}{H_3C-CO-ONa} + KCl$$

Reaction Mechanism

Generation of iodine

$$\underset{\text{Sodium hypochlorite}}{NaOCl} + \underset{\text{Potassium iodide}}{KI} + H_2O \longrightarrow \underset{\text{Iodine}}{I_2} + KCl + NaOH$$

Formation of iodoform

$$\underset{\text{Acetone}}{H_3C-CO-CH_2-H} \xrightarrow[-H_2O]{^-OH} \underset{\text{Nucleophile}}{H_3C-CO-CH_2^-} \xrightarrow[-I]{I_2} H_3C-CO-CH_2I \xrightarrow[-I]{I_2} \underset{\text{Triiodomethyl ketone}}{H_3C-CO-C-I_3}$$

Step 1 Step 2 Step 3 (Step 1 & 2) 2 times

$$\longrightarrow H_3C-CO-C-I_3 \xrightarrow{^-OH} H_3C-C(O^-)(OH)-C-I_3 \longrightarrow \underset{\text{Iodoform}}{CHI_3} + \underset{\text{Acetate}}{H_3C-CO-O^-}$$

Step 4 Step 5

Procedure:

Method 1

Chemical Required: Acetone, Potassium iodide (10%), Sodium hypochlorite (2 M), Methanol.

1. Place acetone (1 mL, 13.4 mmol), aqueous potassium iodide solution (40 mL, 10%) into a flask.

2. Add sodium hypochlorite solution (20 mL, 2 M) to the flask and mix the contents well.

   (*sodium hypochlorite addition should be continued till it forms yellowish solid of iodoform*)
3. Filter the crude iodoform by filtration and wash it with cold water.
4. Allow the mixture to stand at room temperature for 10 min.
5. Purify the crude iodoform by boiling with methanol (~25 mL).
6. Filter the hot solution through a fluted filter paper into a conical flask.
7. Cool the filtrate and allow to crystallize the iodofom (it crystallizes rapidly).
8. The melting point of pure iodoform is 119 °C.

Method 2

Chemical Required: Acetone, Potassium iodide, Iodine, Sodium hydroxide (10%), Methanol.

1. Place acetone (10 mL, 134 mmol), sodium hydroxide solution (10 mL, 10%) into a flask.

   (*sufficient sodium hydroxide removes the brown colour formed initially*)
2. Prepare a solution of potassium iodide by dissolving potassium iodide (8 g, 48 mmol) and iodine (4 g, 16 mmol) with water (50 mL) in a beaker.
3. Add the potassium iodide solution drop wise to the flask with shaking.
4. Filter the crude iodoform by filtration and wash it with cold water.
5. Allow the mixture to stand at room temperature for 10 min.
6. Purify the crude iodoform by boiling with methanol (~25 mL).
7. Filter the hot solution through a fluted filter paper into a conical flask.
8. Cool the filtrate and allow to crystallize the iodofom (it crystallizes rapidly).
9. The melting point of pure iodoform is 119 °C.

KEY POINTS

- Chemical conversion of methyl ketones into trihalomethane using and the hypohalites (OX^{-}) in the alkaline condition is known as haloform reaction.
- Iodoform (antiseptic) can be prepared from acetone using sodium hypoiodate.
- Iodoform test is useful in the qualitative and quantitative determination of methyl ketones.

18

Hantzsch 1,4-Dihydropyridine Synthesis

Arthur Hantzsch (1881) reported the synthesis of 1,4-dihydropyridines (1,4-DHPs). It involves the multicomponent reaction (MCR) of arylaldehyde, β-ketoester and nitrogen donor (e.g., ammonium acetate) to produce 1,4-dihydropyridines in one-pot. This reaction is catlaysed by concentrated hydrochloric acid in ethanol medium. Hence, this reaction is named as Hantzsch 1,4-dihydropyridine (1,4-DHP) synthesis.

β-Ketoester + Arylaldehyde ($ArCHO$) + CH_3COONH_4 (Ammonium acetate) + β-Ketoester $\xrightarrow[C_2H_5OH]{HCl}$ 4-Aryl-1,4-dihydropyridine

Substrates

1) Aryl/heteroaryl aldehydes (e.g., Benzaldehyde, Furfuraldehyde)
2) β-Ketoester (e.g., Ethyl acetoacetate, methyl acetoacetae)
3) Nitrogen donors (e.g., Ammonium acetate, Ammoniun carbonate)

The use of solid supports, microwave activation, ultrasonication, nanoparticles, ionic liquids, and lewis acids as catalysts improved the yields.

Reaction mechanism

Several plausible reaction mechanisms for the 1,4-dihydropyridines (1,4-DHPs) synthesis were proposed. It is also concluded that the reaction conditions and reactants determines the type of reaction pathway. Baeyer and Knoevenagel proposed reaction mechanism is widely accepted. It involves two step reactions:

1) Knoevenagel condensation
2) Michael addition

Knoevenagel condensation

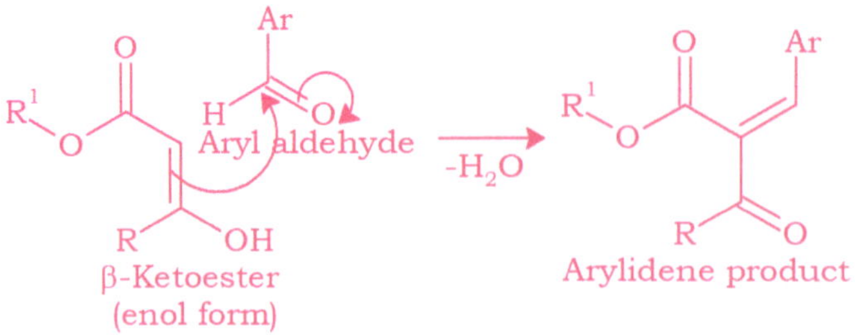

R1 O O; H Ar O; Aryl aldehyde; β-Ketoester (enol form); R OH; $-H_2O$; Arylidene product

Michael addition

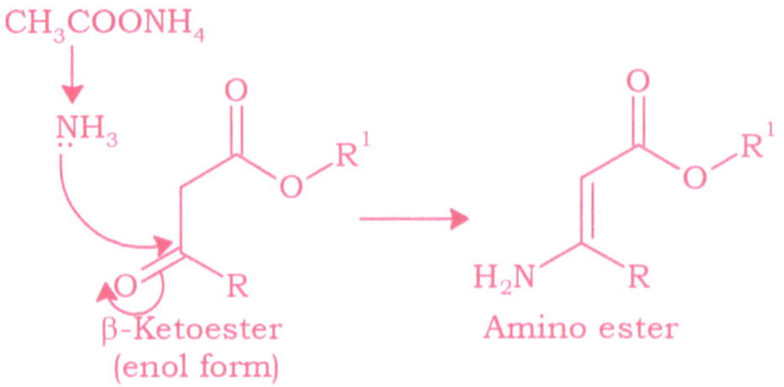

CH_3COONH_4; NH_3; β-Ketoester (enol form); H_2N; Amino ester

Condensation

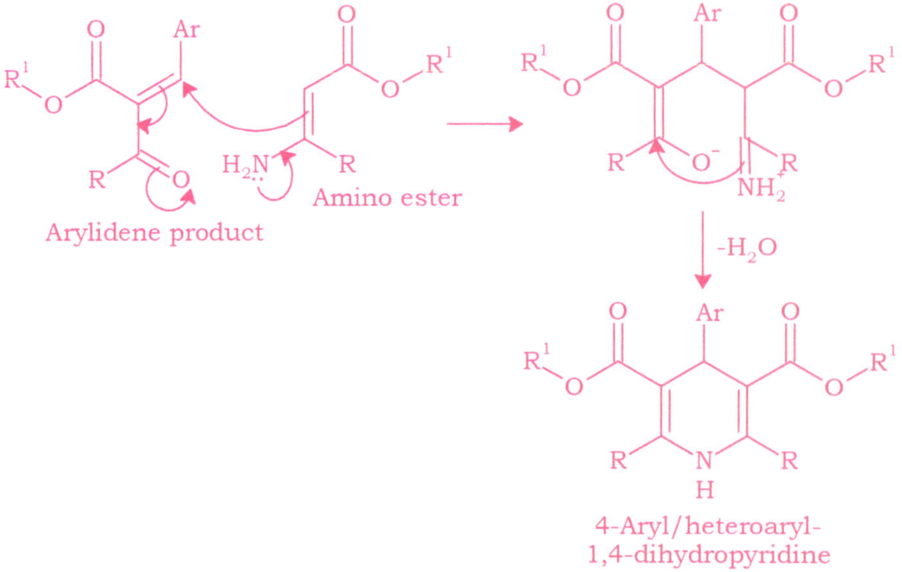

Arylidene product; Amino ester; $-H_2O$; 4-Aryl/heteroaryl-1,4-dihydropyridine

Pharmaceutical Applications

1,4-Dihydropyridines (1,4-DHPs) are known as calcium channel modulators. Cardiovascular agents, such as nifedipine and amlodipine contain 1,4-DHP scaffold.

1,4-Dihydropyridine derivatives possess a variety of biological activities, such as vasodilator, bronchodilator, anti-atherosclerotic, antitumor, geroprotective, hepatoprotective, and anti-diabetic activity. Extensive studies have revealed the neuroprotective, anti-platelet, cerebral anti ischemic and chemosensitizer effect (tumor therapy) of 1,4-DHPs.

β-Ketoester + Arylaldehyde + CH_3COONH_4 Ammonium acetate + β-Ketoester → 4-Aryl-1,4-dihydropyridine

Drug name	R	R[1]	R[2]	R[3]	R[4]
Nifidipine	$-CH_3$	$-CH_3$	$-CH_3$	$-CH_3$	$2-NO_2$
Felodipine	$-CH_3$	$-C_2H_5$	$-CH_3$	$-CH_3$	2,3-Cl
Nitrendipine	$-CH_3$	$-C_2H_5$	$-CH_3$	$-CH_3$	$3-NO_2$
Amlodipine	$-CH_2OCH_2CH_2NH_2$	$-C_2H_5$	$-CH_3$	$-CH_3$	2-Cl

18.1 Preparation of Nifedipine

IUPAC Name: Dimethyl 2,6-dimethyl-4-(2(nitrophenyl)-1,4-dihydropyridine-3,5-dicarboxylate

Mol wt: 346.3 g/mol

Principle: Nifedipine, can be synthesized through Hantzsch 1,4-dihydropyridine (1,4-DHP) synthesis. The condensation of 2-nitrobenzaldehyde with methyl acetoacetate and ammonium acetate in ethanol medium produces nifedipine. The reaction can be catalysed using tetra-*n*-butylammonium bromide (TBAB).

Methyl acetoacetate + 2-Nitrobenzaldehyde + CH_3COONH_4 Ammonium acetate + Methyl acetoacetate $\xrightarrow[\Delta]{C_2H_5OH,\ TBAB}$ Nifedipidine

Procedure:

Chemicals Required: 2-Nitrobenzaldehyde, Methyl acetoacetate, Ammonium acetate, Ethanol, Tetra-*n*-butylammonium bromide.

1. Place methyl acetoacetate (1.1 mL, 10 mmol), 2-nitrobenzaldehyde (1.51 g, 10 mmol), ammonium acetate (1.54 g, 20 mmol), and ethanol (5 mL) in a round bottom flask.
2. Add tetra-*n*-butylammonium bromide (TBAB, 1.43 g) to the flask and stir the mixture at 60 °C for 5 h.
3. Pour the reaction mixture into beaker containing ethanol (2 mL) and crushed ice (10 g) and keep aside for 1 h.
4. Isolate the precipitated nifedipine under vacuum and dry.
5. Purify the nifedipine by recrystallization with ethanol.
6. The melting range of pure nifedipine is 170 to 173 °C.

KEY POINTS

- Multicomponent condensation of arylaldehyde, β-ketoester and nitrogen donor (e.g., ammonium acetate) produces 1,4-dihydropyridines, and this reaction is named as Hantzsch 1,4-dihydropyridine (1,4-DHP) synthesis.
- The reaction mechanism involves two steps namely Knoevenagel condensation and Michael addition.
- 1,4-Dihydropyridines (1,4-DHPs) are well known class of calcium channel modulators.
- Nifedipine and amlodipine are the very widely used 1,4-DHPs in the cardiovascular management therapy.

19

Hydrolysis

Hydrolysis

Hydrolysis is a chemical process of cleaving a molecule into two parts (double decomposition). In common, the hydrolysis reaction occurs with acid or base in water. A compound (AB) gets hydrolyzed into AH and BOH. This reaction is exact reverse of esterification. Carboxylic acids can be prepared by hydrolysis of acid derivatives (esters/ amides/anhydrides).

- Ester hydrolysis generates acid and alcohol.

$$\underset{\text{Ester}}{R\text{-}COO\text{-}R^1} + H_2O \longrightarrow \underset{\text{Acid}}{R\text{-}COOH} + \underset{\text{Alcohol}}{R^1\text{-}OH}$$

- Amides can be hydrolyzed to carboxylic acids and ammonia or amines by acid hydrolysis or base hydrolysis.

$$\underset{\text{Amide}}{R\text{-}CO\text{-}NH_2} + H_2O \longrightarrow \underset{\text{Acid}}{R\text{-}COOH} + \underset{\text{Ammonia}}{NH_3}$$

$$\underset{\text{Amide}}{R\text{-}CO\text{-}NH\text{-}R^1} + H_2O \longrightarrow \underset{\text{Acid}}{R\text{-}COOH} + \underset{\text{Amine}}{R^1\text{-}NH_2}$$

The reaction conditions for amide hydrolysis are more severe than ester hydrolysis, because amides are less reactive than esters.

Hydrolysis involves several steps

Slowest: Formation of a covalent bond between the oxygen atom of water molecules and the carbon atom of the ester.

Rapid: The carbon-oxygen bond of the ester beaks and hydrogen ion becomes detached from the water and attaches to nascent alcohols.

Mechanism for ester hydrolysis

- **Acid catalyzed hydrolysis**

  Protonation of carbonyl oxygen: The carbonyl oxygen of the ester (>C=O) abstracts proton from hydronium ion (acid). This generates the protonated form of ester.

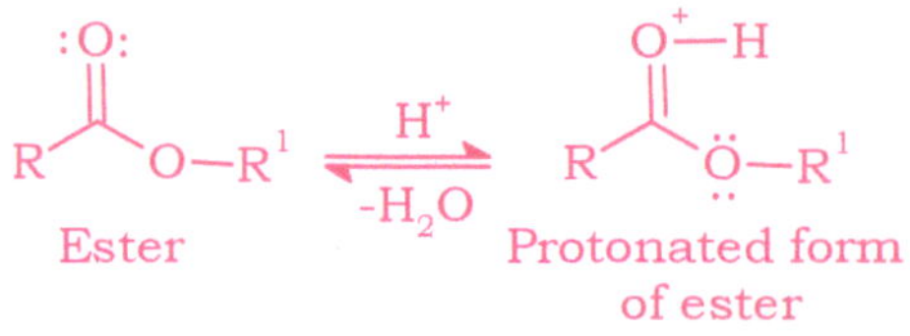

Nucleophilic addition of water to carbonyl carbon: Water molecules attack the carbonyl carbon (nucleophilic attack) and generates oxonium ion.

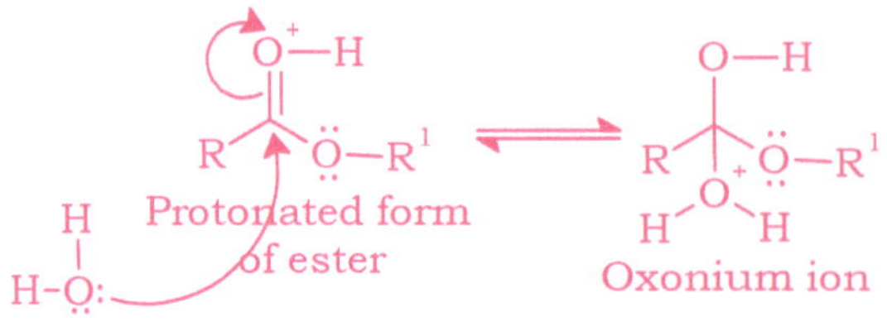

Deprotonation of oxonium ion (neutralization): Water molecules abstract the proton (hydrogen) from the oxonium ion and form the tetrahedral intermediate.

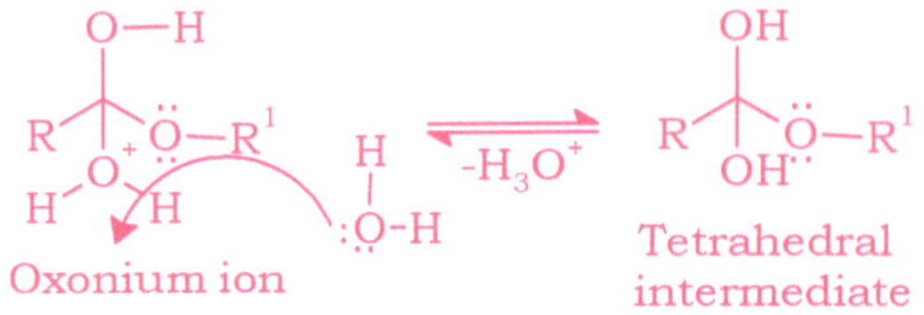

Protonation of tetrahedral intermediate: Proton (acid) addition at etheric oxygen of the tetrahedral intrtermediate oxonium ion and release of water.

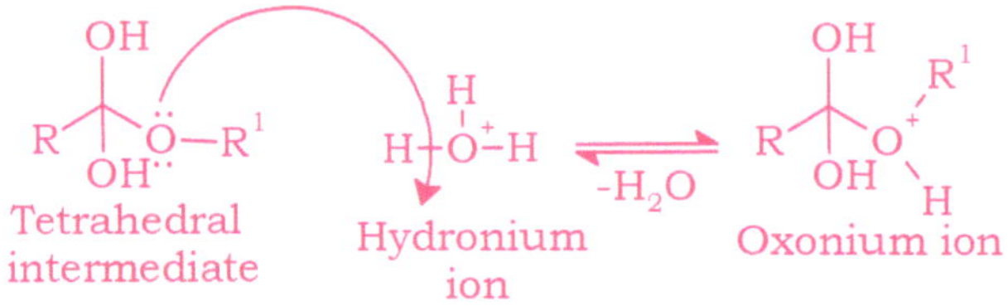

Dissociation of the oxionium ion: The oxonium ion dissociates to form protonated carboxylic acid and alcohol (phenol).

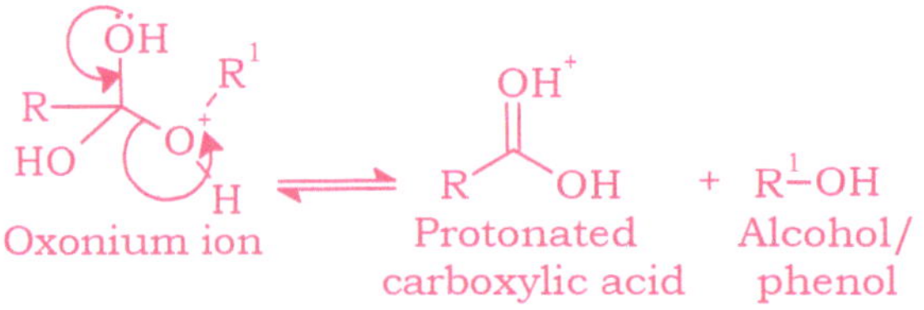

Generation of carboxylic acid: Water molecules abstract the proton from the protonated carboxylic acid and generate the carboxylic acid.

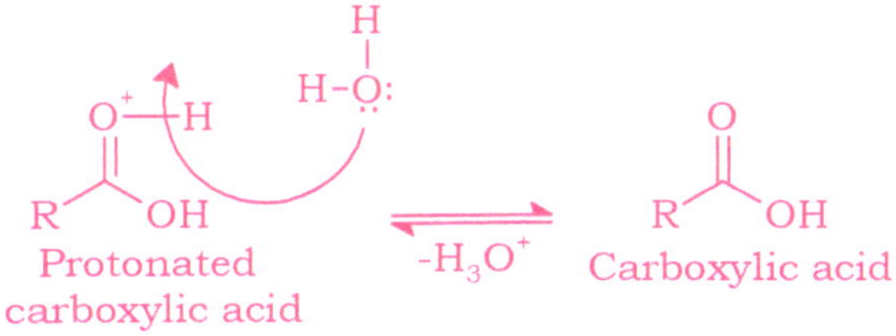

Protonated carboxylic acid $\underset{-H_3O^+}{\rightleftharpoons}$ Carboxylic acid

- **Base catalyzed ester hydrolysis**

  Nucleophilic attack: The hydroxide nucleophile (base) attacks at the electrophilic carbon of an ester (>C=O). This generates the anionic tetrahedral intermediate. The anionic portion of the tetrahedral intermediate abstracts the hydrogen (proton) from the water. This breaks the π bond and creates tetrahedral intermediate.

  Ester $\rightleftharpoons$ Anionic tetrahedral intermediate $\rightleftharpoons$ Tetrahedral intermediate

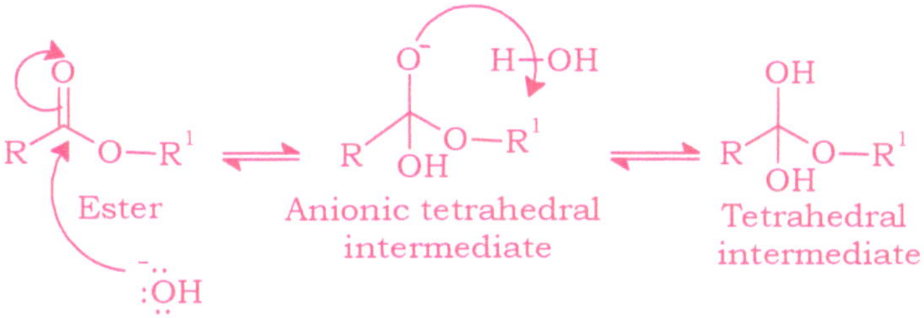

  Formation of alkoxide/phenoxide: The base abstracts the proton from tetrahedral intermediate and generates carboxylic acid and alkoxide/phenoxide.

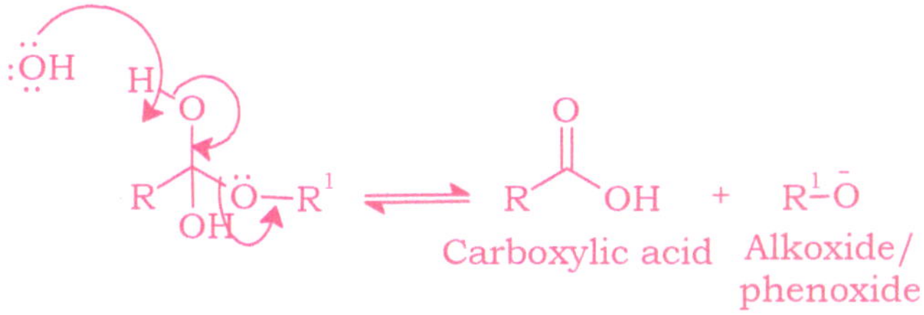

  $\rightleftharpoons$ Carboxylic acid + $R^1\text{-}O^-$ Alkoxide/phenoxide

  Formation of alcohol/phenol: The acid transfers the proton to the alkoxide (or phenoxide) and generates corresponding alcohol (or phenol).

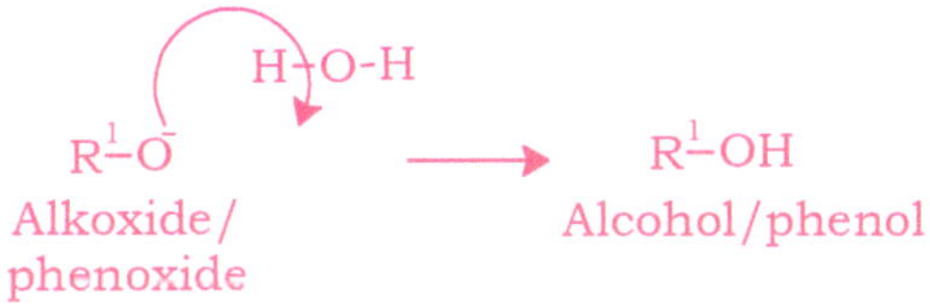

  $R^1\text{-}O^-$ Alkoxide/phenoxide $\longrightarrow$ $R^1\text{-}OH$ Alcohol/phenol

The ester hydrolysis reactions are classified into following categories:

Unimolecular		*Bimolecular*	
Nomenclature	*Characteristics*	*Nomenclature*	*Characteristics*
AAC1	Tetrahedral inrtermediate	AAC2	Tetrahedral inrtermediate
AAL1	Stable carbonium ion	AAL2	Unlikely
BAC1	Unlikely	BAC2	Tetrahedral inrtermediate
BAL1	Stable carbonium ion	BAL2	Ring cleavage at lactone (relieves strain)

1: unimolecular hydrolysis; **2**: bimolecular hydrolysis; **A**: acid catalyzed hydrolysis; **B**: base catalyzed hydrolysis; **AC**: cleavage at acyl carbon; **AL**: cleavage at alkyl carbon;

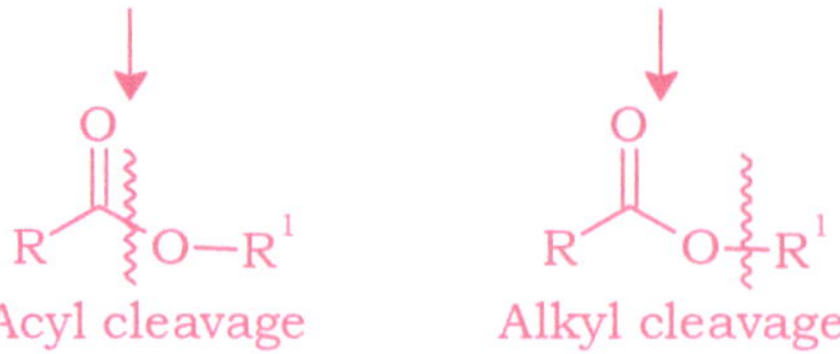

19.1 Preparation of Benzoic Acid

Traditional Name: Dracyclic acid, Carboxy benzene, Phenylformic acid

IUPAC Name*:* Benzoic acid **Mol wt**: 122.12 g/mol

Principle: Base hydrolysis of benzamide produces benzoic acid. This reaction is analogous to ester saponification. Benzamide upon hydrolysis mediated by sodium hydroxide (base) produces benzoic acid (hydrolysis product). Sodium hydroxide (base) drives the reaction to completion and forms sodium benzoate (salt of sodium benzoate) and evolves ammonia. Sodium benzoate upon acid hydrolysis produces benzoic acid.

Benzamide $\xrightarrow[HCl]{NaOH}$ Benzoic acid + NH_3 + NaCl

Reaction Mechanism

Benzamide ($^-$OH) ⇌ intermediate $\xrightarrow[-NH_3]{NaOH}$ Sodium benzoate $\xrightarrow[-NaCl]{HCl}$ Benzoic acid

Procedure:

Chemicals Required: Benzamide, Sodium hydroxide (10%), Hydrochloric acid.

1. Place benzamide (1 g, 8.3 mmol) into a round bottom flask.
2. Add aqueous sodium hydroxide (15 mL, 10%) to the flask and attach reflux condenser.
3. Boil the reaction mixture for 30 min (until no ammonia gas evolves, litmus paper test).
4. Cool the hot reaction mixture by placing in an ice-bath.
5. Acidify the mixture with hydrochloric acid under stirring.
6. Benzoic acid separates out in acidic condition (acid converts soluble sodium benzoate into insoluble benzoic acid).
7. Filter the crude benzoic acid precipitate under suction, wash the residue with ice-cold water and dry.
8. Purify the crude benzoic acid by recrystallization with hot water.
9. The melting point of pure benzoic acid is 121 °C.

KEY POINTS

- Hydrolysis is a double decomposition, which cleaves molecules (e.g., esters, amides) into two parts.
- Ester hydrolysis is reverse of esterfication.
- Hydrolysis can be effeted using acid or base catalysts.

20

Knoevenagel Condensation

Emil Knoevenagel (1898) reported the synthesis of α,β-unsaturated carboxylic acid. Hence this reaction is known as Knoevenagel condensation. This condensation resembles aldol condensation. It has significant role in fine chemical industry. The organic base catalyzed condensation of carbonyl compounds (aldehydes and ketones) with activated methylene groups generates arylidene derivatives. Piperidine is most useful base catalyst.

Carbonyl compound + Active methylene compound $\xrightarrow[\text{Base}]{\Delta}$ α,β-Unsaturated compound

Reaction Mechanism

The reaction proceeds through the following steps.

Step 1 Michael addition: Nucleophilic addition of active methylene group to the carbonyl compound.

Active methylene compound $\xrightarrow{-BH}$ Activated methylene compound (+ Carbonyl compound) → ... $\xrightarrow[-B]{BH}$ ... →

Step 2 Formation of α,β-unsaturated compound.

→ ... $\xrightarrow{-BH}$ ... → α,β-Unsaturated compound

Step 3 Formation of α,β-unsaturated carboxylic acid.

α,β-Unsaturated compound —Δ, 150 to 200 °C→ α,β-Unsaturated carboxylic acid

Catalysts

Base catalysts are preferable. However other catalysts also proved efficient.

Solid catalysts	Piperidine, Potash alum, Sodium acetate, Urea, Thiourea, Metal oxides, Tetrahydropyrrole, Ethylenediamine diacetate (EDDA)
Ionic catalysts	Ethylammonium nitrate (EAN), 1,2,3,3-Tetramethyl guanidine lactate [TMG] [Lac], 1-Butyl-3methyl imidazolium chloride ([bmim]Cl)
Phase transfer catalysts	Polyethylene glycol 300 (PEG300), Tetrabutylammonium bromide (TBAB), Tetrabutylammonium hydroxide (TBAH)

Solvents

- Toluene
- Ionic liquids
- Ethyl ammonium nitrate (EAN)
- Ethyl acetate

Pharmaceutical applications

- The anthelmintic drug pyrantel pamoate preparation involves Knoevenagel condensation.

Thiophene-2-carbaldehyde + Cyanoacetic acid → Knoevenagel product (CH=CH-CN) ⇉ Pyrantel

- The preparation of sulindac (anti-inflammatory drug) involves Knoevenagel condensation.

2-Methyl-1*H*-indenyl-acetic acid + 4-(Methylthio) benzaldehyde ⇉ Sulindac

- The anti-coagulant drug acenocoumarin preparation requires Knoevenagel condensation product as an intermediate.

NO_2 OHC 4-Nitro -benzaldehyde + O H_3C CH_3 Acetone → NO_2 CH_3 O 4-Nitrophenyl-butenone (Knoevenagel product) —Benzo pyran-4-ol→ O NO_2 OH CH_3 O Acenocoumarin

- Ethosuximide (anti-convulsant) drug preparation undergoes Knoevenagel condensation.

CH_3 H_5C_2 O Butanone + NC O OC_2H_5 Ethyl cyanoacetate → CH_3 O H_5C_2 OC_2H_5 CN Knoevenagel product → CH_3 H_3C O N O H Ethosuximide

20.1 Preparation of 4-(benzylidene)-5-methyl-2,4-dihydro-3*H*-pyrazol-3-one

Mol wt: 186.21 g/mol

Principle: 4-(Benzylidene)-5-methyl-2,4-dihydro-3*H*-pyrazol-3-one can be prepared from 5-methyl-2,4-dihydro-3*H*-pyrazol-3-one by Knoevenagel condensation. The condensation of ethyl acetoacetate and hydrazine hydrate, produces 5-methyl-2,4-dihydro-3*H*-pyrazol-3-one.

Preparation of 5-methyl-2,4-dihydro-3H-pyrazol-3-one

O O H_3C OC_2H_5 Ethyl acetoacetate + $NH_2NH_2.H_2O$ Hydrazine hydrate —C_2H_5OH→ N NH H_3C O 5-Methyl-2,4-dihydro-3*H*-pyrazol-3-one

Preparation of 4-benzylidene-5-methyl-2,4-dihydro-3H-pyrazol-3-one

N NH H_3C O 5-Methyl-2,4-dihydro-3H-pyrazol-3-one + CHO Benzaldehyde —Gla CH_3COOH / Anhydrous CH_3COONa→ N NH H_3C O 4-Benzylidene-5-methyl-2,4-dihydro-3*H*-pyrazol-3-one

Reaction Mechanism

5-Methyl-2,4-dihydro-3*H*-pyrazol-3-one

Base

Benzaldehyde

4-Benzylidene-5-methyl-2,4-dihydro-3*H*-pyrazol-3-one

Procedure

***Step 1*:** Preparation of 5-methyl-2,4-dihydro-3*H*-pyrazol-3-one

Chemicals Required: Ethyl acetoacetate, Hydrazine hydrate, Ethanol.

1. Add hydrazine hydrate (2 mL, 40 mmol) in ethanol (4 mL) dropwise with stirring to ethyl acetoacetate (2.6 g, 20 mmol) loaded in a flask.
2. Stir the reaction mixture for 1 h maintaining the temperature at 60 °C.
3. Cool the mixture to room temperature and place in an ice bath to effect the crystallization.
4. Filter the separated solid by filtration and wash with ice cold ethanol.
5. Recrystallize the product with ethanol.
6. The melting range of the pure 5-methyl-2,4-dihydro-3*H*-pyrazol-3-one is 202 to 205 °C.

***Step 2*:** Preparation of 4-(benzylidene)-5-methyl-2,4-dihydro-3*H*-pyrazol-3-one

Chemicals Required: 5-Methyl-2,4-dihydro-3*H*-pyrazol-3-one, Benzaldehyde, Glacial acetic acid, Sodium acetate (anhydrous), Ethanol.

1. Place 5-methyl-2,4-dihydro-3*H*-pyrazol-3-one (1.86 g, 10 mmol), benzaldehyde (1 mL, 10 mmol), anhydrous sodium acetate (0.82 g, 10 mmol) and glacial acetic acid (10 mL) in a round bottom flask.
2. Attach reflux condenser and reflux the reaction mixture for 10 h.
3. Cool the mixture to room temperature and pour on to crushed ice.

4. Isolate the solid separated through vacuum filtration.
5. Purify the product by recrystallization with ethanol.
6. The melting range of the pure 4-(benzylidene)-5-methyl-2,4-dihydro-3*H*-pyrazol-3-one is 239 to 240 °C.

20.2 Preparation of 5-Arylidene Thiazolidine-2,4-dione

Mol wt: 205.23 g/mol

Principle: Arylidene thiazolidinedione is an important pharmacophore in the drug discovery. The base catalyzed condensation of thiazolidine-2,4-dione with arylaldehydes generates 5-arylidene thiazolidinedione derivatives. Piperidine is most useful base catalyst. This is typical example for Knovenagel condensation.

Preparation of Thiazolidine-2,4-dione

Thiourea + Chloroacetic acid --HCl--> Thiazolidine-2,4-dione

Preparation of 5-benzylidene-thiazolidine-2,4-dione

Thiazolidine-2,4-dione + Benzaldehyde --Piperidine--> 5-Benzylidene-thiazolidine-2,4-dione

Reaction Mechanism

Thiazolidine-2,4-dione

Piperidine

Benzaldehyde

Gla CH_3COOH

$-H_2O$

5-Benzylidene-thiazolidine-2,4-dione

Procedure

Step 1: Preparation of thiazolidine-2,4-dione

Chemicals Required: Thiourea, Chloroacetic acid, Water.

1) Place chloroacetic acid (0.095 g, 1 mmol), thiourea (0.114 g, 1.5 mmol) concentrated hydrochloric acid (2 mL) and water (5 mL) into a round bottom flask (50 ml) and mix it well (~5 min).
2) Stir the mixture for 1 h at room temperature
3) Reflux the mixture for 3 h.
4) Allow the hot mixture to cool, continue the stirring procedure.
5) Isolate the crystals and wash with water to remove the unreacted reactants.
6) The melting range of the product is 124 to 125 °C.

Step 2: Preparation of 5-benzylidene-1,3-thiazolidine-2,4-dione

Chemicals Required: Thiazolidine-2,4-dione, Benzaldehyde, Toluene, Piperidine.

1) Place thiazolidine-2,4-dione (0.117 g, 1 mmol), benzaldehyde (0.106 g, 1 mmol) and toluene (4 mL) in to a round bottom flask.
2) Add two drops of piperidine and attach reflux condenser fixed with Dean-Starks apparatus.
3) Reflux the mixture for 6 h.
4) Purify the product by recrystallization with aqueous ethanol (70%).
5) The melting point of pure 5-benzylidene-1,3-thiazolidine-2,4-dione is 240 to 242 °C.

KEY POINTS

- The condensation of carbonyl compounds (aldehydes and ketones) with activated methylene groups generates arylidene derivatives, this reaction is known as Knoevenagel condensation.
- Knoevenagel condensation resembles aldol condensation.
- Chemical synthesis of pyrantel pamoate (anthelmintic), sulindac (anti-inflammatory), acenocoumarin (anti-coagulant) and ethosuximide (anti-convulsant) involves Knoevenagel condensation.

21

Mannich Reaction

The condensation of compounds containing active hydrogen atom (e.g., β-keto esters), formaldehyde and ammonia or amines (1° or 2°) is known as Mannich reaction. The amines should be preferentially in its salt form. The reaction is generally catalyzed by acid (e.g., hydrochloric acid) and produces β-amino-carbonyl compound (Mannich Base). Tertiary amines will not undergo this reaction.

$$R-CO-CH_3 + H_2C{=}O + R^1-NH(R^2).HCl \xrightarrow{HCl} R-CO-CH_2-CH_2-\overset{+}{N}H(R^1)-R^2\ Cl^-$$

Active hydrogen compound; Formaldehyde; Amine; Alkylamino substituted propionone hydrochloride

General mechanism

Generation of methylene alkylamine

Ammonia or amines activate the formaldehyde and generate intermediate enamine through nucleophilic addition. The dehydration reaction produces Schiff base (methylene dimethylamine).

$$O{=}CH_2 \underset{H^+}{\rightleftharpoons} H\overset{+}{O}{=}CH_2 + HN(R^1)(R^2) \rightleftharpoons HO-CH_2-\overset{+}{N}(R^1)(R^2)-H \longrightarrow H_2C{=}\overset{+}{N}(R^2)-R^1$$

Methylene alkylamine

Nitriles, acetylenes, aliphatic nitro compounds, α-alkyl pyridines and imines contain active hydrogen are the good substrates. Electron rich heterocycles such as furan, pyrrole, thiophene and indole also act as substrates.

Formation of mannich base

This electrophilic schiff base reacts with compound containing active hydrogen (acidic) through electrophilic addition reaction. The condensation between acetophenone (active hydrogen compound), formaldehyde and dimethylamine hydrochloride is a typical example. This condensation produces β-dimethylamino propiophenone (Mannich base).

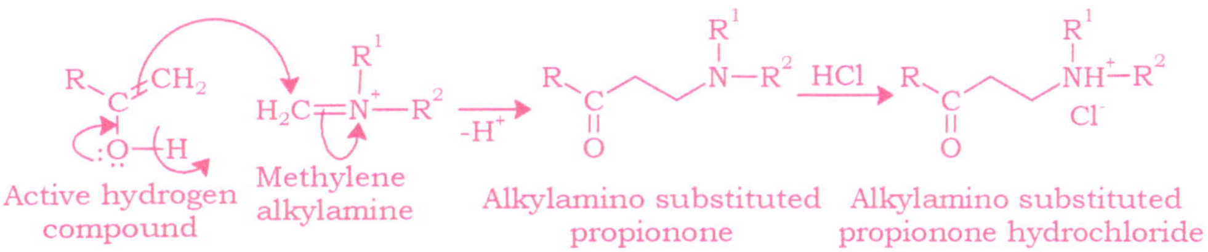

Active hydrogen compound
Methylene alkylamine
Alkylamino substituted propionone
Alkylamino substituted propionone hydrochloride

Pharmaceutical Applications

The product of Mannich reaction, 1,3-amino alcohols are called as Michael acceptors, which finds important role in the medicinal chemistry. Mannich reaction is involved in the synthesis of several pharmaceuticals, natural products and polymers.

1. Propoxyphen (anti-inflammatory and antitussive drug) can be prepared from propiophenone by Mannich reaction.

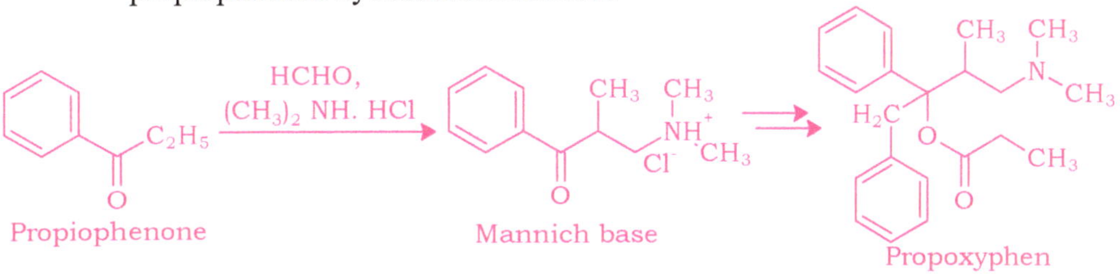

HCHO, $(CH_3)_2$ NH. HCl

Propiophenone
Mannich base
Propoxyphen

2. Furfuryl alcohol can be converted in to a antiulcer drug, ranitidine through Mannich reaction.

HCHO, $(CH_3)_2$ NH. HCl

Furfuryl alcohol
Mannich base
Ranitidine

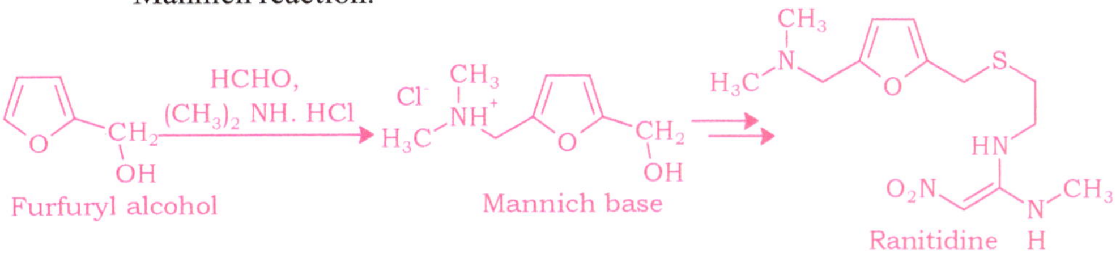

3. Triprolidine (anti-histamine) preparation involves the Mannich reaction.

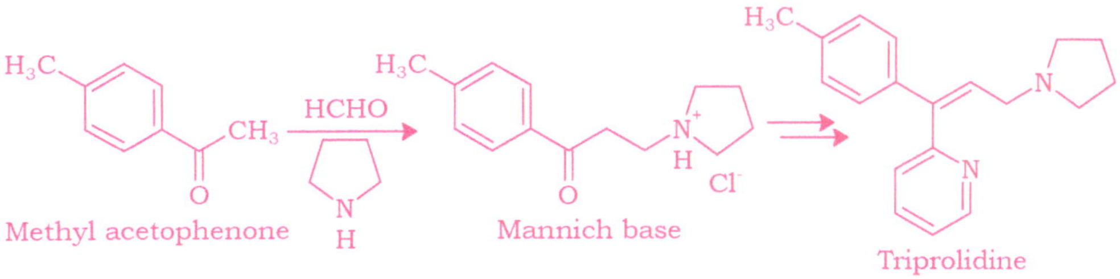

HCHO

Methyl acetophenone
Mannich base
Triprolidine

4. Benzhexol (antispasmodic) can be prepared from acetophenone through Mannich reaction.

HCHO

Acetophenone
Mannich base
Benzhexol

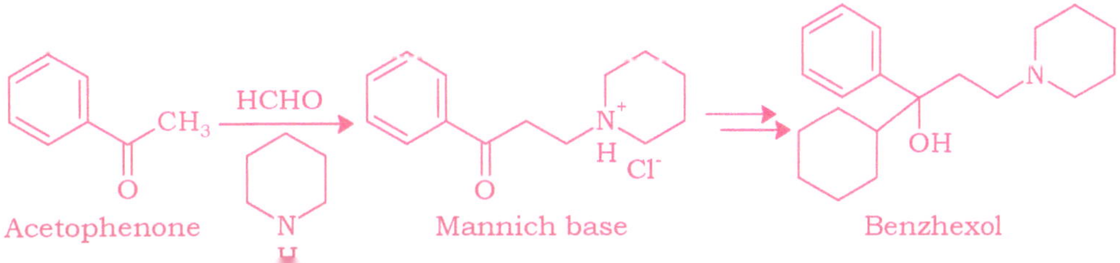

21.1 Preparation of Dimethylamino Propiophenone Hydrochlride

Traditional Name: Dimethylamino propiophenone

IUPAC Name: 3-(Dimethylamino)-1-phenypropan-1-one

Mol wt: 177.25 g/mol

Principle: Acetophenone condenses with formaldehyde and dimethylamine hydrochloride to form β-dimethylamino propiophenone hydrochloride. This reaction is a typical example for the Mannich reaction and product is known as Mannich base. The reaction proceeds in the presence of ethanol.

Acetophenone + $H_2C{=}O$ (Formaldehyde) + $(H_3C)_2NH.HCl$ (Diemethylamine hydrochloride) $\xrightarrow{HCl}$ Dimethylamino propiophenone hydrochloride

Reaction Mechanism

Generation of methylene dimethylamine

$O{=}CH_2 \underset{H^+}{\rightleftharpoons} HO{=}\overset{+}{C}H_2$ + $HN(CH_3)_2$ ⇌ $HO{-}CH_2{-}\overset{+}{N}H(CH_3)_2$ ⟶ $H_2C{=}\overset{+}{N}(CH_3)_2$ (Methylene dimethylamine)

Formation of Mannich base

Acetophenone (enol form) + Methylene dimethylamine $\xrightarrow{-H^+}$ Dimethylamino propiophenone $\xrightarrow{HCl}$ Dimethylamino propiophenone hydrochloride

Procedure:

Chemicals Required: Acetophenone, Paraformaldehyde, Dimethylamine hydrochloride, Hydrochloric acid, Acetone and Ethanol.

1. Place dry dimethylamine hydrochloride (2.7 g, 33 mmol), powdered para formaldehyde (1 g, 33 mmol) and acetophenone (3 mL, 25 mmol) into a round bottom flask.
2. Add ethanol acidified with drop of hydrochloric acid (4 mL, 95%) to the flask.
3. Reflux the mixture by placing on a water bath for 2 h.
   (*the reaction mixture becomes clear and homogeneous*).
4. Filter the yellowish reaction mixture through a hot water funnel.
5. Transfer the warm filtrate to flask and dilute with acetone (20 mL).
6. Cool the mixture to room temperature and place it in a refrigerator overnight.
7. Filter the crystals formed under vacuum, wash with acetone (1 mL) and dry at 40-50 °C.
8. Purify the product by recrystalization with the mixture of hot ethanol and acetone (1:5).
   (*Acetone should be addded slowly to the hot ethanol solution*)
9. Isolate the solid by vacuum filtration and dry at 70 °C.
10. The melting range of pure dimethylamino propiophenone hydrochloride is 155 to 156 °C.

KEY POINTS

- The condensation of compounds containing active hydrogen atom (e.g., β-keto esters), formaldehyde and ammonia or amines (1° or 2°) is known as Mannich reaction.
- The reaction undergoes nucleophilic addition, Schiff base formation and hydrolysis to generate Mannich base.
- Propoxyphen (anti-inflammatory, antitussive), ranitidine (antiulcer), triprolidine (anti-histamine) and benzhexol (antispasmodic) synthesis involves Mannnich reaction.

22

Oxidation

The combination of molecules and oxygen is the most natural reaction. It is referred as oxidation. The loss of electrons in an atom increases its oxidation number (valence) and transforms it into more oxidized state.

The chemical interaction between oxygen molecules and all the different substances are known as oxidation reactions. The process of oxidation involves either loss of one or more electrons (de-electronation) and loss of hydrogen's from the molecular entity, and addition of oxygen to the molecular entity.

Types of oxidation reactions

***Type 1**: Simple composition reactions:* It involves the addition of oxygen to the molecule.

$$\underset{\text{Acetaldehyde}}{H_3C{-}\overset{H}{C}{=}O} \xrightarrow{(O)} \underset{\text{Acetic acid}}{H_3C{-}\underset{\underset{O}{\|}}{C}{-}OH}$$

Type 2: Dehydrogenation: This kind of oxidation removes hydrogens from the molecule.

$$\underset{\text{Ethanol}}{H_3C{-}CH_2\text{-}OH} \xrightarrow{(O)} \underset{\text{Acetaldehyde}}{H_3C{-}\overset{H}{C}{=}O} + H_2O$$

***Type 3: Addition of oxygen and dehydrogenation (combination of type 1 and 2)*:** The kind of oxidation reaction, where both involves both the addition of oxygen to the molecule and removal of hydrogen from the molecule occurs.

$$\underset{\text{Methane}}{CH_4} \xrightarrow{(O)} \underset{\text{Formaldehyde}}{H_2C{=}O} + H_2O$$

Common Oxidants

Oxidant	Chemical functions
Chromium oxidants	
Collins reagent 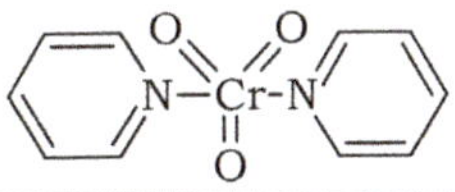	The solution of chromium trioxide (CrO_3) and two molecules of pyridine (Sarett reagent) in methylene chloride is called as Collins reagent. This reagent oxidizes primary alcohols to aldehydes and secondary alcohols to ketones. The excess of reagent (stoichiometric quantities) is essential. This reagent does not affect the labile groups.
Pyridinium chlorchromate (PCC, Corey's reagent) 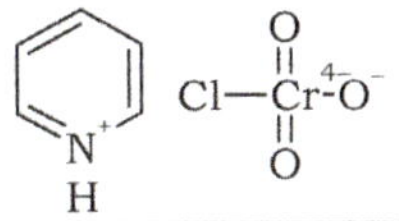	It oxidizes primary alcohols to aldehydes, and secondary alcohols to ketones. More acidic than pyridinium dichloride and Collins reagent. This reagent is not suitable for molecules containing acid labile groups. Buffering the reagent with ethyl acetate protects the acid labile groups.
Pyridinium dichromate 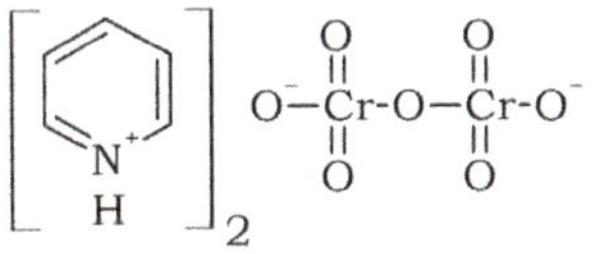	It oxidizes primary alcohols to either aldehydes or carboxylic acids and secondary alcohols to ketones. This reagent is less acidic than pyridinium chlorchromate (PCC) and more acidic than Collins reagent.
Jones reagent CrO_3, H_2SO_4	A solution of chromium trioxide (CrO_3) in dilute sulphuric acid is known as Jones reagent. It oxidizes primary alcohols to carboxylic acids and secondary alcohols to ketones. This reagent is not suitable for the oxidation of molecules containing acid labile groups.
Ruthenium oxidants	
Tetra-n-propylammonium perruthenate (TPAP; tee-pap) 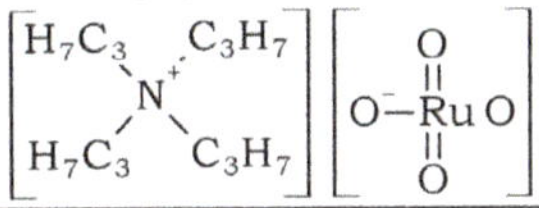	It oxidizes primary alcohols to aldehydes (oxidation to carboxylic acid is rare) more rapidly and secondary alcohols to ketones. The N-methylmorpholine-N-oxide (NMO) is useful in recycling this reagent.
Manganese oxidants	
Manganese dioxide MnO_2	This mild oxidant, oxidizes allylic, propargylic and benzylic alcohols to aldehydes and ketones.
Potassium permanganate $KMnO_4$	It is a powerful oxidant. Aqueous medium promotes the permanganate mediated oxidations, where as organic solvents tampers the oxidation potential. It oxidizes benzylic position of aromatic system to carboxylic acid. Non-chemoselectiveness is the limiting factor.
Peracids (epoxidation oxidants)	
Perbenzoic acid 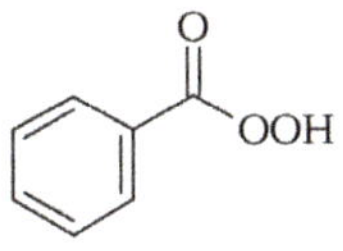	It is a simple peroxy acid, useful in the generation of epoxides.
meta-Chloroperbenzoic acid 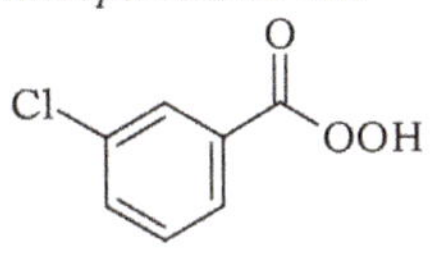 *meta-Nitroperbenzoic acid* 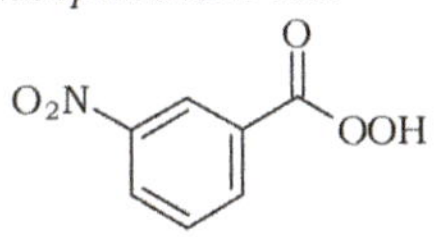	It is an electrophilic oxidant. It oxidizes olefins and reacts preferentially with electron rich carbon-carbon double bonds (C=C).

Oxidant	Chemical functions
Peracids (epoxidation oxidants)	
Perphthalic acid 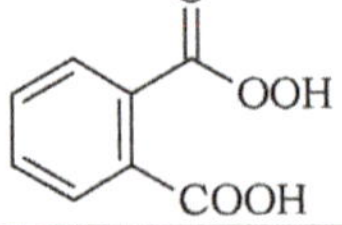 (structure: O, OOH, COOH)	It is useful in the epoxidation and formation of alkene oxide.
Per trifluroacetic acid CF_3COOOH	It is useful in the synthesis of peptides.
Miscellaneous	
Dimethyl sulphoxide $(CH_3)_2SO_2$	It is a very mild oxidant. It is useful in the Swern oxidation and in the Nicolau's synthesis of rapamycin.
Iodine I_2	Hypervalent iodine reagent (+3 and +5 oxidation state of iodine), (Dess-Martin Periodinane (DMP)) oxidizes primary alcohol to aldehyde (not to carboxylic acid) and secondary alcohol to ketones.
Sodium chlorite NaO(OCl)	It oxidizes alcohol to carboxylic acid more efficiently. The use of resorcinol (electrophile scavenger) along with the sodium chlorite prevents the oxidation of olefin functionalities.
Lead tetraacetate $Pb(OCOCH_3)_4$	It is a strong oxidizing agent and a source for acetyloxy groups.
Sodium periodate $NaIO_4$	Sodium periodate is useful in the conversion of 1,2-diols into two corresponding aldehydes and further into carboxylic acid.
Osmium tetroxide OsO_4	It oxidizes olefins into 1,2-diol in presence of pyridine. It occurs through 1,3-cycloaddition formation of osmic ester (osmylation) and hydrolysis of osmic ester.
Hydrogen peroxide H_2O_2	Hydrogen peroxide (simple peroxide) is a strong oxidizer. Higher oxidation capacity of hydrogen peroxide provides bleaching property.
Fenton reagent $H_2O_2 + FeSO_4$ / $Fe\ (OCOCH_3)_2$	The mixture of hydrogen peroxide and ferrous sulphate/ferrous acetate is known as Fenton reagent. It can be used for the hydroxylation of arenes and oxidation of barbituric acid to alloxan.
Selenium dioxide SeO_2	Selenium dioxide commonly oxidizes C-H bonds attached to various activating groups. Aldehydes, ketones and olefins are oxidized with high yields under mild conditions. Alcohols, amines, phenols and mercaptans are oxidized with poor yields under vigorous conditions. Alkanes, ethers and allyl halides undergo oxidation only in severe reaction conditions.
Ozone O_3	A triatomic molecule containing three oxygen atoms. It is a powerful oxidizing agent. The reaction is rapid with increased temperature and pressure.
Dimethyldioxirane 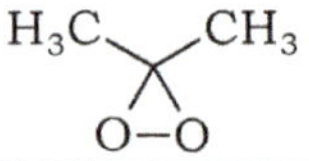 (structure: H_3C, CH_3, O–O)	It is a powerful, selective and electrophilic oxidant. It oxidizes unreactive olefins under mild conditions.
N-Bromo succinamide (NBS) 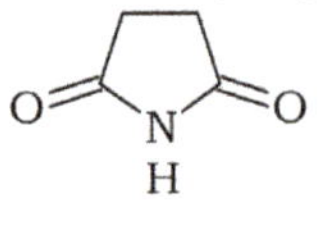 (structure: O, N, H, O)	It mediates oxidations in the presence of UV light and peroxides. The oxidative reaction takes place through free radical mechanism. It oxidizes primary alcohols into aldehydes, and secondary alcohols into ketones. N-Bromosuccinamide in aqueous dimethoxyethane selectively oxidizes the secondary alcohols without affecting the primary alcohol. It converts amino acids into aldehydes through oxidative decarboxylation and deamination.

Important oxidation reactions

Osmylation: The osmium tetroxide oxidizes olefins through 1,3-cycloaddition and forms osmic ester (unstable intermediate). The ester upon hydrolysis generates 1,2-diol, and this reaction is known as Osmylation.

Upjohn dihydroxylation: *Syn*-selective preparation of 1,2-diol from alkenes by the use of osmium tetroxide along with *N*-methyl morpholine-*N*-oxide.

Swern oxidation: The mixture of dimethyl sulfoxide and oxalyl chloride generates dimethylchlorosulphonium *in situ*. It oxidizes primary alcohols into aldehydes and secondary alcohols into ketones. This reaction proceeds even under very mild conditions and avoids the use of toxic metals (chromium).

$$R-CH_2OH \xrightarrow{(O)} R-C(=O)-OH$$

Primary alcohol → Carboxylic acid

$$R-CH(OH)-R^1 \xrightarrow{(O)} R-C(=O)-R^1$$

Secondary alcohol → Ketone

Rubottom oxidation: It involves the oxidation of silyl enol ethers into β-hydroxy ketones using *m*-chloroperbenzoic acid (mCPBA) as an oxidant.

Ozonolysis: The oxidative cleavage of reaction of alkenes into aldehydes, ketones and carboxylic acid mediated by ozone is called as ozonolysis. In general, it requires dichloromethane as a medium and temperature –78 °C.

- Reductive workup with zinc in acetic acid/dimethyl sulphide produces ketones and aldehydes.
- Oxidative workup with hydrogen peroxide forms carboxylic acid.

$$R(R_1)C{=}C(R_2)R_3 \xrightarrow{O_3} R(R_1)C{=}O + O{=}C(R_2)R_3$$

Alkene → Aldehyde + Ketone

Oppenauer oxidation: The aluminium-catalyzed hydride shift from the α-carbon of an alcohol into the carbonyl carbon of ketone is known as Oppenauer oxidation.

$$R{-}CH(OH){-}R^1 + R^2{-}C({=}O){-}R^3 \xrightarrow{Al(OR)_3} R{-}C({=}O){-}R^1 + R^2{-}CH(OH){-}R^3$$

Secondary alcohol + Ketone → Ketone + Secondary alcohol

Jones oxidation: The oxidation of primary alcohols into carboxylic acid and secondary alcohols into ketones by using cromic acid (sodium/potassium chromate and sulphuric acid) is known as Jones oxidation.

$$R{-}CH_2OH \xrightarrow{H_2CrO_4} R{-}C({=}O){-}OH$$

Primary alcohol → Carboxylic acid

$$R{-}CH(OH){-}R^1 \xrightarrow{H_2CrO_4} R{-}C({=}O){-}R^1$$

Secondary alcohol → Ketone

Jacobsen-Katsuki epoxidation: The enantioselective formation of epoxides from substituted olefins (prochiral allylic alcohols) mediated by the mixture of Mn-Salen catalyst (Jacobsen's catalyst) and sodium hypochlorite is known as Jacobsen-Katsuki epoxidation.

$$RCH{=}CHR_1 \xrightarrow[NaOCl]{\text{Mn-Salen catalyst}} \text{R(H)C–C(H)R}_1 \text{ (epoxide, O bridge)}$$

Alkene → Epoxide

Prilezhaev reaction: Alkenes upon epoxidation by peracid (*meta*-chloroperbenzoic acid, peracetic acid, magnesium mono-perphthalate) forms oxirane (epoxide). This reaction is called as Prilezhaev reaction.

$$R(H)C{=}C(R_1)R_2 \xrightarrow{\text{Peracid}} \text{R(H)C–C(R}_1\text{)R}_2 \text{ (O bridge)}$$

Alkene → Oxirane (Epoxide)

Dess-Martin oxidation: A selective and very mild oxidation of alcohols into aldehydes or ketones by Dess-Martin periodinane (DMP, hyper valent iodine) is known as Dess-Martin oxidation.

R–CH(OH)–R[1] —DMP→ R–C(=O)–H + R–C(=O)–R[1]

Secondary alcohol → Aldehyde + Ketone

Baeyer-Villiger oxidation: The conversion of ketones into esters and cyclic ketones into lactones by oxidative cleavage mediated through *m*CPBA/hydrogen peroxide.

Ketone —mCPBA, H_2O_2→ Ester

Sommelet reaction: Arylalkyl halides upon reaction with hexamethylene tetramine (hexamine) forms an arylalkyl quaternary salt. This intermediate upon oxidation produces aryl aldehyde.

$Ar-CH_2-X$ (Aryl alkylhalide) + Hexamethylene tetramine (Hexamine) → $Ar-CH_2-N^+$ (Quanternary salt) —H_2O→ Aryl aldehyde

Sarett oxidation: The oxidation of primary alcohols into aldehydes and secondary alcohols into ketones by Collins reagent (CrO_3-pyridine) is known as Sarett oxidation.

Pharmaceutical Applications

1) Cortisone (anti-inflammatory agent) can be prepared from 3α, 21-diacetoxy pregnane-1,2-dione by osmium tetraoxide mediated oxidation reaction. The reduction of cortisone produces hydrocortisone.

—OsO_4→ —CrO_3, Na_2SO_3→ Cortisone

2) Sulindac (NSAID) preparation involves the sodium periodate ($NaIO_4$) mediated oxidation in the final step.

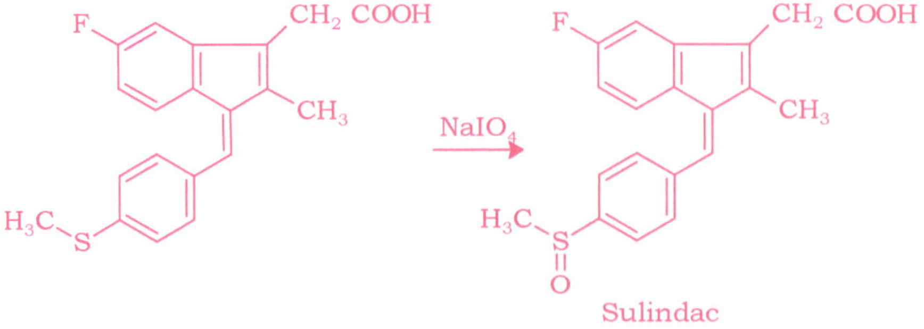

F, CH_2 COOH, CH_3, H_3C–S — $NaIO_4$ → F, CH_2 COOH, CH_3, H_3C–S(=O)

Sulindac

3) N-Bromosuccinamide mediated oxidation is required in the preparation of carbamazepine (anticonvulsant drug).

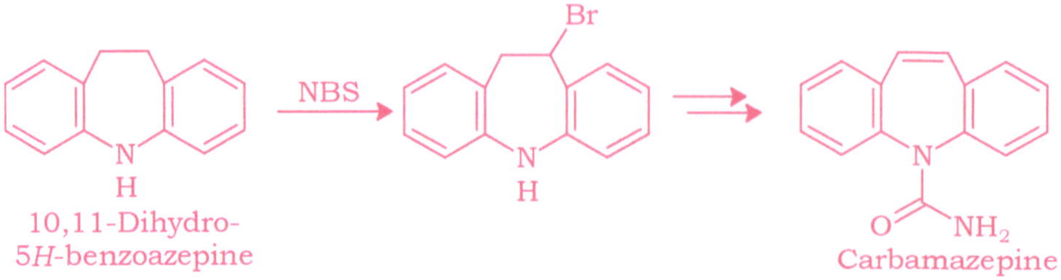

10,11-Dihydro-5*H*-benzoazepine — NBS → (Br, N–H) ⇉ Carbamazepine (N, O, NH_2)

4) Preparation of Vitamin A_1 and A_2 by using potassium permanganate, N-bromo succinamide and lithium aluminium hydride (LAH).

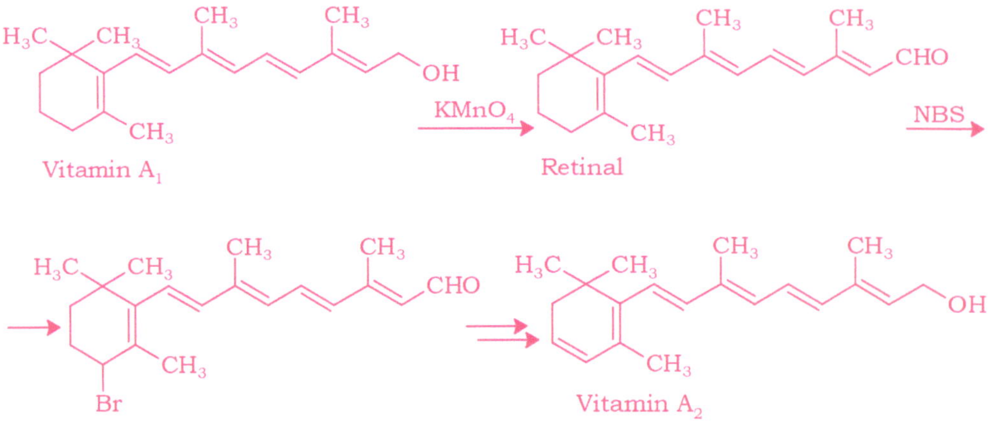

Vitamin A_1 (H_3C, CH_3, CH_3, CH_3, CH_3, OH) — $KMnO_4$ → Retinal (H_3C, CH_3, CH_3, CH_3, CH_3, CHO) — NBS →

→ (H_3C, CH_3, CH_3, CH_3, CH_3, CHO, Br) ⇉ Vitamin A_2 (H_3C, CH_3, CH_3, CH_3, CH_3, OH)

5) Preparation of azatadine (antihistamine) using peracid.

22.1 Preparation of Benzil

Traditional Name: Diphenylethanedione, Diphenylglyoxal, Bibenzoyl

IUPAC Name: 1,2-Diphenylethane-1,2-dione **Mol wt**: 210. 23 g/mol

Principle: Benzil can be prepared by the oxidation of benzoin. Concentrated nitric acid is useful as oxidizing agent. Benzoin contains secondary alcohol and keto group. The secondary alcohol of the benzoin can be oxidized. The resulting product is called as benzil. The oxidation can be effected by using chlorine, iodine and electrolytical methods. Ammonium acetate-copper(II)acetate, ammonium chlorochromate-alumina, bismuth(III)nitrate-copper(II)acetate, clayfen, copper sulphate in pyridine, modified Fehling solution ($CuSO_4$ in pyridine), lithium nitrate in acetic anhydride, hydrogen peroxide, ferric(III)chloride, nickel acetate, sodium hydride in tetra hydrofuran (THF), thalium nitrate and Nano-MgO and ytterbium(III)nitrate are some of the important oxidizing agents useful.

Reaction Mechanism

Procedure:

Chemicals Required: Benzoin, Concentrate nitric acid, Ethanol.

1. Place benzoin (1 g, 4.7 mmol) and concentrated nitric acid (5 mL) into a round bottom flask.
2. Heat the reaction mixture for 90 min (1.5 h) by placing in a water bath. (*until the evolution of nitrogen oxides ceases*)
3. Pour the reaction mixture into a beaker containing cold water (20 mL).
4. Stir well to crystallize the oil into yellow solid (crude benzil).
5. Isolate the crude benzil by vacuum filtration, wash with water and dry.
6. Purify the crude benzil by recrystallization with ethanol.
7. The melting range of pure benzil is 94 to 96 °C.

***Note*:** Carry out the reaction in fume hood to avoid the breathing of evolved nitrogen oxides.

22.2 Preparation of Benzoic Acid

Traditional Name: Carboxybenzene, Dracyclic acid, Phenylformic acid

IUPAC Name: Benzoic acid **Mol wt**: 122. 12 g/mol

Principle: Benzyl chloride upon permanganate (potassium permanganate) oxidation in alkaline medium produces benzoic acid. In alkaline medium, permanganate functions as a powerful oxidizing agent. Alternatively, benzyl chloride oxidation can be effected by using dilute nitric acid. But the reaction proceeds very slow.

Cl $\xrightarrow[Na_2CO_3]{KMnO_4}$ OH $\xrightarrow[Na_2CO_3]{KMnO_4}$ O, H

Benzyl chloride Benzyl alcohol Benzaldehyde

$KMnO_4$
Na_2CO_3

O, OH+ $HMnO_3$

Benzoic acid

Benzyl chloride gets oxidized and forms benzyl alcohol. In the next step, benzyl alcohol oxidizes into benzaldehyde. Further oxidation converts the benzaldehyde into benzoic acid. Potassium permanganate gets reduced into manganese oxide, which produces brownish precipitate (upon oxiding the benzyl chloride) along with benzoic acid. Addition of sodium sulphite solution dissolves brownish manganese dioxide alone. This facilitates the appearance of colourless crystals of benzoic acid.

Reaction Mechanism

Step 1 Formation of manganate: Potassium permanganate dissociates and generates manganate ion (MnO_4^-). The manganese ion (MnO_4^-) is very stable in alkaline medium (sodium carbonate provides alkaline environment).

$$KMnO_4 \longrightarrow K^+ + MnO_4^-$$

Step 2 Oxidation of benzyl chloride into benzaldehyde: Chlorinated alkyl group of benzyl chloride offers positive inductive effect and increases the susceptibility of oxidation. Manganate ion attacks benzyl chloride (nucleophilic substitution) and forms benzaldehyde.

Step 3 Oxidation of benzaldehyde into benzoic acid: Benzaldehyde undergoes oxidation by manganate ion to give benzoic acid.

Procedure:

Chemicals Required: Benzyl chloride, Sodium carbonate (anhydrous), Potassium permanganate, Concentrated hydrochloric acid, Sodium sulphite.

1. Place anhydrous sodium carbonate (2.5 g, 23.59 mmol) and potassium permanganate (5 g, 31.64 mmol) into a round bottom flask containing cold water (100 mL).
2. Add benzyl chloride (2.5 mL, 22.7 mmol) to the flask slowly with stirring to produce clear solution.

3. Attach reflux condenser to the flask and boil the mixture, until the liquid running from the condenser contains no oily drops of benzyl chloride (~1½ h).

   (*violet colour of permanganate changes to brown precipitate of manganese dioxide*)
4. Cool the reaction mixture under running water and shake vigorously to avoid the formation of lumps.
5. Add concentrated hydrochloric acid (25 mL) to the mixture to precipitate the benzoic acid.
6. Add sodium sulphite solution (50 mL, 20%) to dissolve the brown precipitate of manganese dioxide. This facilitates the appearance of colourless precipitate of benzoic acid.
7. Isolate the crude benzoic acid through vacuum filtration, wash the solid with cold water (several times) and dry.
8. Purify the crude benzoic acid by recrystallization with hot water.
9. The melting point of pure benzoic acid is 121 °C .

KEY POINTS

- The reaction of molecules and oxygen increases the oxidation number (valence) of atoms and is referred as oxidation.
- Jones reagent, potassium permanganate and hydrogen peroxide are the well known oxidizing agents.
- Oppenauer oxidation and Jones oxidation are very important oxidation reactions.
- Chemical synthesis of cortisone (anti-inflammatory), sulindac (NSAID), carbamazepine (anticonvulsant), Vitamin A and azatadine (antihistamine) involves different oxidation reactions.

23

Paal-Knorr Pyrazole Synthesis

The condensation of β-diketones (1,3-dicarbonyl compounds) and hydrazines generates pyrazole derivatives. This condensation reaction is known as Paal-Knorr Pyrazole synthesis.

$H_2N{-}NH_2$ Hydrazine + β-Diketone (1,3-dicarbonyl compound) ⟶ Pyrazole

β-Ketoaldehydes and β-ketoesters can be used in place of β-diketones (1,3-dicarbonyl compounds).

- β-Ketoaldehydes produce isomer mixture.
- β-Ketoesters produce pyrazolone (e.g., antipyrine synthesis).

Reaction Mechanism

The nitrogen of the hydrazine attacks carbonyl carbon and forms imine intermediate. The nitrogen of hydrazine also attacks other carbonyl carbon and forms second imine intermediate. The imine intermediate upon dehydrogenation forms pyrazole product. Reaction of semicarbazide or amino guanidines with acetyl acetone gives 1-carbamido or 1-carboxamide derivatives, which on hydrolysis and decarboxylation gives 3,5-dimethyl pyrazole. It can be also prepared from 1,2-pentanedien-4-one and hydrazine hydrate.

β-Diketone (1,3-dicarbonyl compound) ⇌ ... + $H_2\ddot{N}{-}NH_2$ Hydrazine ⟶ ... ⟶ $\xrightarrow{-H_2O}$ ... ⟶ ... $\xrightarrow{-H_2O}$ 3,5-Dimethyl-1*H*-pyrazole

Pharmaceutical Applications

Celecoxib (anti-inflammatory), zaleplon (sedative and hypnotic), sildenafil (treat erectile dysfunction), zoniporide (cardioprotective) and acomplia (anti-obesity) are the important pharmaceuticals containing pyrazole nucleus. β-Pyrazol-1-yl-alanine is present in water melon seeds.

1) The antiinflammatory drug antipyrine can be synthesized through Paal-Knorr Pyrazole synthesis.

Phenylhydrazine + Ethyl acetoacetate → 5-Methyl-2-phenyl-1,2-dihydro-3*H*-pyrazol-3-one $\xrightarrow[\text{NaOH}]{(CH_3)_2SO_4}$ Antipyrine

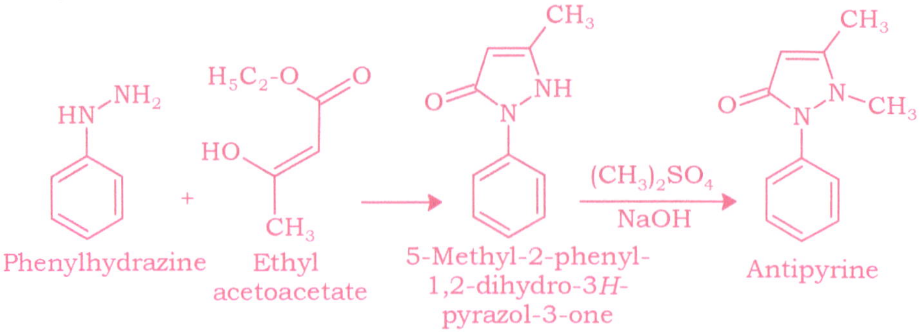

2) The analgesic and antipyretic drug propyphenazone can be synthesized through Paal-Knorr Pyrazole synthesis.

Phenylhydrazine + Ethyl acetoacetate → 5-Methyl-2-phenyl-1,2-dihydro-3*H*-pyrazol-3-one ⇉ Propyphenazone

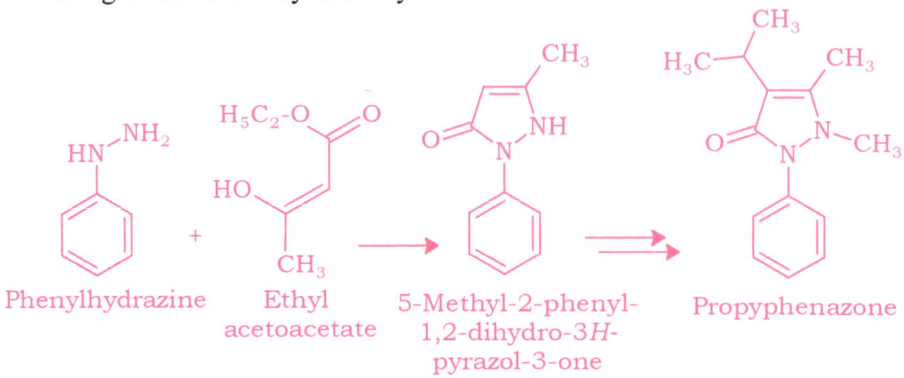

3) The anti-rheumatic drug metamizol can be synthesized through Paal-Knorr Pyrazole synthesis.

Phenylhydrazine + Ethyl acetoacetate → 5-Methyl-2-phenyl-1,2-dihydro-3*H*-pyrazol-3-one ⇉ Metamizol

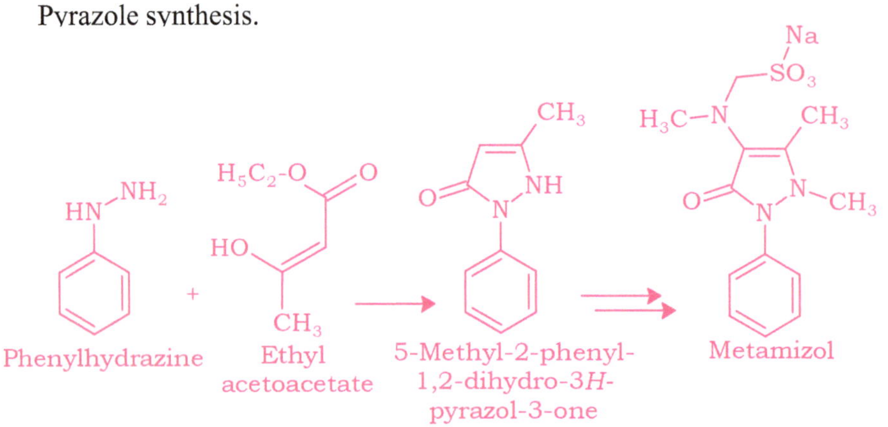

4) The uricosuric drug sulphinpyrazone can be synthesized through Paal-Knorr Pyrazole synthesis.

1,2-Diphenyl hydrazine + Diethyl (2-(phenylsulphanyl) ethylpropanedione → Sulphinpyrazone

5) The anti-inflammatory drug phenylbutazone can be synthesized through Paal-Knorr Pyrazole synthesis.

1,2-Diphenyl hydrazine + Diethyl butylpropanedione → Phenylbutazone

23.1 Preparation of 3,5-Dimethyl-1*H*-Pyrazole

IUPAC Name: 3,5-Dimethyl-1H-pyrazole **Mol wt**: 96. 13 g/mol

Principle: The condensation of acetyl acetone (2,4-pentanedione) with hydrazine hydrate in aqueous alkali produces 3,5-dimethylpyrazole. Hydrazine hydrate is violent and produces abnoxious vapour (CNS irritant). Hence, hydrazine sulphate is preferred for the condensation.

$$H_2N{-}NH_2.H_2SO_4 + H_3C{-}CO{-}CH_2{-}CO{-}CH_3 \xrightarrow{NaOH} \text{3,5-Dimethyl-1}H\text{-pyrazole}$$

Hydrazine sulphate Acetyl acetone 3,5-Dimethyl-1*H*-pyrazole

Acetyl acetone exists in *keto-enol* tautomeric form. The lone pair of electrons present in the nitrogen of hydrazine sulphate attacks enolic carbon of acetyl acetone. This forms 5-substituted pentane-2-one, and on cyclization eliminates two water molecules and produces 3,5-dimethylpyrazole.

Acetyl acetone

$H_2\ddot{N}-NH_2.H_2SO_4$
Hydrazine sulphate

$-H_2O$ $-H_2O$

3,5-Dimethyl-1*H*-pyrazole

Procedure:

Chemicals Required: Acetyl acetone, Hydrazine sulphate, Sodium hydroxide (2.5 M), Ether, Potassium carbonate.

1. Place hydrazine sulphate (1.3 g, 10 mmol) and sodium hydroxide solution (8 mL, 2.5 M) into a flask and mix the contents well.
2. Equip the flask with thermometer, magnetic stirrer and dropping funnel.
3. Immerse the flask in an ice-bath to reduce the temperature to 15 °C.
4. Add acetyl acetone (1 mL, 10 mmol) dropwise with stirring, maintaining the temperature (15 °C).
5. Continue the stirring for further 1 h at 15 °C, dimethylpyrazole separates while stirring.
6. Add water (10 mL) to the mixture to dissolve the inorganic salts (sodium sulphate) formed during the reaction.
7. Transfer the contents to a separating funnel and extract with ether (5 mL, three times).
8. Combine the ethereal layers and dry over anhydrous potassium carbonate.
9. Evaporate the ether to obtain pale yellow solid dimethylpyrazole.
10. The melting range of pure dimethylpyrazole is 107 to 108 °C.

23.2 Preparation of 5-Methyl-2-phenyl-1,3-dihydropyrazol-3-one (intermediate of antipyrine)

IUPAC Name: 5-Dimethyl-2-phenyl-1,2-dihydropyrazol-3-one

Mol wt: 174.20 g/mol

Principle: The condensation of ethyl acetoacetate and phenylhydrazine produces 5-methyl-2-phenyl-pyrazole-5-one. This upon methylation (*N*-alkylation) with dimethyl sulphate forms antipyrine. The *enol* form of the ethyl acetoacetate readily condenses with phenylhydrazine and forms 5-methyl-2-phenyl-1,3-dihydro-pyrazol-3-one.

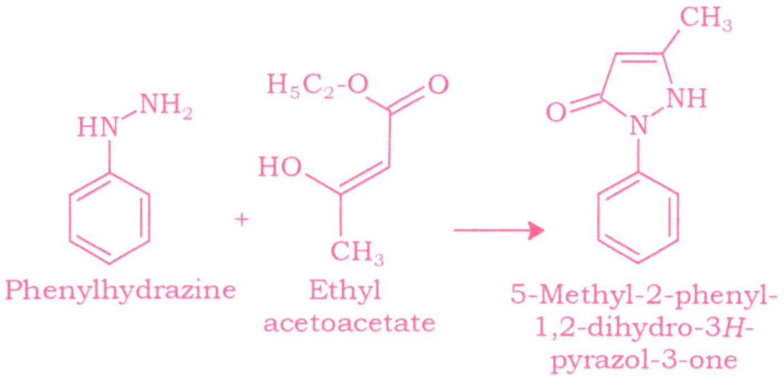

Phenylhydrazine + Ethyl acetoacetate → 5-Methyl-2-phenyl-1,2-dihydro-3*H*-pyrazol-3-one

Reaction Mechanism

Keto-enol tautomerism in ethyl acetoacetate: Inductive effect on the two carbonyl group (keto and carboxylic) of the ethyl acetoacetate, increases the acidity of the carbon-hydrogen (>C-H) bond of active methylene group. This favours the dissociation of hydrogen atom from active methylene group and abstraction of the hydrogen by keto group.

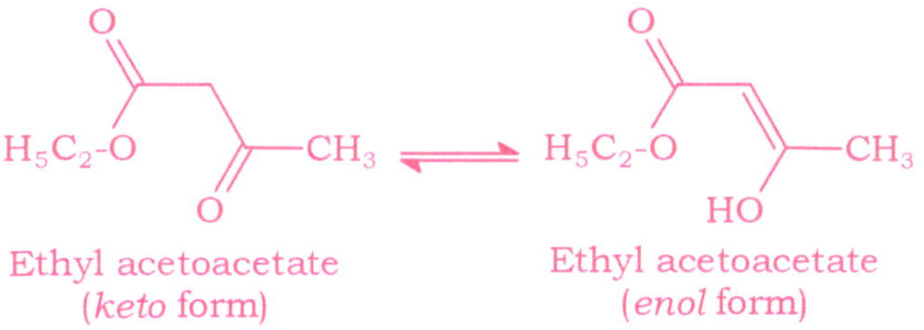

Ethyl acetoacetate (*keto* form) ⇌ Ethyl acetoacetate (*enol* form)

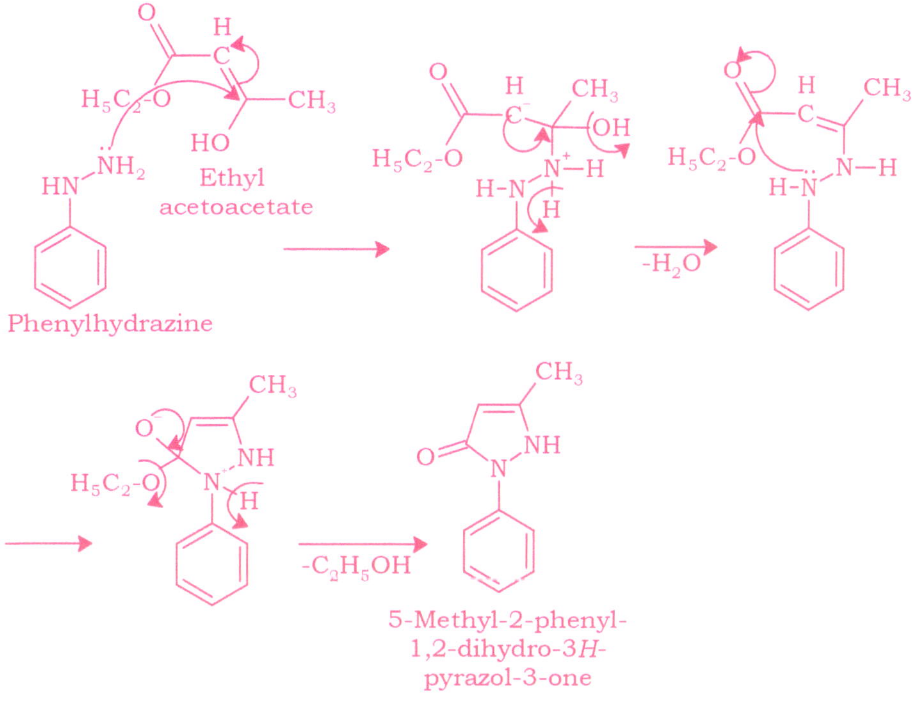

Ethyl acetoacetate + Phenylhydrazine → → $-H_2O$ →

→ $-C_2H_5OH$ → 5-Methyl-2-phenyl-1,2-dihydro-3*H*-pyrazol-3-one

Procedure:

Chemicals Required: Ethyl acetoacetate, Phenylhydrazine, Diethyl ether, Ethanol, water.

1. Mix distilled ethyl acetoacetate (2 mL, 16 mmol) and phenylhydrazine (1.5 mL, 15 mmol) in a china dish.
2. Heat the mixture in a fume cupboard for 2 h (stir with glass rod).
3. Cool the red syrup, add diethyl ether (4 mL) and stir the mixture vigorously.
4. Keep the mixture aside for 15 min and filter the solid (vacuum filtration).
5. Wash the filtered solid with diethyl ether (to remove unreacted reactants and impurities) and dry.
6. Purify the crude product by recrystallization with hot water (or ethanol-water mixture (1:1)).
7. The melting point of pure 5-methyl-2-phenyl-1,2-dihydropyrazol-3-one is 127 °C.

KEY POINTS

- The condensation of β-diketones and hydrazines generates pyrazole derivatives, and the reaction is known as Paal-Knorr Pyrazole synthesis.
- The reaction proceeds through the formation of imine intermediate and dehydrogenation of imine forms pyrazole.
- Antipyrine (anti-inflammatory), propyphenazone (analgesic and antipyretic), metamizol (anti-rheumatic), sulphinpyrazone (uricosuric) and phenylbutazone (anti-inflammatory) synthesis occurs through Paal-Knorr Pyrazole synthesis.

24

Paal-Knorr Pyrrole Synthesis

The cyclization of acetonyl acetone and ammonia/primary amines produces 2,5-dimethylpyrrole. This cyclization reaction is known as Paal-Knorr Pyrrole synthesis. Ammonium carbonate and ammonium acetate can be substituted with ammonia for a nitrogen donor function. Primary amines (aliphatic and aromatic) also can be used in place of ammonia. This cyclization produces N-substituted 2,5-dimethylpyrrole.

$(NH_4)_2CO_3$

1,4-dicarbonyl compound → 2,5-Disubstituted pyrrole

The substituent groups R and R_1 can be symmetric or asymmetric. The use of substituted amines generates N-substituted pyrroles.

Reaction Mechanism

1,4-dicarbonyl compound (*keto* form) ⇌ 1,4-dicarbonyl compound (*enol* form)

$(NH_4)_2CO_3 \longrightarrow NH_3$

1,4-dicarbonyl compound

$-H_2O$

$-H_2O$

2,5-Disubstituted pyrrole

Pharmaceutical Applications

Pyrrole nucleus is present in wide range of natural and synthetic drugs.

1. Synthesis of pyrvinium pamoate (anthelmintic drug).

Acetonyl acetone + Aniline → 2,5-Dimethyl-1-phenyl pyrrole → Pyrvinium pamoate (.1/2 Pamoate)

2. Synthesis of tolmetin (COX-2 inhibitor).

Butanedial + $H_2N—CH_3$ (Methylamine) → 1-Methylpyrrole → Tolmetin

24.1 Preparation of (2,5-Dimethylpyrrole)

Traditional Name:

IUPAC Name: 2,5-Dimethylpyrrole **Mol wt**: 95.14 g/mol

Principle: The condensation of acetonyl acetone and ammonium carbonate generates 2,5-dimethylpyrrole. This reaction is typical example for Paal-Knorr Pyrrole synthesis. The lone pair of electrons present in the nitrogen of ammonia attacks enolic carbon of acetonyl acetone. The intermediate product 5-amino-hexane-2-one, upon further cyclization produces 2,5-dimethylpyrrole.

Acetonyl acetone + $(NH_4)_2CO_3$ → 2,5-Dimethyl pyrrole

Reaction Mechanism

1,4-dicarbonyl compound (*keto* form) ⇌ 1,4-dicarbonyl compound (*enol* form)

$(NH_4)_2CO_3 \longrightarrow NH_3$

1,4-dicarbonyl compound

$-H_2O$

$-H_2O$

2,5-Dimethyl pyrrole

Procedure:

Chemicals Required: Acetonyl acetone, Ammonium carbonate, dichloromethane, sodium sulphate.

1. Place acetonyl acetone (1 mL, 8.5 mmol) and ammonium carbonate (1.9 g, 20 mmol) into the round bottom flask.
2. Attach air condenser and heat the mixture at 100 °C (until effervescence stops, ~60–90 min).
3. Ammonium carbonate sublimes in the condenser, hence it should be pushed back into the flask using glass rod.
4. Replace air condenser with reflux condenser after the effervescence ceases and reflux the mixture for 30 min at 115 °C.
5. Dissolve the solid sublimed on the condenser with hot water (2 mL) and cool the solution.
6. Separate the upper yellow layer and extract the lower layer with dichloromethane (2 mL).
7. Combine the two layers and dry over anhydrous sodium sulphate.
8. Distil the mixture and collect the 2,5-dimethylpyrrole at 78 to 80 °C.

KEY POINTS

- The cyclization of acetonyl acetone and ammonia/primary amines produces 2,5-dimethylpyrrole and the reaction is known as Paal-Knorr Pyrrole synthesis.
- Ammonium carbonate and ammonium acetate can be substituted with ammonia.
- Pyrvinium pamoate (anthelmintic) and tolmetin (COX-2 inhibitor) synthesis occurs through Paal-Knorr Pyrrole synthesis.

25

Paal-Knorr Thiophene Synthesis

Thiophene is an important building block in pharmaceuticals. The 1,4-dicarbonyl compounds cyclize (cyclo-dehydration reaction) with sulphur sources and produces thiophene derivatives through sulphurization. This reaction is known as Paal-Knorr Thiophene synthesis. The most important sulphur source for the sulphurization reactions are phosphorous pentasulphide (P_2S_5) or Lawesson's reagent. Phosphorous pentasulphide and Lawesson's reagent also act as dehydrating agents. The preparation of 2,5-dimethylthiophene from acetonyl acetone is the typical example of Paal-Knorr Thiophene synthesis. The reaction forms furan first and then gets converted into thiophene. Toxic hydrogen sulphide (H_2S) will form as a side product regardless of a sulphur source.

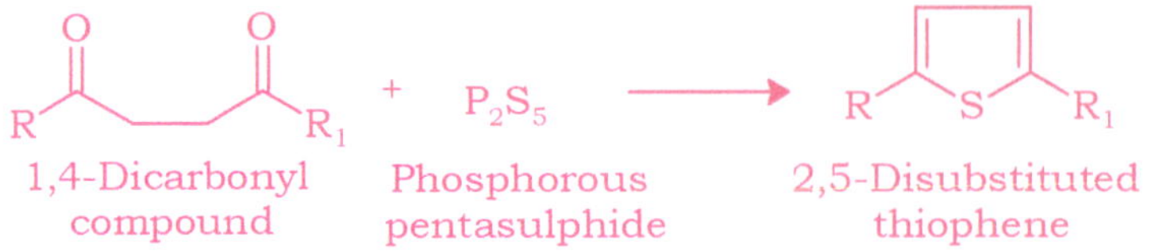

1,4-Dicarbonyl compound + P_2S_5 (Phosphorous pentasulphide) ⟶ 2,5-Disubstituted thiophene

The substituent groups R and R_1 can be symmetric or asymmetric.

Reaction Mechanism

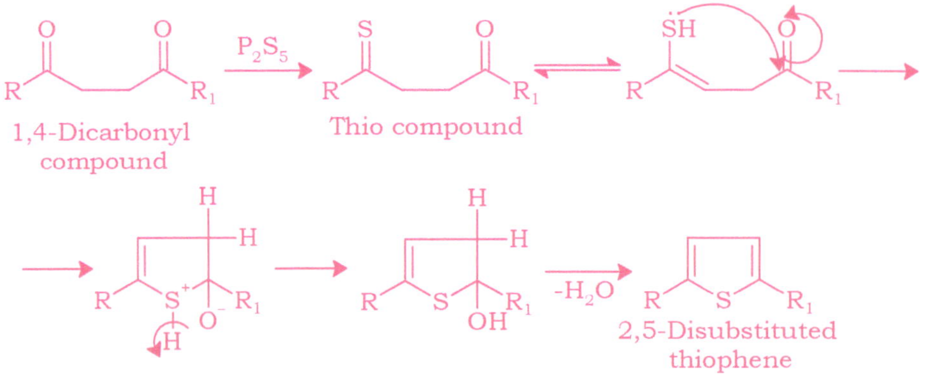

1,4-Dicarbonyl compound $\xrightarrow{P_2S_5}$ Thio compound ⇌ ⟶ ⟶ $\xrightarrow{-H_2O}$ 2,5-Disubstituted thiophene

Thiophene also can be synthesized by Gewald reaction, Volhard-Erdmann cyclization, Victor-Meyor method, Hinsberg synthesis and Fiesselmann thiophene synthesis.

Pharmaceutical Applications

Many thiophene derivatives were identified as chemotherapeutic agents. Thiophene fused heterocyclic systems produces enhanced pharmacological activity. Thienopyrimidines, structural analogues of purines are potential nuleic acid antimetabolites.

25.1 Preparation of 2,5-Dimethylthiophene

Traditional Name:

IUPAC Name: 2,5-Dimethylthiophene **Mol wt**: 112.19 g/mol

Principle: The 2,5-dimethylthiophene can be prepared by cyclizing the sulphurated acetonyl acetone (1,4-dicarbonyl compound). Phosphorous pentasulphide (P_2S_5) is useful in sulphurating acetonyl acetone. It also acts as dehydrating agent. This reaction is typical example for Paal-Knorr Thiophene reaction.

Acetonyl acetone + P_2S_5 (Phosphorous pentasulphide) $\xrightarrow{\Delta}$ 2,5-Dimethyl thiophene

Reaction Mechanism

Acetonyl acetone by the action of phosphorous pentasulphide (sulphurizing agent) forms thioketone. Thioketone form of acetonyl acetone upon cyclization in the presence of phosphorous pentasulphide produces 2,5-dimethylthiophene.

Acetonyl acetone $\xrightarrow{P_2S_5}$ Thio compound ⇌ (enethiol) → (cyclic sulphonium intermediate) → (2-hydroxy-2,5-dimethyl-2,3-dihydrothiophene) $\xrightarrow{-H_2O}$ 2,5-Dimethyl thiophene

Procedure:

Chemicals Required: Acetonyl acetone (hexane-2,5-dione), Phosphorus pentasulphide, Diethyl ether, Sodium carbonate, Magnesium sulphate.

1. Place phosphorous pentasulphide (4.6 g, 21 mmol) into a round bottom flask.

2. Add the first lot of acetonyl acetone (2 mL, 17 mmol) dropwise to the flask.
3. Attach Leibig-type (reflux) condenser to the flask and heat the reaction mixture with small flame until the exothermic reaction commences.
4. Remove the flame and add second lot of acetonyl acetone (7 mL, 60 mmol) dropwise to the flask.
5. Immerse the flask into a cold-water bath, if the exothermic reaction becomes vigorous.
6. After the complete addition, reflux the reaction mixture for 1 h.
7. Cool the reaction mixture into the room temperature and pour into beaker containing ice cold water (20 mL).
8. Extract the aqueous mixture with diethyl ether (5 mL, four times).
9. Combine the ether extracts and wash with anhydrous sodium carbonate solution followed by water.
10. Dry the organic layer by passing through anhydrous magnesium sulphate and distill to isolate 2,5-dimethylthiophene.
11. The boiling range of pure 2,5-dimethylthiophene is 135 to 136 °C.

Precautions:

- Phosphorous pentasulphide (P_2S_5) produces skin and eye irritation.
- Phosphorous pentasulphide (P_2S_5) cause shortness of breath, pulmonary edema, dizziness, headache and seizures.
- It is an explosive chemical, hence should be handled in fume-cupboard.

KEY POINTS

- The cyclization of 1,4-dicarbonyl compounds through sulphurization produces 2,5-disubstitutedthiophene and the reaction is known as Paal-Knorr Thiophene synthesis.
- Phosphorous pentasulphide and Lawesson's reagent are reagents for sulphurization.
- Phosphorous pentasulphide (P_2S_5) produces irritation (skin and eye), shortness of breath and pulmonary edema, hence utmost care should be taken during the reaction (fume cupboard operation is must).

26

Pechmann Reaction

Coumarin is an important synthon in the medicinal chemistry research. The most convenient method of synthesizing coumarin is Pechmann reaction. The condensation of phenol and β-ketoester produces coumarin. This reaction is known as Pechmann reaction. This reaction can be catalyzed by using acid condensing agents. It includes sulphuric acid, phosphorous pentoxide, aluminium chloride, trichloroacetic acid and polyphosphoric acid.

Phenol + β-Ketoester $\xrightarrow[-R^1\text{-}OH]{H^+}$ Coumarin

- Polyhydric phenols, such as resorcinol (containing two hydroxyl groups *meta* to each other) undergoes the condensation with great ease.
- Polyphosphoric acid and trifluoroacetic acid are most effective acid condensing agents and produce higher yields.
- Sulphuric acid is less effective comparatively. It requires careful temperature control.

Reaction Mechanism

The inductive effect caused by two carbonyl oxygens of the β-ketoester weakens the C-H bond and dissociates H-atom to generate a stable anion. The acidity of the >C-H bond produces tautomeric mixture of *keto* and *enol* form.

β-Ketoester (*keto* form) ⇌ β-Ketoester (*enol* form)

Formation of coumarin

The *enol* form of the β-ketoester readily condenses with phenol and renders coumarin.

Phenol β-Ketoester $-H_2O$ $-R^1$-OH Coumarin

Perkin, Knoevenagel, Reformatsky and Wittig reactions, also can synthesize coumarins.

Pharmaceutical Applications

1. Preparation of umbelliferone (antioxidant)

Resorcinol + Formyl acetic acid $\xrightarrow{H_2SO_4}$ Umbelliferone

26.1 Preparation of 7-Hydroxy-4-Methylcoumarin

Traditional Name: Hymecromone, 4-Methyl umbelliferone

IUPAC Name:

Mol wt: 176.17 g/mol

Principle: The condensation of resorcinol and ethyl acetoacetate using acidic condensing agent produces 7-hydroxy-4-methylcoumarin. This reaction is known as Pechmann reaction. Polyphosphoric acid is an effective acid condensing reagent. Sulphuric acid also useful, but less effective and requires tempearature control. Acid condensing agents mediates the *trans*-esterification and *keto-enol* tautomerism (β-ketoester).

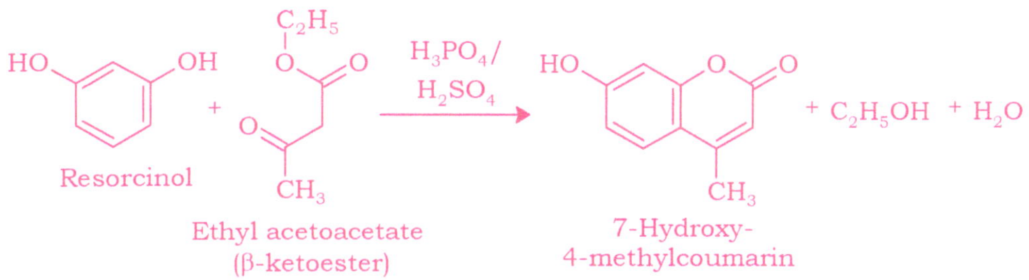

Resorcinol + Ethyl acetoacetate (β-ketoester) $\xrightarrow{H_3PO_4/H_2SO_4}$ 7-Hydroxy-4-methylcoumarin + C_2H_5OH + H_2O

Reaction Mechanism

The inductive effect caused by two carbonyl oxygens of the ethyl acetoacetate (β-ketoester) weakens the C-H bonds and dissociates H-atom to generate a stable anion. The acidity of the >C-H bond produces tautomeric mixture of *keto* and *enol* form.

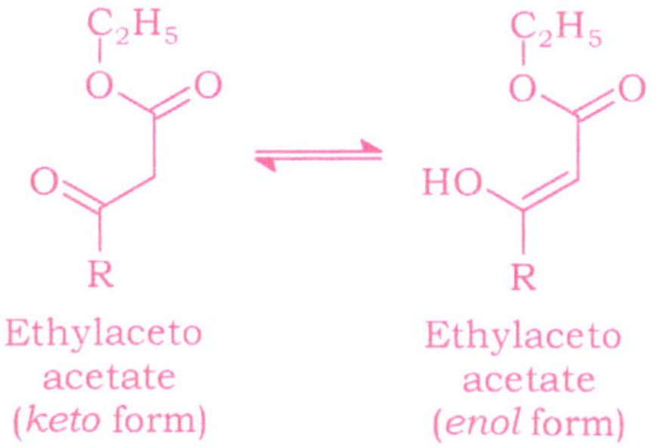

Ethylaceto acetate (*keto* form) ⇌ Ethylaceto acetate (*enol* form)

Formation of coumarin

The *enol* form of the ethyl acetoacetate readily condenses with resorcinol and renders 7-hydroxy-4-methylcoumarin.

Resorcinol + Ethyl acetoacetate (β-ketoester) → $\xrightarrow{-H_2O}$ → $\xrightarrow{-C_2H_5OH}$ 7-Hydroxy-4-methylcoumarin

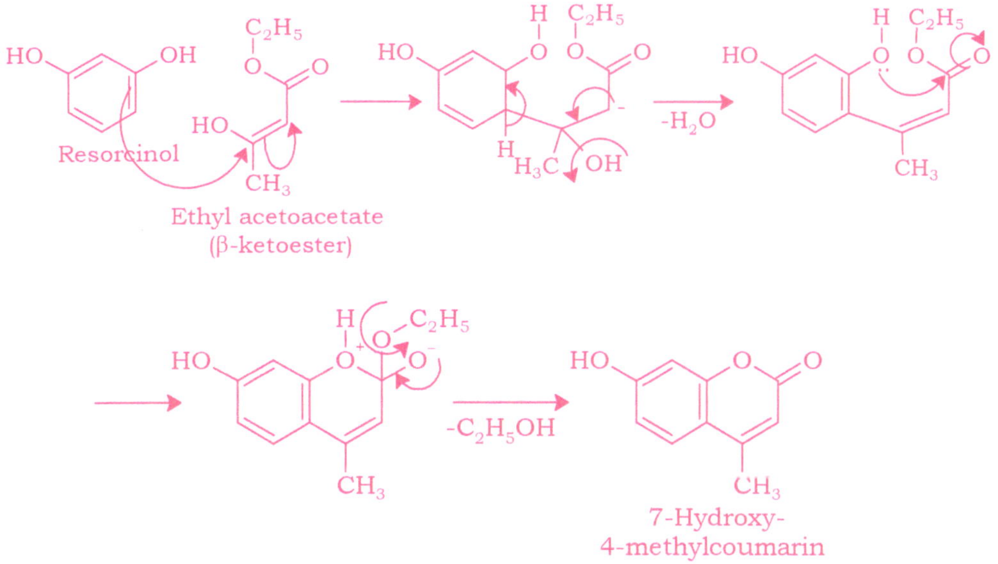

Procedure:

Method 1 (*using sulphuric acid as acid condensing agent*)

Chemicals Required: Resorcinol, Ethyl acetoacetate, Sulphuric acid, Sodium hydroxide (10%), Hydrochloric acid.

1. Place sulphuric acid (10 mL) in a beaker and stir mechanically by placing in an ice-salt bath to reduce the temperature of acid below 10 °C.
2. Mix powdered resorcinol (1 g, 9 mmol) and ethyl acetoacetete (1.3 mL, 10 mmol) by stirring to produce solution.
3. Add the mixture of resorcinol and ethyl acetoacetate, drop-wise with stirring to the beaker containing cold sulphuric acid.

   (*maintain the temperature below 10 °C using ice-salt bath, during the addition*)
4. Stir the acidic mixture for 30 min.
5. Pour the stirred acidic reaction mixture into the beaker containing crushed ice (20 g).
6. Isolate the yellowish solid by vacuum filtration and wash the solid with cold water (3 mL, three times).
7. Dissolve the solid in cold sodium hydroxide (15 mL, 5% w/v)
8. Filter the alkaline solution and neutralize the filtrate with dilute sulphuric acid (alternatively hydrochloric acid) with vigorous stirring.
9. Isolate the crude solid product by filtration and dry.
10. Purify the crude product by recrystallization with ethanol.
11. The melting point of pure 7-hydroxy-4-methylcoumarin is 185 °C.

Method 2 (*using polyphosphoric acid as acid condensing agent*)

Chemicals Required: Resorcinol, Ethyl acetoacetate, Phosphoric acid, Sodium hydroxide (10%), Hydrochloric acid, ethanol.

1. Mix powdered resorcinol (1 g, 9 mmol) and ethyl acetoacetete (1.3 mL, 10 mmol) in a flask by stirring to produce solution.
2. Add polyphosphoric acid (12.3 g, 36.4 mmol) to the flask containing mixture of resorcinol and ethyl acetoacetate in small quantities.
3. Stir the mixture (mechanical) and heat for 20 min, maintaining the temperature in the range of 75 to 80 °C.
4. Pour the reaction mixture into the beaker containing ice-cold water.
5. Isolate the yellowish precipitate through vacuum filtration, wash with cold water and dry.
6. Purify the crude 7-hydroxy-4-methylcoumarin by recrystallization with ethanol.
7. The melting point of pure 7-hydroxy-4-methylcoumarin is 185 °C.

26.2 Preparation of Umbelliferone

Traditional Name: Hydrangine, Skimmetine, β-Umbelliferone

IUPAC Name: 7-Hydroxycoumarin **Mol wt**: 360.31 g/mol

Principle: Umbelliferone is a natural fluorescence indicator dye. It can be prepared by Pechmann reaction. The preparation involves the condensation of malic acid and resorcinol in the presence of sulphuric acid. Sulphuric acid acts as acid condensing agent and dehydrating agent. The malic acid generates formyl acetic acid *in situ*, which condenses with resorcinol to generate umbelliferone.

Resorcinol + Malic acid $\xrightarrow[120\ °C]{H_2SO_4}$ Umbelliferone

Malic acid can be substituted with fumaric acid or maleic acid for the preparation.

Reaction Mechanism

Malic acid $\xrightarrow{H_2SO_4}$ Formyl acetic acid; Resorcinol + Formyl acetic acid → … $\xrightarrow{-H_2O}$ … $\xrightarrow[-H_2O]{H_2SO_4}$ Umbelliferone

Procedure:

Chemical Required: Malic acid, Resorcinol, Concentrated sulphuric acid, Ethanol, Dilute acetic acid.

1) Grind malic acid (27 g, 20 mmol) and resorcinol (22 g, 20 mmol) into fine powder and transfer the powder into the reaction flask.

2) Add concentrated sulphuric acid (6 mL) to the flask.
3) Heat the flask to liquefy the mixture.
   (*the liquid solidifies in a few minutes (light yellow mass) and melt quickly. Stop the heating as soon as liquefaction is complete*).
4) Pour the hot liquid into a beaker containing ice-cold water (25 mL).
5) Allow the aqueous mixture to stand at room temperature.
6) The umbelliferone precipitates in the water.
   (*it may take three days tom complete the precipitation*).
7) Purify the crude product by recrystallization with ethanol.
8) Further recrystallization with with dilute acetic acid is desirable.
9) The melting point of the pure umbelliferone is 225 °C.

KEY POINTS

- The condensation of phenol and β-ketoester produces coumarin, and this reaction is known as Pechmann reaction.
- Coumarins are important synthons in the medicinal chemistry research.
- The antioxidant molecule umbelliferone can be synthesized through Pechmann reaction.

27

Perkin Synthesis

The condensation of aromatic aldehydes with anhydrides of aliphatic acids containing two α-hydrogen atoms produce β-aryl-acrylic acid (α,β-unsaturated acid). This condensation reaction is known as Perkin synthesis. The sodium salt of aliphatic acid, corresponding to the anhydride catalyzes (basic catalyst) the reaction.

$$\underset{\text{Aromatic aldehyde}}{Ar\text{-}CHO} + \underset{\text{Aliphatic anhydride}}{R\text{-}H_2C\text{-}CO\text{-}O\text{-}CO\text{-}CH_2\text{-}R} \xrightarrow[\Delta]{\text{Base catalyst}} \underset{\substack{\beta\text{-aryl-acrylic acid} \\ (\alpha,\beta\text{-unsaturated acid})}}{Ar\text{-}HC{=}C(R)\text{-}COOH}$$

Base catalysts: In case of acetic anhydride (anhydride of acetic acid), sodium acetate acts as a catalyst. Base catalysts include sodium acetate, potassium acetate, salts of carboxylic acid, carbonates of alkali metals and triethyl amines.

The condensation of two carbonyl compounds containing at least one α-hydrogen generates α, β-unsaturated system. This reaction is known as aldol condensation. But the use of anhydride (enoalte form) in the condensation is known as Perkin synthesis.

Reaction Mechanism

Enolate anion of the acetic anhydride attacks aromatic aldehyde and forms C=C bond. The reaction involves intermolecular aldol-type condensation followed by dehydration. Perkin condensation will not take place with aliphatic aldehydes.

Aldol condensation

$$\underset{\text{Aliphatic anhydride}}{R\text{-}HC(H)\text{-}CO\text{-}O\text{-}CO\text{-}CH_2R} + \underset{\text{Base}}{B^-} \xrightarrow{-BH} \underset{\text{Nucleophile}}{R\text{-}HC^-\text{-}CO\text{-}O\text{-}CO\text{-}CH_2R} + \underset{\text{Aromatic aldehyde}}{Ar\text{-}CHO} \longrightarrow R\text{-}C(H)(CH(Ar)O^-)\text{-}CO\text{-}O\text{-}CO\text{-}CH_2R \longrightarrow$$

Perkin synthesis

Enolization

$-R\text{-}CH_2COO^-$

β-aryl-acrylic acid
(α,β-unsaturated acid)

The condensation of acetic anhydride with benzaldehyde in presence of base catalyst produces cinnamic acid (α, β-unsaturated acid). This synthesis is useful in the generation of β-acrylic acids (cinnamic acid and its derivatives). This reaction is typical example for Perkin condensation. The condensation of benzaldehyde with cyclic anhydrides, such as succinic anhydrides gives lactone. This is considered as a special case of Perkin synthesis.

Pharmaceutical Applications

1. Perkin condensation helps in the addition of two carbon atoms to the side chain of an aromatic ring.
2. Used in the preparation of x-ray contrast media - iopanoic acid (iodo aromatics).

3-Nitro benzadehyde + Butanoic anhydride $\xrightarrow[\Delta]{C_3H_7COONa}$ → 1) Ni/H_2 2) ICl → Iopanoic acid

3. Synthesis of sulindac (anti-inflammatory drug).

4-Fluoro benzadehyde + Propanoic anhydride $\xrightarrow[\Delta]{C_2H_5COONa}$ → Sulindac

27.1 Preparation of Cinnamic Acid

Traditional Name: Cinnamylic acid, Phenylacrylic acid.

IUPAC Name: 3-Phenyl-prop-2-enoic-acid **Mol wt**: 164.16 g/mol

Principle: The condensation of acetic anhydride with benzaldehyde generates cinnamic acid (β-aryl-acrylic acid, α,β-unsaturated acid). Potassium acetate (salt of acetic acid) acts as base catalyst for this condensation reaction. This reaction is a typical example for Perkin synthesis.

Benzaldehyde + Acetic anhydride $\xrightarrow[\Delta]{CH_3COOK}$ Cinnamic acid (β-aryl-acrylic acid) + CH_3COOH + H_2O

Reaction Mechanism

The potassium acetate (base) abstracts the proton from methyl group of acetic anhydride to generate nucleophile. The nucleophile attacks positively charged carbon of carbonyl group of benzaldehyde (due to electromeric effect) and forms intermediate. The reaction involves intermolecular aldol-type condensation followed by dehydration. This intermediate on heating eliminates water molecule and on hydrolysis removes acetate to yield cinnamic acid.

Aldol condensation

CH_3COO^- H–H_2C Acetic anhydride CH_3 → $-CH_3COOH$ H_2C^- Nucleophile CH_3 → Benzaldehyde H

Perkin synthesis

CH_3 → CH_3 → CH_3 →

Enolization → CH_3 OH → $-CH_3COO^-$ OH O

Cinnamic acid
(β-aryl-acrylic acid)

Procedure:

Chemicals Required: Benzaldehyde, Acetic anhydride, Potassium acetate, Concentrated hydrochloric acid, Sodium carbonate, Ethanol.

1. Place freshly distilled benzaldehyde (2 mL, 20 mmol), distilled acetic anhydride (2.8 mL, 29 mmol) and finely powdered freshly fused potassium acetate (1.2 g, 12 mmol) into a dry round bottom flask.
2. Mix well the contents and attach air condenser fitted with calcium guard tube (prevents the moisture entrapment) to the flask.
3. Heat the mixture in an oil bath for 1 h, maintaining the temperature at 160 °C (alternatively sand bath can be used).
4. Continue the heating for 3 h by maintaining the temperature in the range of 175 to 180 °C.
5. Pour the hot mixture into a round bottom flask containing water (10 mL).
6. Add saturated sodium carbonate solution with shaking until a drop of withdrawn solution turns red litmus into distinct blue.
7. Distill (steam distillation) the solution to separate the unreacted benzaldehyde (distillate should be clear) and discard the distillate.

8. Cool the residual solution and filter to remove resinous materials.
9. Acidify the filtrate by adding concentrated hydrochloric acid slowly and with vigorous stirring (*until the evolution of carbon dioxide ceases*).
10. Cool the acidified mixture, filter the precipitate, wash with cold water and dry.
11. Purify the crude product by recrystallization with hot water (or aqueous ethanol mixture; 3:1).
12. The melting point of pure cinnamic acid is 133 °C.

***Note*:**

1. *Fused potassium acetate*: Potassium acetate acts as a catalyst. Heat potassium acetate in a porcelain dish to liquify in a small flame and remove the residual water. Powder the solid and store in tightly stoppered bottle.
2. Sodium acetate, potassium carbonate and triethylamine also can be used, in place of potassium acetate. But it requires additional 4 h heating.
3. Sodium hydroxide should not be used in place of sodium carbonate to neutralize as it may generate benzoic acid.

27.2 Preparation of O-Acetoxycinnamic Acid

Traditional Name: β-Arylacrylicacid

IUPAC Name: 3(2'- Acetoxyphenyl)2-propenoic acid **Mol wt**: 222.19 g/mol

Principle: The condensation of acetic anhydride with salicylaldehyde in presence of triethylamine gives *ortho*-acetoxycinnamic acid. Triethylamine acts as a base catalyst and generates a nucleophile.

CHO, OH, Salicylaldehyde + H_3C–CO–O–CO–CH_3 Acetic anhydride $\xrightarrow[\Delta]{\text{Triethyl amine}}$ CH=CH-COOH, O–CO–CH_3 *Ortho*-Acetoxy cinnamic acid (β-Aryl acrylic acid) + CH_3COOH + H_2O

Reaction Mechanism

Aldol condensation

Triethylamine $(H_3C)_3N^-$ H–H_2C–CO–O–CO–CH_3 Acetic anhydride $\rightarrow$ $-(H_3C)_3NH$; H_2C^-–CO–O–CO–CH_3 Nucleophile (attacks CHO of salicylaldehyde, H, OH) $\rightarrow$ O⁻, OH $\rightarrow$

Perkin synthesis

CH_3 OH OH OH

Enolization

ortho-Hydroxy cinnamic acid

$- CH_3COO^-$

H_3C CH_3 Acetic anhydride

ortho-Acetoxycinnamic acid

Procedure

Chemicals Required: Salicylaldehyde, Acetic anhydride, Triethylamine, Sodium bicarbonate, Dilute hydrochloric acid (1:1).

1. Place salicylaldehyde (2.1 g, 7 mmol), anhydrous triethylamine (2 mL, 14.33 mmol) and acetic anhydride (5 mL, 52 mmol) into a round bottom flask.
2. Mix well the contents and attach reflux condenser fitted with calcium guard tube (prevents the moisture entrapment) to the flask.
3. Reflux the mixture gently for 12 h.
4. Cool the contents to room temperature and distill (steam distillation).
5. Discard the distillate (unreacted salicylaldehyde).
6. Add sodium bicarbonate slowly to the flask containing residue (red litmus test).
7. Cool the contents by placing in an ice bath and filter.
8. The crude solid product is coumarin (preserve it separately).
9. Acidify the filtrate with dilute hydrochloric acid (1:1) to precipitate the product (Congo red test).
10. Purify the crude product (*o*-acetoxycinnamic acid) by recrystallization with propanol (70%).
11. The melting range of pure *o*-acetoxycinnamic acid is 153 to 154 °C.

27.3 Preparation of Coumarin

IUPAC Name: 2H-Chrom-2-one, 2H-benzopyran-2-one

Mol wt: 146.15 g/mol

Principle: The spontaneous cyclization of *ortho*-hydroxycinnamic acid (Perkin synthesis product) under triethylamine (base) catalyzed condition generates coumarin.

Salicylaldehyde + $(CH_3CO)_2O$ Acetic anhydride --(Triethyl amine, Δ; $-CH_3COOH$, $-H_2O$)--> *Ortho*-Hydroxy cinnamic acid --($NaHCO_3$)--> Coumarin

Reaction Mechanism

Aldol condensation

Triethylamine $(H_3C)_3N$ + Acetic anhydride → $-(H_3C)_3NH$ → Nucleophile + Salicyladehyde →

Perkin synthesis

→ → → →

Enolization → $-CH_3COO^-$ → *ortho*-Hydroxy cinnamic acid →

Coumarin

Procedure

Chemicals Required: Salicylaldehyde, Anhydrous triethylamine, Acetic anhydride, Calcium oxide, Sodium bicarbonate, Charcoal

Experimental steps

1. Place salicylaldehyde (2.2 g, 7 mmol), anhydrous triethylamine (2 mL, 14.33 mmol) and acetic anhydride (5 mL, 52 mmol) into a round bottom flask.
2. Mix well the contents and attach reflux condenser fitted with calcium guard tube (prevents the moisture entrapment) to the flask.
3. Reflux the mixture gently for 12 h.
4. Cool the contents to room temperature and distill (steam distillation).
5. Discard the distillate (unreacted salicylaldehyde).
6. Add sodium bicarbonate slowly to the flask containing residue (red litmus test).
7. Cool the contents by placing in an ice bath and filter.
8. The crude solid product is coumarin (preserve it separately).
9. Boil the crude coumarin (isolated solid product) with water (200 mL) and charcoal (200 mg).
10. Filter the hot solution and concentrate the filtrate (~80 mL).
11. Cool the concentrate and collect the solid product crystallizing out.
12. Purify the crude coumarin by recrystallization with methanol.
13. The melting range of pure coumarin is 68 to 69 °C.

KEY POINTS

- The condensation of aromatic aldehydes with aliphatic anhydrides produce β-aryl-acrylic acid (α,β-unsaturated acid), this reaction is known as Perkin synthesis.
- The condensation with cyclic anhydrides generates lactone.
- Preparation of iopanoic acid (x-ray contrast media) and sulindac (anti-inflammatory drug) involves Perkin synthesis.

28

Phillips Reaction

Five membered ring containing nitrogen atoms at 1st and 3rd positions is known as imidazole. Naturally occurring imidazoles and synthetic imidazoles have most important therapeutic importance. Benzimidazole, a heterocyclic compound, consists of the fusion of benzene and imidazole rings.

The condensation between formic acid and *ortho*-phenylenediamine using hydrochloric acid as catalyst produces benzimidazole. This reaction is known as Phillips reaction. The acid catalyzed condensation of *o*-phenylenediamines with acids (aliphatic/aromatic) generates 2-subtituted benzimidazoles. Mineral acids, such as hydrochloric acid are useful catalysts.

NH_2 NH_2 + R–C(=O)–OH $\xrightarrow[\Delta]{H^+}$ 2-Substituted benzimidazole (N, NH, R)

ortho-Phenylene diamine   Aliphatic acid   2-Substituted benzimidazole

This method produces good yields with aliphatic acids (acetic acid). Reaction in sealed tube increases the yield for aromatic acids (e.g., benzoic acid).

Reaction Mechanism

One of the amine nitrogen of *ortho*-phenylenediamine undergoes acylation with aliphatic acid in the presence of mineral acid catalyst and produces N-acylated compound. The second amine nitrogen of *ortho*-phenylenediamine acylate with acyl group carbonyl carbon of N-acylated compound. This acylation reaction leads to ring closure and generates benzimidazole.

NH_2 NH_2 + R–C(=O)–OH $\xrightarrow[\Delta]{H^+}$ (NH_2, O^-, N^+, H, H, R, OH) $\xrightarrow{-H_2O}$ (NH_2, O, N, H, R) $\longrightarrow$

ortho-Phenylene diamine   Aliphatic acid

2-Substituted benzimidazole

Pharmaceutical Applications

1. The most prominent benzimidazole compound in nature is N-ribosyl-dimethyl benzimidazole, which serves as an axial ligand for cobalt in vitamin B_{12}.
2. Preparation of thiabendazole (antiparasite).

ortho-Phenylene diamine + Thiazole-4-carboxylic acid $\xrightarrow[\Delta]{H^+}$ Thiabendazole

3. Preparation of clemizole (antihistamine).

ortho-Phenylene diamine + HOOC-CH_2-Cl (Chloroacetic acid) $\xrightarrow[\Delta]{H^+}$ 2-(Chloromethyl)-1*H*-benzimidazole $\rightarrow$ Clemizole

28.1 Preparation of Benzimidazole

Traditional Name: Benzoimidazole, 1,3-Benzodiazole, Azindole, 3-Azaindole

IUPAC Name: 1*H*-Benzimidazole **Mol wt**: 118.14 g/mol

Principle: The condensation of *o*-phenylenediamine with formic acid catalyzed by the hydrochloric acid produces benzimidazole. This reaction is a typical example for Phillips reaction. The amine nitrogens of *ortho*-phenylenediamine undergoes acylation with formic acid in the presence of mineral acid catalyst. The second acylation leads to ring closure and generates benzimidazole with the elimination of water molecules.

ortho-Phenylene diamine + H-COOH Formic acid —HCl, Δ→ Benzimidazole

Reaction Mechanism

ortho-Phenylene diamine + Formic acid —HCl, Δ→ … —$-H_2O$→ … → … → … —H^+, $-H_2O$→ Benzimidazole

Procedure:

Chemicals Required: *ortho*-Phenylenediamine, Formic acid, Hydrochloric acid (4 N), Charcoal, Sodium hydroxide.

1. Transfer *o*-phenylenediamine (1.08 g, 10 mmol) into the round bottom flask.
2. Add formic acid (0.64 mL, 90%) and catalytic amount of hydrochloric acid (2 drops, 4 N) to the flask.
3. Place the flask on a water bath and heat the contents for 2 h, maintaining the temperature at 100 °C.
4. Cool the reaction mixture to room temperature.
5. Neutralize the mixture with sodium hydroxide solution (10% w/v) with constant stirring (litmus paper test).
6. Filter the solid product and wash with ice cold water to remove water soluble salts.
7. Dissolve the product in boiling water (16 mL), add charcoal (400 mg) and heat for 15 min.
8. Filter in hot condition, cool to 10 °C, wash with cold water and dry.
9. Purify the crude benzimidazole by recrystallization with boiling water.
10. The melting range of pure benzimidazole is 171 to 172 °C.

KEY POINTS

- The acid catalysed condensation of formic acid and *ortho*-phenylenediamine produces benzimidazole and the reaction is known as Phillips reaction.
- Mineral acids, such as hydrochloric acid are useful catalysts.
- Thiabendazole (antiparasite) and clemizole (antihistamine) synthesis involves Philips reaction.

29

Quinoxaline Synthesis

Quinoxaline is a ring complex made up of benzene ring and pyrazine ring (also called as benzopyrazine). In general, quinoxaline can be prepared by cyclocondesation reaction of *ortho*-phenylenediamines with 1,2-diketones. Substituted quinoxaline can be prepared by replacing diketones with α-ketonic acids, α-chloroketones, α-aldehyde alcohols and α-ketone alcohols. The condensation reaction between *ortho*-phenylenediamine and benzil in ethanol medium generates 2,3-diphenyl quinoxaline.

ortho-Phenylene diamine + Diketones → 2,3-Disubtituted quinoxalines

Reaction Mechanism

One of the amine nitrogen of *ortho*-phenylenediamine undergoes acylation with 1,2-diketones and produces N-acylated compound. The second amino group acylate with second carbonyl carbon and through ring closure generates quinoxaline.

ortho-Phenylene diamine + Diketones → ... → $\xrightarrow[-\ H_2O]{\Delta}$ 2,3-Disubtituted quinoxaline

Pharmaceutical Applications

Quinoxalines are used as dyes and pharmaceuticals. The antibiotics, such as eolaquindox, cabadox, amiloride, chinomycin, levomycin, actinomysin and actinoleutin contains quinoxaline nucleus.

29.1 Preparation of 2,3-Diphenylquinoxaline

IUPAC Name: 2,3-Diphenylbenzopyrazine **Mol wt**: 282.34 g/mol

Principle: The condensation of *ortho*-phenylenediamine and benzil in the presence of ethanol produces 2,3-diphenylquinoxaline. One of the amine nitrogen of *ortho*-phenylenediamine undergoes acylation with benzil keto group and produces N-acylated compound. The second amino group acylate with second keto carbon and through ring closure generates 2,3-diphenylquinoxaline.

NH_2, NH_2 + O, O —C_2H_5OH→ N, N

ortho-Phenylene diamine Benzil 2,3-Diphenylquinoxaline

Reaction Mechanism

NH_2 O, NH_2 O → H H O^- N^+ O NH_2 → H OH N O NH_2 →

ortho-Phenylene diamine Benzil

→ H N OH, N H OH —Δ, $-H_2O$→ N, N

2,3-Diphenylquinoxaline

Procedure:

Chemicals Required: Benzil, *ortho*-phenylenediamine, Ethanol.

1. Place benzil (1 g, 5 mmol) into a round bottom flask and dissolve with ethanol (4 mL).
2. Prepare the solution of *ortho*-phenylenediamine (0.55 g, 5 mmol) in ethanol (4 mL).
3. Warm both the solutions and add the warm ethanolic solution of *ortho*-phenylenediamine into the flask containing warm solution of ethanolic benzil.
4. Warm the mixture by placing in water bath for 30 min.
5. To the warm mixture add water until a slight cloudiness persists and allow it to cool.
6. Filter the resulting mixture and dry.
7. Purify the crude product by recrystallization with aqueous ethanol.
8. The melting range of pure 2,3-diphenylquinoxaline is 125 to 126 °C.

KEY POINTS

- The cyclocondesation reaction of *ortho*-phenylenediamines with 1,2-diketones generates quinoxalines.
- 1,2-Diketones can be replaced with α-ketonic acids, α-chloroketones, α-aldehyde alcohols and α-ketone alcohols to generate structurally different quinoxalines.
- The antibiotics, such as eolaquindox, cabadox, amiloride, chinomycin, levomycin, actinomysin and actinoleutin contain quinoxaline nucleus.

30

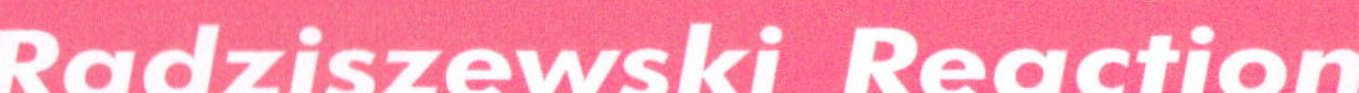

Radziszewski Reaction

Five membered ring containing nitrogen atoms at 1st and 3rd positions is known as imidazole. Naturally occurring imidazoles and synthetic imidazoles have most important therapeutic importance.

The condensation of α-dicarbonyl compounds, aldehydes (aliphatic and aromatic) and two equivalent of ammonium acetate (or amines) in alcohol produce 2,4,5-tri-subtitued/1,2,4,5-tetra-substituted imidazoles. This reaction is known as Radziszewski reaction. Glyoxal condenses with formaldehyde and ammonia to generate imidazole. The use of acetaldehyde in place of formaldehyde produces a 2-methylimidazole.

α–Diketone + Ar—CHO (Aryl/heteroaryl aldehyde) + CH_3COONH_4 (Ammonium acetate) ⟶ 2,4,5-Trisubstituted imidazole

The conventional synthesis offers very lower yields and requires longer reaction path. Modified protocols utilizing catalysts, such as ionic liquids, organic acids, mineral acids, inorganic salts, etc., provide improved yields. Polyethylene glycol-400 (PEG400) is a notable catalyst.

Reaction Mechanism

CH_3COONH_4 → NH_3; α-Diketone $\xrightarrow{-H_2O}$ Schiff base of α-diketone

Arylaldehyde + NH_3 $\xrightarrow{-H_2O}$ Schiff base of arylaldehyde

Schiff base of α-diketone + Schiff base of arylaldehyde ⟶ ⟶ $\xrightarrow{-H_2O}$ 2,4,5-Trisubstituted imidazole

Pharmaceutical Applications

Molecule name and Structure	Uses
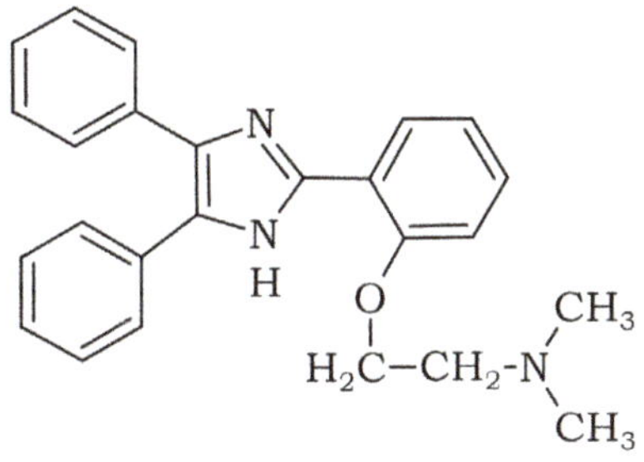 Trifenagrel	Platelet aggregation inhibitor
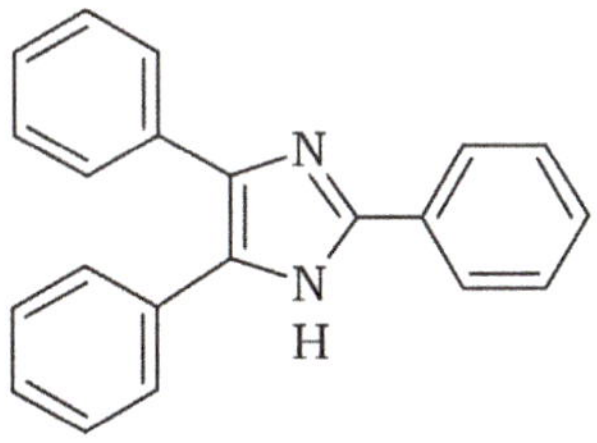 Lophine	Chemiluminescent (analytical reagent for metal detection)

30.1 Preparation of 4,5-Diphenylimidazole

Traditional Name: 4,5-Diphenylglyoxaline

IUPAC Name: 4,5-Diphenyl-1*H*-imidazole **Mol wt**: 220.28 g/mol

Principle: The condensation of benzil, hexamine and ammonium acetate in glacial acetic acid produces 4,5-diphenylimidazole. This condensation reaction is an example of Radziszewski reaction. Hexamine is a precursor for formaldehyde (special form of ammonia). Hexamine hydrolyses to formaldehyde and ammonia by thermal effect *in situ*. This slows down reaction compared with reaction using formaldehyde. The formaldehyde reacts with ammonium acetate and forms formamide (methanimine), which offer carbon and nitrogen atoms for the ring formation.

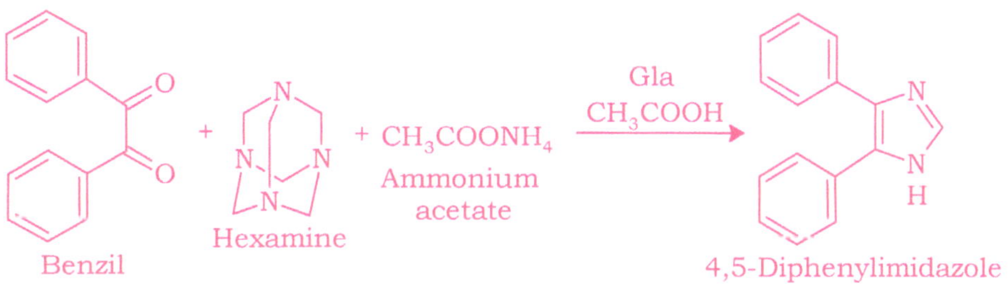

Benzil + Hexamine + CH_3COONH_4 Ammonium acetate $\xrightarrow[CH_3COOH]{Gla}$ 4,5-Diphenylimidazole

Reaction Mechanism

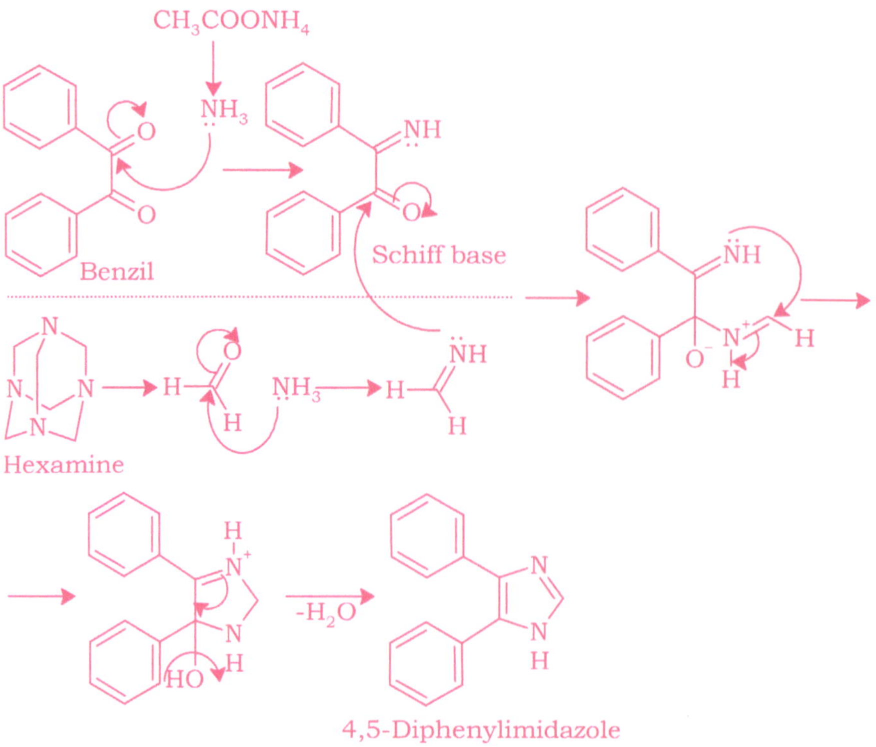

CH_3COONH_4

Benzil

Schiff base

Hexamine

$-H_2O$

4,5-Diphenylimidazole

Procedure:

Chemicals Required: Benzil, Hexamine, Ammonium acetate, Glacial acetic acid, Ammonium hydroxide, Charcoal, Ethanol.

1. Place benzil (1.1 g, 5 mmol), hexamine (13 g, 93 mmol), ammonium acetate (3 g, 39 mmol) and glacial acetic acid (25 mL) in a round bottom flask.
2. Attach reflux condenser to the flask and heat the contents for 1 h maintaining the temperature 118 °C.
3. Pour the hot reaction mixture into beaker containing water (20 mL).
4. Add charcoal to the mixture and boil to remove the turbidity (*if any formed*).
5. Cool the reaction mixture to room temperature.
6. Filter the mixture and make the filtrate alkaline with ammonium hydroxide (neutralizes unreacted acetic acid and ammonium acetate).
7. Filter the solid product, wash with water (several times), and dry.
8. Purify the crude product by recrystallization with ethanol.
9. The melting range of 4,5-diphenylimidazole is 228 to 230 °C.

Precautions:

- Hexamine is sensitive to skin and causes allergic reactions (irritation, reddening and blistering).
- Use protective gloves and dust masks to protect against the allergic effects.

30.2 Preparation of 2, 4, 5-Triphenylimidazole

Traditional Name: Lophine

IUPAC Name: 2,4,5-Triphenyl-1*H*-imidazole **Mol wt**: 296.37 g/mol

Principle: The condensation of benzil, benzaldehyde and ammonium acetate produces 2,4,5-triphenylimidazole. This reaction is a typical example of Radziszewski reaction. Glacial acetic acid and Polyethylene glycol-400 (PEG400) mixture acts as catalyst for this reaction and enhance the product yield.

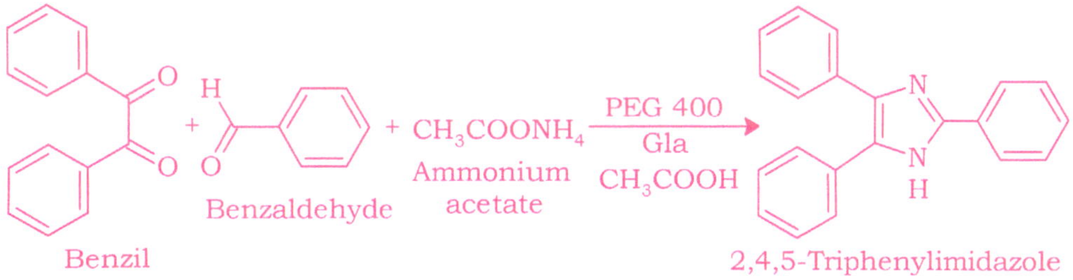

Reaction Mechanism

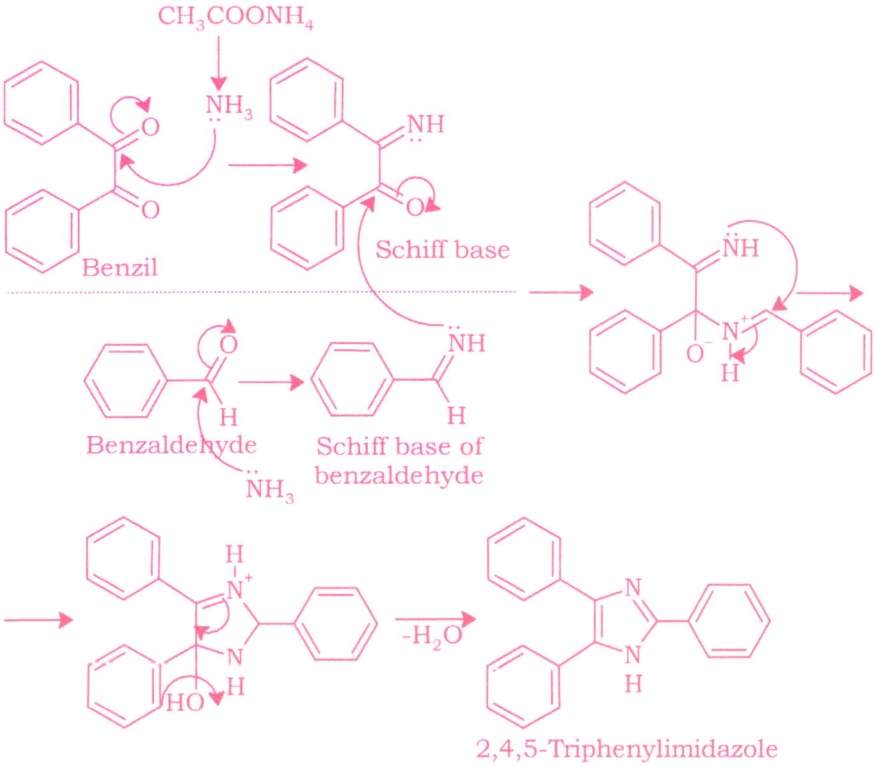

Procedure:

Chemicals Required: Benzil, Benzaldehyde, Ammonium acetate, Glacial acetic acid, Polyethylene glycol 400 (PEG 400) and Ethanol.

1. Place benzil (2.1 g, 10 mmol), benzaldehyde (1.1 mL, 10 mmol) and ammonium acetate (2 g, 25 mmol) into a round bottom flask.
2. Add glacial acetic acid (10 mL) and PEG 400 (5 g) to the flask.
3. Attach condenser and heat the mixture with stirring for 5 h maintaining the temperature at 118 °C.
4. Pour the reaction mixture into the beaker containing cold water (500 mL).
5. Isolate the precipitate formed through vacuum filtration, wash with cold water and dry the crude product.
6. Purify the crude product by recrystallization with ethanol.
7. The melting range of pure 2,4,5-triphenylimidazole is 267 to 269 °C.

Note: The reaction is applicable for any other aryl/heteroaryl aldehydes.

KEY POINTS

- The condensation of α-dicarbonyl compounds, aldehydes and ammonia to produce 2,4,5-tri-subtitued/1,2,4,5-tetra-substituted imidazoles is known as Radziszewski reaction.
- Ammonia can be substituted with ammonium salts or amines and hexamine.
- Hexamine causes irritation, reddening and blistering, hence use of protective mechanism is very much essential.

31

Reduction

Reduction is a chemical transformation in which a chemical system gains electrons. In reduction, addition of hydrogen to a compound or subtraction of oxygen from a compound results (opposite to oxidation).

Reduction with subtraction of oxygen

$$\underset{\text{Ketone}}{R-\overset{\overset{\large O}{||}}{C}-R} \longrightarrow \underset{\text{Alkane}}{R-CH_2-R}$$

Reduction with addition of hydrogen

$$\underset{\text{Ketone}}{R-\overset{\overset{\large O}{||}}{C}-R} \longrightarrow \underset{\text{Alcohol}}{R-\overset{\overset{\large OH}{|}}{C}H-R}$$

The chemical reagent useful in the reduction process is known as reducing agent. Hydrogen gas, hydrazine, dihydronaphthalene, dihydroanthracene, isopropanol and formic acid are some of the useful hydrogen sources.

Reduction (hydrogenation) differs from protonation or hydride addition. In reduction, products are uncharged (neutral). But on protonation, products receive charge.

Types of reductions

1. Catalytic reduction.
2. Metal hydride reduction.
3. Dissolving metal reduction.

31.A Catalytic Reduction

Reduction is a chemical reaction between molecular hydrogen and olefinic compounds usually in presence of a catalyst. Reduction (hydrogenation) has three components, the unsaturated substrate, the molecular hydrogen and catalyst. It reduces or saturates olefinic compounds. An addition of molecular hydrogen to the olefinic bond in the presence of a catalyst is known as catalytic reduction (hydrogenation). Non-catalytic reduction reaction requires very higher temperature.

$$\underset{\text{Alkene}}{R{-}CH{=}CH_2} + H_2 \xrightarrow{\text{Catalyst}} \underset{\text{Alkane}}{R{-}CH_2{-}CH_3}$$

The chemical conversion of styrene into ethylbenzene using platinum supported on carbon is a typical example.

$$\underset{\text{Styrene}}{C_6H_5{-}CH{=}CH_2} + H_2 \xrightarrow{\text{Pt/C}} \underset{\text{Ethylbenzene}}{C_6H_5{-}CH_2{-}CH_3}$$

The catalytic reduction conditions cannot reduce the aromatic ring system (hydrogenation). It requires special conditions (dissolving metal reduction).

Mechanism

The hydrogen and the organic compound addition onto the surface of the catalyst, at first stage. It establishes, metal catalyst-carbon (organic compound) and metal-hydrogen bond in the next step. The transfer of hydrogen from the metal-hydrogen associate to the organic compound. This facilitates the release of organic compound from the catalyst surface and catalyst regeneration.

Catalysts

- ***Lindlar's catalyst:*** Mixture of Palladium-Barium sulphate (Pd-$BaSO_4$) partially poisoned with quinoline is known as Lindlar's catalyst. Mixture of Palladium-Calcium carbonate (Pd-$CaCO_3$) partially poisoned with lead acetate is also known and Lindlar's catalyst.
- ***Wilkinson's catalyst:*** Chlorotris (triphenylphosphine)rhodium ($RhCl(PPh_3)_3$; coordination compound) is known as Wilkinson's catalyst. It catalyzes the hydrogenation of alkenes in homogenous solution.
- ***Adam catalyst:*** Platinum-platinum oxide ($PtO_2.H_2O$; Platinum (IV) oxide hydrate) is known as Adam's catalyst.
- ***Nickel:*** A finely divided nickel is a powerful catalyst for the reduction of multiple bonds present in aliphatic, alicyclic and aromatic compounds.
- ***Zinc***: Zinc is an important metal catalyst for the reduction of organic molecules. The following combinations are useful.
  - o Zinc and hydrochloric acid (Zn-HCl).
  - o Zinc and acetic acid (Zn-CH_3COOH).
  - o Zinc and sodium hydroxide (Zn-NaOH).
  - o Zinc-copper couple and ethanol (Zn-Cu/C_2H_5OH)

Platinum, palladium, rhodium and ruthenium are highly active metal catalysts. Tin also acts as a reducing agent (mild).

Important Reactions

Rosenmund reduction: The reduction of acid chlorides into aldehydes by the use of Lindlar's catalyst (Pd/C) in boiling xylene condition is known as Rosenmund reduction. It is useful in the reduction of triple bonds into double bonds (half saturation) and prevents further reduction (full saturation).

$$\underset{\text{Acid chloride}}{R-\overset{O}{\overset{\|}{C}}-Cl} + H_2 \xrightarrow{Pd\text{-}BaSO_4/C} \underset{\text{Aldehyde}}{R-\overset{O}{\overset{\|}{C}}-H} + HCl$$

Clemmensen reduction: It involves deoxygenation of aldehydes and ketones into alkanes by amalgamated zinc in presence of hydrochloric acid.

$$\underset{\text{Carbonyl compound}}{R-\overset{O}{\overset{\|}{C}}-R^1} + H_2 \xrightarrow{Zn\text{-}Hg,\ HCl} \underset{\text{Alkane}}{R-CH_2-R^1}$$

Sabatier-Senderens reduction: Catalytic reduction of organic compounds in their vapour phase mixed with hydrogen by passing over finely divided nickel at 200 to 300 °C is known as Sabatier-Senderens reduction.

$$\underset{\text{Alkene}}{>C=C<} + H_2 \xrightarrow[200\text{-}300\ °C]{Ni} \underset{\text{Alkane}}{H-\overset{|}{\underset{|}{C}}-\overset{|}{\underset{|}{C}}-H}$$

Staudinger reduction: Conversion of azides into amines by hydrogenation (mild reduction), using triphenyl phosphine (PPh_3) is called as Staudinger reduction.

$$\underset{\text{Azide}}{R-N_3} + H_2 \xrightarrow{PPh_3} \underset{\text{Amine}}{R-NH_2}$$

Corey-Bakshi-Shibata reduction: It involves enantioselective reduction of ketones into alcohols by borane and chiral oxazaborolidine catalyst.

$$\underset{\text{Ketone}}{R-\overset{O}{\overset{\|}{C}}-R} \xrightarrow{\text{Catalyst}} \underset{\text{Alcohol}}{R-\overset{OH}{\overset{|}{C}H}-R}$$

Pharmaceutical Applications

1. Synthesis of phenylbutazone (non-steroidal anti-inflammatory drug).

Nitrobenzene —Pd/C [H]→ 1,2-Diphenylhydrazine —Diethyl-*n*-butyl melonate→ Phenylbutazone

2. Synthesis of ibuprofen (non-steroidal anti-inflammatory drug).

Isobutyl acetophenone —Pd/C [H]→ Isobutyl phenylethanol ⇉ Ibuprofen

3. Synthesis of salbutamol (anti-asthmatic drug).

Intermediate (penultimate) —Pd/C [H]→ Salbutamol

31.1 Preparation of Benzhydrol

Traditional Name: Hydroxydiphenyl methane, Diphenylcarbinol
IUPAC Name: Diphenylmethanol **Mol wt**: 184.23 g/mol

Principle: Benzophenone upon reduction by zinc dust and alcoholic sodium hydroxide forms benzhydrol (secondary alcohol). Metallic zinc serves as a source of electrons (electron donor). Alcoholic sodium hydroxide (reducing agent) liberates nascent hydrogen, thus acts as source of hydrogen. Both benzophenone and nascent hydrogen adsorbs on the surface of the zinc. The high reactive nascent hydrogen reduces benzophenone into benzhydrol (diphenylmethanol).

O
Zn dust
C_2H_5OH
OH
Benzophenone
Benzhydrol

Reaction Mechanism

H^+
O
O^-
OH
OH
Benzophenone
Zn
($2e^-$)
H^+
Benzhydrol

Procedure:

Chemicals Required: Benzophenone, Zinc powder, Sodium hydroxide, Ethanol.

1. Place benzophenone (1 g, 5.5 mmol), sodium hydroxide (1 g, 25 mmol) in ethanol (10 mL) and zinc powder (1.5 g) into a round bottom flask.
2. Mix the reactants well, attach a reflux condenser to the flask and stir the reaction mixture. This elevates the temperature slowly to 70 °C.
3. Warm the reaction mixture on a water bath for ~ 90 min (if requires).
4. Cool the flask to 60 °C (~ 3 h) and filter the reaction mixture under vacuum.
5. Wash the residue with hot ethanol (2 mL, two times).
6. Pour the filtrate into a beaker containing ice-cold water (50 mL).
7. Acidify with concentrated hydrochloric acid (2.5 mL).
8. Viscous oil separates out and solidifies a white crystalline mass on cooling (after standing overnight).
9. Isolate the solid through vacuum filtration and dry.
10. Purify the crude benzhydrol by recrystallization with hot ethanol.
11. The melting point of the pure benzhydrol is 65 °C.

Note: The dry zinc dust is inflammable. Hence, do not allow the filtered zinc mass to dry. Prevent the contact with combustible material and destroy it by treating with mineral acid.

31.2 Preparation of Vanillyl Alcohol

IUPAC Name: 4-(Hydroxymethyl)-2-methoxyphenol

Mol wt: 154.16 g/mol

Principle: Vanillyl alcohol can be prepared by reducing the vanillin. The sodium borohydride (reducing agent) reduces the aldehyde group of the vanillin and generates vanillyl alcohol.

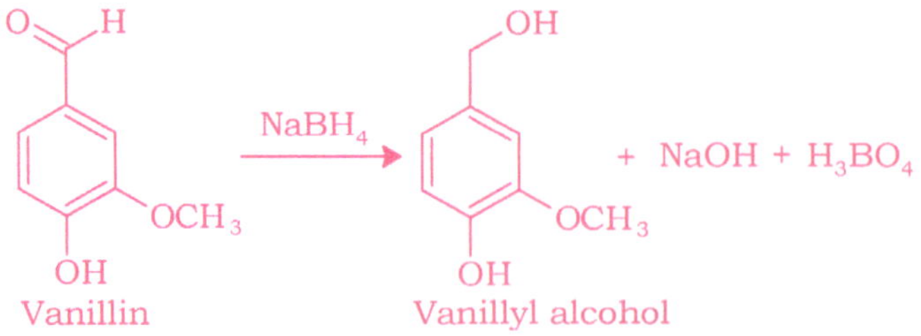

Vanillin $\xrightarrow{NaBH_4}$ Vanillyl alcohol + NaOH + H_3BO_4

Reaction Mechanism

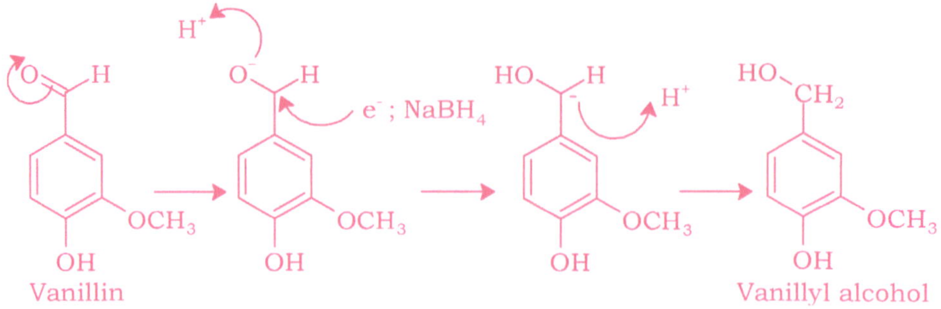

Vanillin → (e⁻; $NaBH_4$) → (H^+) → Vanillyl alcohol

Procedure

Chemical Required: Vanillin, Ethanol, Sodium borohydride, Sodium hydroxide (1 M), Hydrochloric acid (6 M).

Experimental steps:

1. Place vanillin (2 g, 13.2 mmol) and ethanol (22 g) into a flat bottom flask loaded with magnetic bead (stir bar).
2. Stir the solution to effect the solution.
3. Place the flask on ice-bath (reaction is exothermic) and add the solution of sodium borohydride dropwise to the flask (~10 min).

   Sodium borohydride solution can be prepared by dissolving the sodium borohydride (0.5 g) in sodium hydroxide (3.8 mL, 1 M)
4. Remove the ice-bath and continue the stirring for 10 min.
5. Cool the mixture by placing in an ice-bath, and add hydrochloric acid (6 M) drop-wise (till the evolution of hydrogen gas ceases) with stirring. Hydrogen gas evolution can be checked by using pH paper.
6. Stir the reaction mixture for further 10 minutes to precipitate vanillyl alcohol.
7. Wash the product with ice-cold water and dry.
8. Purify the product by recrystallization with ethanol.
9. The melting point of the pure vanillyl alcohol is 225 °C.

31.B Metal Hydride Reduction

The reduction reactions mediated by the hydride donors are known as hydride reductions. The hydride donors are metal hydrides, such as lithium aluminum hydride and sodium borohydride. Hence, this reaction is known as metal hydride reduction.

- ***Lithium aluminum hydride ($LiAlH_4$):*** It is the most versatile reducing agent used in fine chemical industries for the reduction of carbonyl compounds (esters, carboxylic acids and amides). Reduction with lithium aluminum hydride (LAH) is usually carried out in etheral solutions. LAH violently react with water and atmospheric moisture and releases inflammable gaseous hydrogen (frothing of hydrogen). This reaction is exothermic, hydrogen can ignite spontaneously and form explosive mixture with air. Destroy the unreacted and excess of LAH by slow careful addition of ethyl acetate (diluted with dry THF) after reaction under nitrogen. LAH on reaction with water releases lithium hydroxide, which is corrosive to skin and eye.

  LAH is most powerful than sodium borohydride. Al-H bond of LAH is weaker than the B-H bond of sodium borohydride. In lithium aluminium hydride, hydrogens bear electron pair and a negative charge. In case of sodium borohydride, a bare proton with no surrounding electrons and positive charge is possible.

- ***Sodium borohydride ($NaBH_4$):*** It is an important and safe hydride used in the separation of uranium salts. It is useful in reducing carbonyl groups (ketones and aldehydes). Sodium borohydride is not effective in reducing carboxylic acids, esters, amides and nitro group.

H_3CO–$C_6H_3(O_2N)$–CHO $\xrightarrow[CH_3OH]{NaBH_4}$ H_3CO–$C_6H_3(O_2N)$–CH_2OH

3-Nitro,4-methoxy benzaldehyde → 3-Nitro,4-methoxy benzylalcohol

The most important other hydrides are listed in the table.

Hydride name	Function
Lithium borohydride ($LiBH_4$)	It reduces lactones into diols. It also reduces aldehydes, ketones, acid chlorides, epoxides and esters.
Magnesium borohydride ($MgBH_4)_2$	It readily reduces esters.
Aluminium borohydride ($Al(BH_4)_3$)	It is a very powerful reagent for the reduction of the lactones, epoxides, carboxylic acids, tertiary amides, nitriles, ketones, aldehydes and esters.
Zinc borohydride ($Zn(BH_4)_2$)	It is a most useful reagent for the reduction of α,β-unsaturated aldehydes and ketones.
Cerium borohydride ($Ce(BH_4)_2$)	It is known as Luche reagent. It is very selective reagent for the reduction of conjucated aldehydes and ketones.
Sodium cyanoborohydride ($NaBH_3CN$)	It readily reduces iodides, bromides and tosylates to hydrocarbons.

Table ***Contd...***

Hydride name	Function
Aluminium hydride (AlH_3)	It readily reduces aldehydes, ketones, carboxylic acid, acid chloride, anhydrides, esters and lactones.
Diisobutylaluminium hydride	This is also known as Dibal/Dibal-H ($([(CH_3)_2CHCH_2]_2\text{-}AlH)_2$. Most widely useful in reducing esters, lactones and nitriles.
Alkoxy and alkyl borohydride	Acyloxy borohydrides [$NaBH_{4\text{-}n}\text{-}(O_2CR)n$] selectively reduces aldehydes and ketones.
Super-hydrid-Lithium triethyborohydride ($LiBH(C_2H_5)_3$)	Lithium hydride reacts with triethylborane and generates super-hydride. Most useful in the reductive dehalogenation of alkyl halides.
Selectrides	Potassium tri-*sec*-butyl borohydride is known as *K*-Selectride and lithium tri-*sec*-butyl borohydride is known as *L*-Selectride. Selectrides reduces aldehydes and ketones into corresponding alcohols.
Diborane (B_2H_6)	The stable dimer of borane is a potent reducing agent for aldhydes, ketones, lactones, epoxides, acids, tertiary amides and nitriles.

Pharmaceutical Applications

Lithium aluminum hydride

1. Lithium aluminum hydride is useful in the chemical conversion of Vitamin A1 into Vitamin A2.

$LiAlH_4$

Vitamin A1 → Vitamin A2

2. Thiamphenicol (antibacterial drug) preparation utilizes lithium aluminum hydride.

$LiAlH_4$

Precursor for thiamphenicol → Thiamphenicol

3. Cyclic amines can be prepared by reducing the lactam ring using lithium aluminum hydride.

$LiAlH_4$ Ether

Lactum → 2,2-Dimethyl pyrollidine

Sodium borohydride

4. D-Sorbitol (alditol) an artificial sweetener for foods can be prepared by reducing D-glucose using sodium borohydride.

CHO / H—OH / HO—H / HO—OH / H—OH / H_2C—OH
D-Glucose

$\xrightarrow{NaBH_4}$

H_2C—OH / H—OH / H—OH / H—OH / H—OH / H_2C—OH
Sorbitol

5. Sodium borohydride is useful in the preparation of intermediate for the ibuprofen (anti-inflammatory drug).

Isobutyl acetophenone $\xrightarrow{NaBH_4}$ Isobutyl phenylethanol $\longrightarrow\longrightarrow$ Ibuprofen

6. Roxaltidine (H_2 blocker, antiulcer drug) preparation requires the intermediate piperdine methylphenol. This intermediate can be prepared by the condensation of piperidine and 3-hydroxybenzaldehyde using sodium borohydride.

Piperidine + Phenol $\xrightarrow{NaBH_4}$ Piperidine methylphenol $\longrightarrow\longrightarrow$ Roxaltidine

31.3 Preparation of 3-Nitrobenzyl Alcohol (*meta*-Nitrobenzyl Alcohol)

IUPAC Name: (3-Nitrophenylmethanol) **Mol wt**: 168.12 g/mol

Principle: Sodium borohydride reduces 3-nitrobenzaldehyde into 3-nitrobenzyl alcohol. Sodium borohydride is chemoselective for the carbonyl groups and do not react with other reducible functional groups. Hence, nitro group present in 3-nitrobenzaldehyde (*m*-nitrobenzaldehyde) remains intact after the reduction with sodium borohydride. Sodium borohydride acts as donar of hydride ion and attacks carbonyl carbon and forms tetrahedral intermediate. The alkoxide upon protonation affords 3-nitrobenzyl alcohol.

O_2N–C₆H₄–CHO $\xrightarrow[CH_3OH]{NaBH_4}$ O_2N–C₆H₄–CH_2OH

3-Nitrobenzaldehyde → 3-Nitrobenzyl alcohol

Reaction Mechanism

3-Nitrobenzaldehyde → (e⁻; $NaBH_4$; H^+) → [H] → 3-Nitrobenzyl alcohol

Procedure:

Chemicals Required: 3-Nitrobenzaldehyde, Sodium Borohydride, Methanol, Sodium hydroxide.

1. Place 3-nitrobenzaldehyde (1.5 g, 10 mmol) into a flask and dissolve with methanol (10 mL).
2. Add the dilute sodium borohydride solution dropwise to the flat bottomed flask maintaining the temperature in between 18 to 25 °C.

   Dissolve sodium borohydride (0.14 g, 3.7 mmol) in sodium hydroxide (2 mL, 2 M).

   Add water (2 mL) to the 0.2 mL solution of sodium borohydride and add sodium hydroxide (2 mL of 2 M). Dilute the solution with water (18 mL).
3. Completion of the reaction can be identified by the treatment of a small portion of reaction mixture with dilute sulphuric acid after the addition of 3/4th of the dilute sodium borohydride solution.
4. Evolution of hydrogen indicates the completion of reduction. If no evolution of hydrogen, continue the addition of sodium borohydride solution.
5. Dilute the reaction mixture with ice-cold water (10 mL).
6. Extract the aqueous mixture with ether (10 mL) and wash the ether layer with water.
7. Dry the organic layer by passing through anhydrous magnesium sulphate.
8. Evaporate the organic layer to collect yellowish oil and cool the oil by placing in an ice-bath to solidify the oil.
9. Isolate the pale yellow solid of 3-nitrobenzyl alcohol.
10. The melting point of pure 3-nitrobenzyl alcohol is 30 °C.

31.4 Preparation of N-(*m*-Nitrobenzyl) Aniline

IUPAC Name: *N*-[(2-Nitrophenyl)methyl]aniline **Mol wt**: 243.23 g/mol

Principle: The reduction of N-(*m*-nitrobenzylidene) aniline (schiff base) with sodium borohydride generates N-(*m*-nitrobenzyl) aniline. Sodium borohydride is chemoselective for carbonyl and olefin groups. Hence, do not reduce the nitro group. Sodium borohydride is stable and safer than lithium aluminium hydride. N-(*m*-Nitrobenzylidene) aniline can be prepared by the reaction between aniline and 3-nitrobenzaldehyde.

$NaBH_4$ / CH_3OH; $N{=}CH$; NO_2; $NHCH_2$; NO_2

N(3-Nitrobenzylidene) aniline N(3-Nitrobenzyl) aniline

Reaction Mechanism

N(3-Nitrobenzylidene) aniline

H^+; $N{=}CH$; NO_2; $N^-{-}C$ H_2; NO_2; H N—C H_2; NO_2

$NaBH_4$; e^- N(3-Nitrobenzyl) aniline

Procedure:

Chemicals Required: N-(3-Nitrobenzylidene) aniline, Methanol, Sodium borohydride.

1. Place N-(3-nitrobenzylidene) aniline (1 g, 4.4 mmol) and methanol (10 mL) into a two necked round bottom flask.

   Note: Refer chapter 33 page no. 241 for the preparation of Schiff base.
2. Attach reflux condenser to the flask loaded with magnetic bead.
3. Warm the solution to about 40 °C on a magnetic stirrer unit and add sodium borohydride (0.17 g, 4.4 mmol) with stirring over a period of 30 min.
4. Reflux the mixture for 15 min, add water (10 mL) and cool.
5. Isolate the solid product separated by filtration and dry.
6. Purify the product by recrystallization with mixture of methanol and water.
7. The melting range of pure N-(3-nitrobenzyl) aniline is 84 to 85 °C.

31.C Dissolving Metal Reduction

The reduction of aromatic compounds with alkali metal in suitable acidic solvent is known as dissolving metal reduction. Alkali metal transfers electron to the organic molecule and acidic solvent supplies protons to the reactive intermediates. Reduction using alkali metals as the electron source are the most important synthetic transformations in organic chemistry.

Water, alcohol and ammonia (also primary and secondary amines) act as acidic solvent and quenches the radical anion. This type of reduction is applicable for the reduction of molecules with polarised groups, such as >C=O, and – CN.

Important Reactions

Bouveault-Blanc reduction: It is the reduction of esters into primary alcohols using absolute ethanol and sodium metal.

$$\underset{\text{Ester}}{R{-}\overset{O}{\overset{\|}{C}}{-}OR^1} \xrightarrow{Na\text{-}C_2H_5OH} \underset{\text{Carboxylic acid}}{R{-}\overset{O}{\overset{\|}{C}}{-}OH} + \underset{\text{Alcohol}}{R^1{-}OH}$$

Meerwein-Ponndorf-Verley (MPV) reduction: Reduction of ketones into corresponding alcohols by aluminium isopropoxide (AIP) in isopropanol is known as Meerwein-Ponndorf Verley (MPV) reduction.

$$\underset{\text{Ketone}}{R{-}\overset{O}{\overset{\|}{C}}{-}R^1} + \underset{\text{Alcohol}}{R^2{-}\overset{OH}{\overset{|}{C}H}{-}R^3} \xrightarrow{\text{Aluminium isopropoxide}} \underset{\text{Alcohol}}{R{-}\overset{OH}{\overset{|}{C}H}{-}R^1} + \underset{\text{Ketone}}{R^2{-}\overset{O}{\overset{\|}{C}}{-}R^3}$$

Pinacol reduction: Reduction of ketones into corresponding alcohols (pinacol) by acidic solvent is known as pinacol reduction.

$$\underset{\text{Ketone}}{R{-}\overset{O}{\overset{\|}{C}}{-}R^1} \longrightarrow \underset{\text{Alcohol}}{R{-}\overset{OH}{\overset{|}{C}H}{-}R^1}$$

Benkeser reduction: Reduction of naphthalene by calcium in diethylamine-dimethylamine is known as Benkeser reduction. It is more suitable for large scale production as it gives better yields.

Naphthalene $\xrightarrow{\text{Ca-DEA-DMA}}$ [bicyclic alkene] + [bicyclic alkene]

Birch reduction: The dissolving metal reductions of aromatic compounds with alkali metal (sodium/lithium), alcohol (ethanol/*t*-butanol) in liquid ammonia is known as Birch reduction.

Benzene $\xrightarrow{Na\text{-}C_2H_5OH}$ 1,4-Cyclohexadiene

Pharmaceutical Applications

Birch reduction

1. In the synthesis of vitamin A2.

β-Ionone $\xrightarrow[\text{Na-}\ C_2H_5OH]{HC{\equiv}CH}$ → → Vitamin A2

2. In the synthesis 17 α-ethinyl estradiol. Allylstrenol, tibolone, spironolactone, medrogestrone and lynestrenol also can be prepared through Birch reduction.

Oestrone $\xrightarrow[\text{Li-}C_2H_5OH]{HC{\equiv}CH}$ 17-α-Ethinylestradiol

3. In the synthesis of epicillin.

Phenylalanine $\xrightarrow[C_2H_5OH]{Li}$ 2,5-Dihydrophenylalanine → → Epicillin

4. Nadolol (antihypertensive, β-blocker) can be prepared from 5,8-dihydronaphthol. It can be prepared by the birch reduction of 1-naphthol.

1-Naphthol $\xrightarrow{\text{Li, Liq } NH_3}$ 5,8-Dihydro 1-naphthol → → Nadolol

31.5 Preparation of 1,4-Dihydrobenzoic acid (cyclohexa-2,5-diene Carboxylic Acid)

IUPAC Name: Cyclohexa-2,5-diene-1-carboxylic acid

Mol wt: 124.13 g/mol

Principle: Sodium metal reduces benzoic acid into 1,4-dihydrobenzoic acid (cyclohexa-2,5-diene carboxylic acid) in presence of ammonia and ethanol. This reduction reaction is a typical example for Birch reduction.

COOH COOH

Na, NH_3

Na-C_2H_5OH

Benzoic acid 1,4-Dihydrobenzoic acid

Reaction Mechanism

Step 1: *Formation of reducing reagent*: Sodium metal (dissolved in liquid ammonia) ionize into sodium ion (Na^+) and forms blue solution, which contains solvated electrons (forms $e^-(NH_3)_n$).

$$Na \xrightarrow{NH_3} Na^+ + e^-[NH_3]_n$$

e^-

Step 2: The aromatic ring system accepts electrons from sodium metal and undergoes reduction (hydrogenation).

The lowest anti-bonding orbital of benzoic acid accepts the electron from the reducing agent and generates radical anion. Further, the radical anion accepts hydrogen (proton) from the ethanol. The reduced form of ammonia ($-NH_2^-$) couples with Na^+ and forms sodium amide.

The molecule turns into radical and accepts another electron to form pentadienyl anion. The pentadienyl anion accepts hydrogen ethanol and forms 1,4-dihydrobenzoic acid.

COOH COOH COOH H COOH

Na $e^-[NH_3]_n$ C_2H_5OH

Benzoic acid H H H

Radical anion Radical

$\xrightarrow{e^-[NH_3]_n}$ Radical anion $\xrightarrow{C_2H_5OH}$ 1,4-Dihydrobenzoic acid

Procedure:

Chemicals Required: Benzoic acid, Sodium metal, Ammonia, Ethanol, Hydrochloric acid (10%), Magnesium sulphate, Saturated sodium chloride solution, Diethyl ether, Ammonium chloride.

Experimental steps

1. Place benzoic acid (1 g, 8 mmol), ethanol (10 mL) and liquid ammonia (60 mL) into the flat bottom flask and stir the mixture.
2. Add sodium metal (0.62 g) in small pieces to the solution with stirring followed by ammonium chloride (1.46 g, 27 mmol).
3. Evaporate the ammonia and dissolve the residual material in ice water (50 mL).
4. Acidify the solution with dilute hydrochloric acid (10%).
5. Extract the acidic mixture with diethyl ether (10 mL, 4 times) and wash the ether layer with saturated sodium chloride solution.
6. Dry the ether layer by passing through the anhydrous magnesium sulphate and concentrate.
7. Distill the pale yellow oil obtained at 96 to 98 °C and collect 1,4-dihydrobenzoic acid.

KEY POINTS

- A chemical transformation of addition of hydrogen to a compound or subtraction of oxygen from a compound is known as reduction.
- Catalytic reduction, metal hydride reduction and dissolving metal reduction are the major groups of reduction reactions.
- Synthesis of non-steroidal anti-inflammatory drugs namely phenyl butazone, ibuprofen, anti-asthmatic drug-salbutamol occurs through catalytic reduction (Pd/C).
- Vitamin A, ibuprofen, roxaltidine and thiamphenicol (antibacterial drug) synthesis involves metal hydride reduction reactions.
- Dissolving metal reduction is important step in the synthesis of nadolol (antihypertensive).

32

Reimer-Tiemann Reaction

The conversion of phenols into salicylaldehyde (2-hydroxybenzaldehyde) by *o*-formylation reaction is generally known as Reimer-Tiemann reaction. This reaction can be divided into normal and abnormal Reimer-Tiemann reactions.

Normal Reimer-Tiemann Reaction: It involves the chemical conversion of phenols into salicylaldehyde (2-hydroxybenzaldehyde, major product) and 4-hydroxybenzaldehyde (minor product). The mixture of chloroform and potassium hydroxide (or sodium hydroxide) is useful as formylating reagent.

Phenol + $CHCl_3$ (Chloroform) + 3KOH ⟶ Salicylaldehyde (Major product) + 4-Hydroxybenzaldehyde (Minor product)

Abnormal Reimer-Tiemann Reaction: Phenols (2 or 4 substituted) produce disubstituted (2,2 or 4,4) cyclohexadienones along with the desired product. This reaction is known as abnormal Reimer-Tiemann reaction.

Cresol + $CHCl_3$ (Chloroform) + 3 KOH ⟶ 5-Methylsalicylaldehyde (Major product) + 4,4-Disubstituted cyclohexadienone

Pyrrole also undergo this reaction because of their relative electron richness. Pyrrole and similar five membered rings produce ring expansion products.

Pyrrole + $CHCl_3$ (Chloroform) + 3 KOH ⟶ Pyrrole-3-carbaldehyde + 3-Chloropyridine

Reaction Mechanism

Step 1: *Formation of dichlorocarbene*: The base (–OH) abstracts the proton of chloroform and forms carbanion. The carbanion gives off chlorine (α-elimination, slow) and generates dichlorocarbene (reactive intermediate).

Cl_3C-H (Chloroform) + OH^- (Base) $\underset{-H_2O}{\overset{H_2O}{\rightleftharpoons}}$ $Cl-\bar{C}-Cl_2$ (Carbanion) $\xrightarrow{\alpha\text{-Elimination}}$ $\overset{+}{C}-Cl_2$ (Dichlorocarbene)

Step 2: *Formation of salicyladehyde*: The *o*-carbon of phenoate attacks dichlorocarbene to produce salicylaldehyde.

Phenol $\xrightarrow{KOH}$ phenoxide + $\overset{+}{C}-Cl_2$ (Dichlorocarbene) → C–Cl_2 adduct (H) → CH·Cl (Cl) → CH–Cl + OH^- (Base) → CH–Cl / OH → CH·OH ⇌ OH / CHO (Salicylaldehyde)

32.1 Preparation of 2-Hydroxynaphthaldehyde (β-Hydroxynaphthaldehyde)

IUPAC Name: 2-Hydroxynaphthalene-1-carbaldehyde

Mol wt: 172.18 g/mol

Principle: Formylation reaction on 2-naphthol generates 2-hydroxynaphthaldehyde. This reaction can be carried out using chloroform and potassium hydroxide. The sodium hydroxide (–OH) abstracts the proton from chloroform and forms carbanion. The carbanion gives off chlorine (α-elimination, slow) and generates dichlorocarbene (reactive intermediate). The *o*-carbon of β-naphthol attacks dichlorocarbene and produces 2-hydroxynaphthaldehyde.

2-Naphthol + $CHCl_3$ (Chloroform) + 3 KOH ⟶ 2-Hydroxynaphthalaldehyde

Reaction Mechanism

Step 1: *Formation of dichlorocarbene*

$Cl_3C{-}H$ (Chloroform) + OH^- (Base) $\underset{-H_2O}{\overset{H_2O}{\rightleftharpoons}}$ $Cl{-}\bar{C}{-}Cl_2$ (Carbanion) $\xrightarrow{\alpha\text{-Elimination}}$ $\overset{+}{C}{-}Cl_2$ (Dichlorocarbene)

Step 2: *Formation of 2-hydroxynaphthaldehyde*

2-Naphthol $\xrightarrow{KOH}$ naphthoxide (O^-) + $\overset{+}{C}{-}Cl_2$ (Dichlorocarbene) → $C{-}Cl_2$, H → $CH{\cdot}Cl$, Cl → $CH{\cdot}Cl$ + OH^- (Base) → $CH{-}Cl$, OH → $CH{\cdot}OH$ ⇌ OH, CHO (2-Hydroxynaphthal aldehyde)

Procedure:

Chemicals Required: 2-Napthol (β-Naphthol), Chloroform, Potassium hydroxide, Ethanol, Hydrochloric acid, Magnesium Sulphate and Ether.

Experimental steps

1. Place 2-naphthol (1 g, 7 mmol) and ethanol (3 mL) into the flat bottomed flask with thermostatic socket.
2. Place magnetic bead and add potassium hydroxide solution (2 g in 4.2 mL of water) with rapid stirring.
3. Heat the mixture (60 to 70 ºC) by placing the flask on a water bath.
4. Add chloroform (1 mL) drop wise.

   (*development of deep blue colour indicates the commencement of reaction*).
5. Remove the flask from water bath and add chloroform (3 mL).
6. Reflux the mixture gently for 1.5 h.

   (*The sodium salt of phenolic aldehyde separates*)
7. Stirr the reaction mixture for 1 h.
8. Acidify the residue/mixture with hydrochloric acid (congo red paper test).
9. Add water to dissolve the separated salt.

10. Extract the remaining oily layer with ether and wash the ether layer with water.
11. Dry the ether layer by passing through anhydrous magnesium sulphate.
12. Evaporate the ether layer and allow the residue to cool to obtain solid product.
13. Purify the 2-hydroxynaphthaldehyde by recrystallization with ethanol.
14. The melting range of pure 2-hydroxynaphthaldehyde is 80 to 81 °C.

KEY POINTS

- The formylation reaction of phenols into salicylaldehyde is known as Reimer-Tiemann reaction.
- The mixture of chloroform and potassium hydroxide (or sodium hydroxide) is the useful formylating reagent.
- Reimer-Tiemann reaction of 2-napthol yields 2-hydroxynapthaldehyde.

33

Schiff Base Synthesis (Nucleophilic Addition Reaction)

Schiff base reaction is specific for carbonyl compounds (aldehydes and ketones). Hugo Schiff (1864) reported the synthesis of Schiff base through the condensation of primary aromatic amine with a carbonyl compound. A Schiff base contains a carbon-nitrogen double bond (-CH=N-), this functionality is known as azomethane and aldimine. A Schiff base derived from aniline is called as anil.

$$RR_1C{=}O + H_2N{-}R_2 \longrightarrow RR_1C{=}N{-}R_2 + H_2O$$

Carbonyl compound + Primary amine → Schiff base

Reaction Mechanism

Formation of carbinolamine: The nucleophilic addition of amino group to the carbonyl group forms an intermediate known as carbinolamine.

$$RR_1C{=}O + H_2\ddot{N}{-}R_2 \longrightarrow R{-}C(O^-)(R_1){-}\overset{+}{N}H_2{-}R_2 \longrightarrow R{-}C(OH)(R_1){-}NH{-}R_2$$

Carbonyl compound + Primary amine → Carbinolamine

Formation of Schiff base: The carbinolamine eliminates water molecule and forms a Schiff base.

$$R{-}C(OH)(R_1){-}NH{-}R_2 \xrightarrow{H^+} R{-}C(\overset{+}{O}H_2)(R_1){-}\ddot{N}H{-}R_2 \xrightarrow{-H_2O} R{-}C(R_1){=}\overset{+}{N}H{-}R_2 \longrightarrow R{-}C(R_1){=}N{-}R_2$$

Carbinolamine → Schiff base

The nucleophilic addition on the nitrogen makes the Schiff base stable imine. Schiff base of aromatic aldehydes having an effective conjugation system are more stable, whereas aliphatic aldehydes are relatively unstable.

Pharmaceutical Applications

1. Schiff bases are useful in the identification and determination of drugs and pharmaceuticals containing carbonyl groups (aldehydes and ketones).
2. Purification and protection of carbonyl or amino groups can be done through Schiff base formation.
3. Schiff bases appear to be an important intermediate in a number of enzymatic reactions involving interaction of an enzyme with an amino or a carbonyl group of the substrate. Fructose-1,6-biphosphate aldolase catalyzed reaction (glycolysis) and metabolism of amino acids generates Schiff base as an intermediate.
4. Maillard reaction is the reaction between amino acids and reducing sugars in the food processing. This reaction proceeds through Schiff base formation.
5. Preparation of mucolytic drug, Ambroxol.

Br, CHO, NH_2, Br — 2-Amino-3,5-dibromo benzaldehyde + OH, NH_2 — 4-Amino cyclohexanol → Br, CH=N—, —OH, NH_2, Br — Ambroxol

6. Preparation of antiprotozoal drug, Nifurtimox.

O_2N, O, CHO — 5-Nitrofurfural + H_2N—N, S, O, O, H_3C — 2-Methyl-1,4-oxithian -4,4-dioxide → O_2N, O, C=N—N, H, S, O, O, H_3C — Nifurtimox

33.1 Preparation of N-(3-Nitrobenzylidene)aniline

Traditional Name: 3-Nitrobenzal-anilin

IUPAC Name: 1-(3-Nitrophenyl)-N-phenylmethanimine

Mol wt: 226.23 g/mol

Principle: N-(3-Nitrobenzylidene)aniline can be prepared by the condensation of 3-nitrobenzaldehyde with aniline. The amino group of aniline attacks (nucleophilic addition) carbonyl carbon of 3-nitrobenzaldehyde and forms carbinolamine as an intermediate. The formed carbinolamine eliminates water molecule and forms N-(3-nitrobenzylidene) aniline (Schiff base).

CHO NH$_2$ HC=N NO$_2$ + $\xrightarrow[\Delta]{C_2H_5OH}$ NO$_2$

3-Nitro benzaldehyde   Aniline   N-(3-Nitrobenzylidene)aniline

Reaction Mechanism

***Formation of carbinolamine*:** The nucleophilic addition of amino group to the carbonyl group forms an intermediate known as carbinolamine.

O H$_2$N H Aniline O$_2$N 3-Nitrobenzaldehyde → O$^-$ H C N$^+$ H H O$_2$N → HO C N H H O$_2$N Carbinolamine

***Formation of Schiff base*:** The carbinolamine eliminates water molecule and forms a Schiff base.

HO C N H H O$_2$N Carbinolamine $\xrightarrow{H^+}$ H$_2$O$^+$ H C N R$_1$ O$_2$N → H C=N$^+$ R$_1$ O$_2$N → C=N H O$_2$N N-(3-Nitrobenzylidene)aniline

Procedure:

***Chemicals Required*:** 3-Nitrobenzaldehyde, Aniline, Ethanol, Methanol.

1. Place 3-nitrobenzaldehyde (1 g, 7 mmol), aniline (0.46 g, 5 mmol) and ethanol (2 mL) in a round bottom flask.
2. Attach reflux condenser and reflux the mixture by placing on the water bath for 20 min.
3. Add water until a slight cloudiness persists and allow it to cool.
4. Stir the separated oil with glass rod to induce the crystallization.
5. Filter and wash the solid with cold aqueous ethanol.
6. Purify the product by recrystallization from aqueous methanol.

7. The melting range of pure N-(3-nitrobenzylidene) aniline is 65 to 66 °C.

(Schiff base can be prepared by heating the components in the absence of solvent at 100 °C for 15 min, cool and then stir the product with methanol to induce crystallization).

KEY POINTS

- The condensation of primary aromatic amine and carbonyl compound generates Schiff base.
- A carbon-nitrogen double bond (-CH=N-) functionality is known as azomethane and aldimine.
- The food processing reaction between amino acids and reducing sugars proceeds through Schiff base formation.
- Schiff bases are useful in the analysis of drugs and pharmaceuticals.
- Preparation of Ambroxol (mucolytic drug) and nifurtimox (antiprotozoal) involves Schiff base reaction.

34

Skraup Synthesis

Zdenko Hans Skraup (Czech-Austrian Chemist, 1880) demonstrated the synthesis of quinoline. The condensation of aniline with glycerol produces quinoline and the reaction is known as Skraup synthesis. Concentrated sulphuric acid acts as dehydrating agent, facilitates the chemical conversion, and produces dihydroquinoline. The oxidizing agents, such as ferrous sulphate, iodine, arsenic and nitrobenzene convert the dihydroquinoline into quinoline through oxidation reaction.

Aniline + Glycerol $\xrightarrow{H_2SO_4}$ Quinoline

Reaction Mechanism

Concentrated sulphuric acid dehydrates glycerol and forms acrolein. Acrolein reacts with aniline through 1,3-addition forms an intermediate, which eliminates water molecule and produces dihydroquinoline. The oxidation of dihydroquinoline produces quinoline.

Formation of acroline

HO–CH₂–CH(OH)–CH₂–OH (Glycerol) $\xrightarrow{H^+}$ HO–CH(H)–CH(OH_2^+)–CH₂–OH $\xrightarrow{-H_2O}$ HO–CH=CH–CH₂–OH $\xrightarrow{H^+}$ H_2O^+–CH=CH–CH₂–OH $\xrightarrow{-H_2O}$ HC^+=CH–CH₂–OH ⟶ H_2C=CH–CH=O (Acroline)

Formation of dihydroquinoline and quinoline

Aniline
Acroline
H^+
$-H^+$
$-H_2O$
H_2SO_4
(O)
Quinoline

Pharmaceutical Applications

1. Synthesis of chloroquine (antimalrial drug).

3-Chloroaniline
Diethyl oxaloacetate
Chloroquine

2. Preparation of anti-malarial drugs, Primaquine and Pamaquine.

4-Methoxy-2-nitroaniline
Glycerol
H_2SO_4
Primaquine: $R = R_1 = H$
Pamaquine: $R = R_1 - C_2H_5$

3. Synthesis of Chlorquinaldol (antiseptic for skin infections).

2-Hydroxyaniline (2-aminophenol) + Crotanaldehyde $\xrightarrow{H_2SO_4}$ 8-hydroxy-2-methylquinoline $\xrightarrow{Cl_2, HCOOH}$ Chlorquinaldol

4. Synthesis of Niacin (vitamin B3).

Quinoline $\xrightarrow{KMnO_4}$ Pyridine-2,3-dicarboxylic acid $\longrightarrow$ Niacin (Vitamin B3)

34.1 Preparation of Quinoline

Traditional Name: 1-Azanaphthalene, Benzopyridine **Mol wt**: 129.16 g/mol

Principle: Quinoline can be synthesized by condensing aniline and glycerol through 1,3-addition reaction in presence of sulphuric acid (dehydrating agent, catalyst).

Aniline + Glycerol $\xrightarrow{H_2SO_4}$ 1,2-dihydroquinoline $\xrightarrow{I_2}$ Quinoline

Concentrated sulphuric acid dehydrates glycerol and forms acrolein. Acrolein reacts with aniline through 1,3-addition forms dihydroquinoline (intermediate). Dihydroquinoline can be converted into quinoline through oxidation reaction. In this chemical synthesis, Iodine acts as oxidizing agent.

Procedure:

Chemicals Required: Aniline, Anhydrous glycerol, Concentrated sulphuric acid, Iodine, Sodium hydroxide, Sodium nitrite, Starch iodide paper, Ether.

Experimental steps

1. Transfer aniline (2 mL, 22 mmol), glycerol (1.3 g, 14 mmol) and iodine (0.1 g) into three necked round bottom flask.
2. Stir the reaction mixture and add sulphuric acid (3.3 mL) dropwise through the condenser. (*temperature raises to ~105 °C*)

3. Heat the reaction mixture by placing in an oil bath and maintain the temperature at 140 °C.
4. The reaction evolves sulphur dioxide vapour and iodine vapour.
5. Continue the heating at 170 °C for 1 h.
6. Cool the mixture and add sodium hydroxide (17 mL, 5 M) to neutralize the mixture.
7. Distil the quinoline from the mixture through steam distillation.
8. Purification of quinoline
   - Add sulphuric acid (2 mL) to the distillate and cool (0-5 °C).
   - Add sodium nitrite solution (0.3 g in water (2 mL)) dropwise (until a drop of reaction mixture gives blue colour with starch-iodide paper or paste).
   - Heat the mixture for 1 h and add solution of sodium hydroxide (1.5 g in 5 mL of water).
   - Distil the extract and extract the distillate with ether.
   - Evaporate the ether layer to isolate the product.
   - The melting range of pure quinoline is 236 to 238 °C.

34.2 Preparation of 8-Hydroxyquinoline

Traditional Name: 1-Azanaphthalene-8-ol, Oxine.

IUPAC Name: Quinolin-8-ol **Mol wt**: 145.16 g/mol

Principle: 8-Hydroxyquinoline can be synthesized by condensing 2-hydroxyaniline (2-aminophenol) and glycerol through 1,3-addition reaction.

2-Hydroxyaniline (2-aminophenol) + Glycerol $\xrightarrow{H_2SO_4}$ (1,2-dihydro-8-hydroxyquinoline) $\xrightarrow{FeSO_4}$ 8-Hydroxyquinoline

Concentrated sulphuric acid dehydrates glycerol and forms acrolein which reacts with 2-hydroxyaniline (2-aminophenol) through 1,3-addition and forms 1,2-dihydro-8-hydroxyquinoline (intermediate). Dihydroquinoline can be converted into 8-hydroxyquinoline through oxidation reaction. In this chemical synthesis, ferrous sulphate acts as oxidizing agent.

Procedure:

Chemicals Required: 2-Hydroxyaniline, Glycerol, Sulphuric acid, Ferrous sulphate.

Experimental steps

1. Transfer concentrated sulphuric acid (2.3 mL), 2-hydroxyaniline (1 g, 9 mmol) and anhydrous glycerol (2.5 g, 27 mmol) into a flask (flask 1).
2. Liquify the mixture present in flask 1 by placing on a steam bath.
3. Place 2-hydroxyaniline (2-aminophenol) (0.7 g, 5 mmol) and ferrous sulphate (0.1 g) into another flask (flask 2).
4. Attach reflux condenser to the flask 2 and heat the contents to 100 - 120 °C.
5. Add the liquid mixture of flask 1 to the flask 2 in small portions; maintaining the temperature between 135 to 150 °C.
6. Reflux the combined mixture at 130 °C for 4 h.
7. Cool the reaction mixture and add sodium hydroxide solution with vigorous stirring to produce the pH 7 (neutralization).
8. Add crushed ice and filter the precipitate.
9. Distil the isolated product under reduced pressure (discard the first 1 mL of the distillate).
10. Cool the distillate to crystallize the product.
11. The melting range of pure 8-hydroxyquinoline is 74 to 75 °C.

Preparation of anhydrous Glycerol:

- Heat glycerol (50 mL) in porcelain dish with stirring maintaining the temperature at 180 °C.
- Reduce the temperature to 100 °C and pour into beaker.
- Keep the beaker in desiccators over sulphuric acid for 24 h, and use for the reaction.

KEY POINTS

- The condensation of aniline with glycerol produces quinoline and the reaction is known as Skraup synthesis.
- Dehydrating agents and oxidizing agents promote the reaction.
- Preparation of anti-malarial drugs, such as chloroquine, primaquine and pamaquine, and chlorquinaldol (antiseptic) occurs through Skraup synthesis.

35

Sulphonamide Synthesis

Sulphonamides, the first antimicrobial drugs produced revolution in antibiotic medicines. The term sulphonamide is a generic name employed for the *para*-aminosulphonamide derivatives. Prontosil is the first sulphonamide discovered and offered strong protection against *Streptococci* infections. The research team of Pasteur Institute discovered the therapeutic potential of sulphanilamide (metabolite of prontosil).

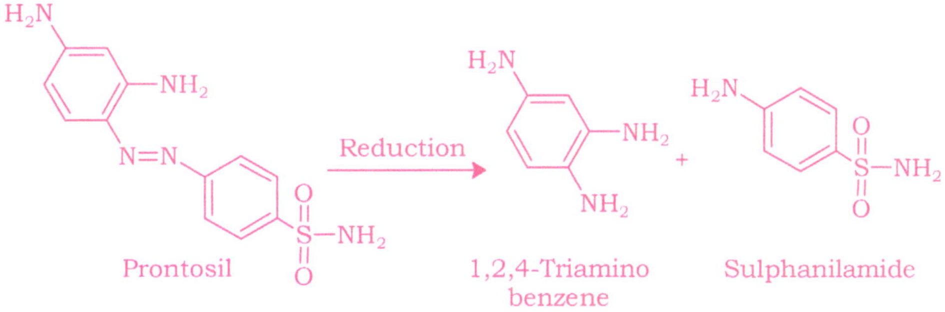

Prontosil —Reduction→ 1,2,4-Triamino benzene + Sulphanilamide

This discovery led to the development of several clinically useful sulphonamides. Sulphonamides are useful in the treatment of urinary tract infection, tonsilitis, burns, conjunctivitis, peptic ulcer and bacillary dysentry. Folic acid is essential for the DNA and RNA synthesis and *para*-aminobenzoic acid, an essential component in the synthesis of folic acid. The sulphanilamides competes with *para*-aminobenzoic acid and inhibits the folic acid synthesis and arrests the bacterial growth.

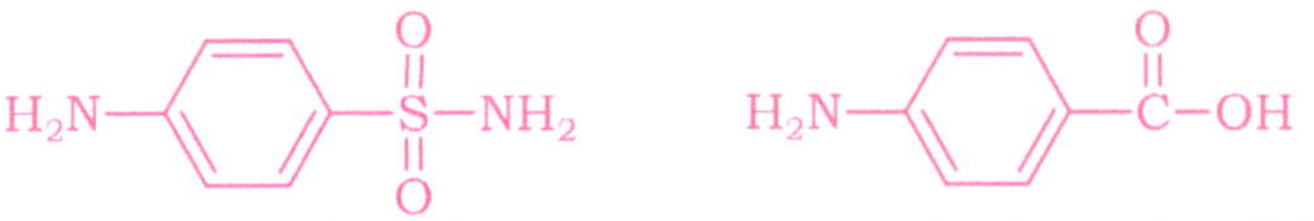

Sulphanilamide   *para*-Aminobenzoic acid

Clinically useful Sulphonamides

1. Sulphonamides having different therapeutic potentials can be synthesised from acetanilide. Chlorosulphonylation, amination with desired reactant followed by hydrolysis produces the sulphonamide of interest.

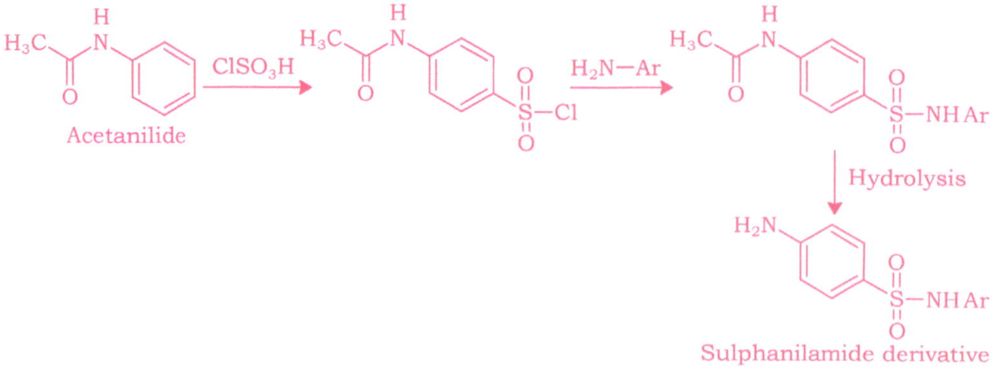

Acetanilide $\xrightarrow{ClSO_3H}$ $\xrightarrow{H_2N-Ar}$ $\xrightarrow{Hydrolysis}$ Sulphanilamide derivative

Drug	Structure	Therapeutic use
Sulphisoxazole	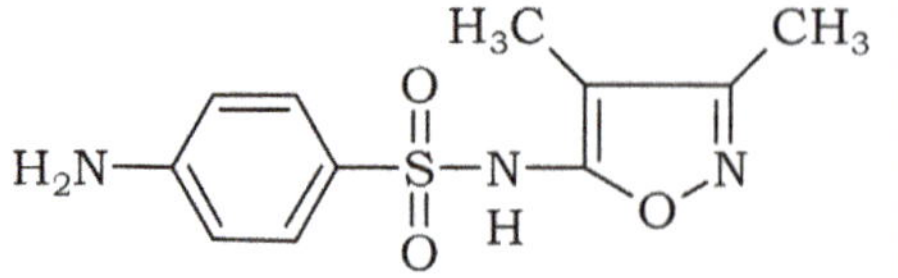	Antibiotic: Otis media
Sulphamethoxazole	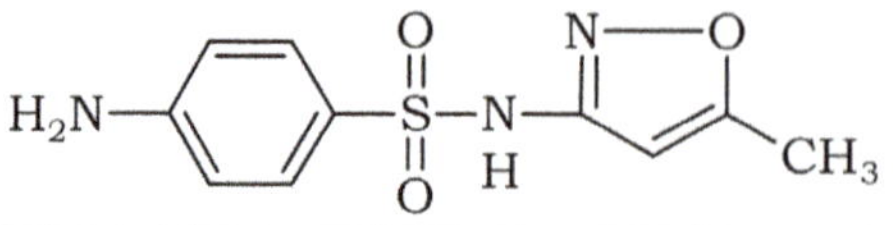	Antibiotic: Sinusitis
Sulphadiazine	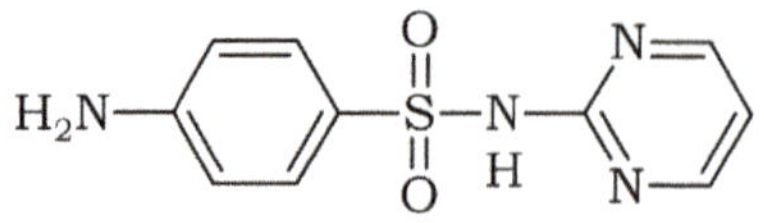	Antibiotic: Urinary tract infection
Silver sulphadiazine	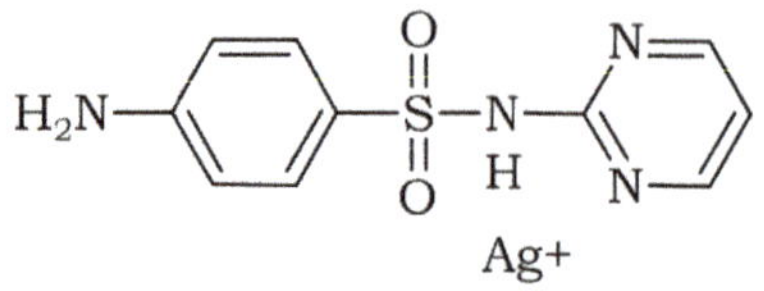 Ag+	Burns

2. Synthesis of diuretic drug, Bumetanide: 4-Chloro-3-nitrobenzoic acid upon chlorosulphonylation, amination and reduction produces bumetanide.

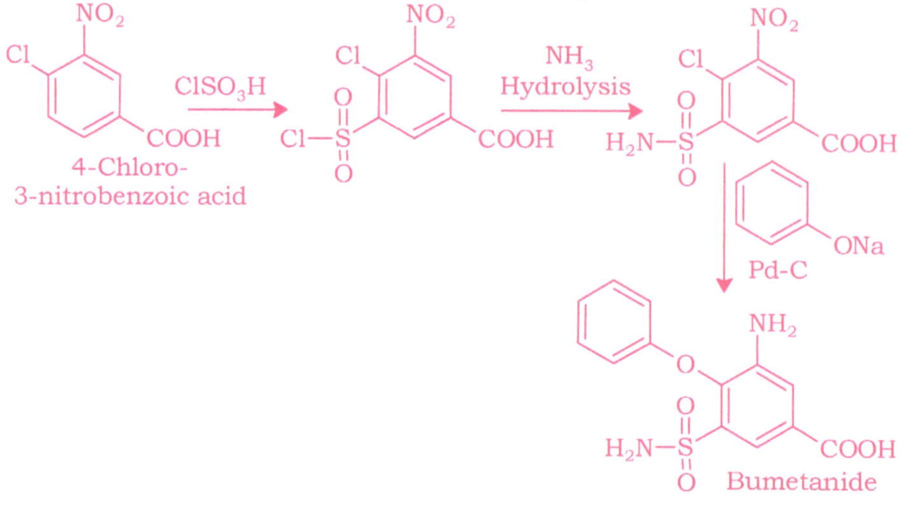

4-Chloro-3-nitrobenzoic acid $\xrightarrow{ClSO_3H}$ $\xrightarrow{NH_3,\ Hydrolysis}$ $\xrightarrow{C_6H_5ONa,\ Pd-C}$ Bumetanide

3. Synthesis of anti-inflammatory drug, piroxicam.

Toluene → ($ClSO_3H$) → → (NH_3, (O)) → Saccharin → Piroxicam

4. Synthesis of diuretic drug, Mafenide: Benzylacetamide upon chlorosulphonylation, amination and hydrolysis produces mafenide.

Benzylacetamide → ($ClSO_3H$) → → (NH_3, Hydrolysis) → Mafenide

35.1 Preparation of Sulphanilamide

IUPAC Name: 4-Aminobenzene sulphonmide **Mol wt**: 161.03 g/mol

Principle: Sulphanilamide can be synthesised from acetanilide through chlorosulphonation using chlorosulphonic acid and sulphonylation with ammonia. At first, acetanilide undergoes chlorosulphonation and forms *p*-acetamido-benzenesulphonyl chloride. In the next step, *p*-acetamidobenzenesulphonyl chloride undergoes amination with ammonia and forms N-acetylated sulphanilamide. Protected amino group (N-acetyl group) prevents the chlorosulphonation of amino group and directs the chlorosulphonation at aromatic ring (4th position). The acid mediated hydrolysis of acetyl group (deacetylation) of N-acetylated sulphanilamide produces sulphanilamide.

Acetanilide → ($ClSO_3H$) → → (NH_3) → → (HCl) → Sulphanilamide

Reaction Mechanism

Step 1: Formation of para-acetamidobenzenesulphonyl chloride (chlorosulphonation)

H_3C O HN Cl—S—OH O O Acetanilide → H_3C O HN + H O S Cl O OH → $-H_2O$ H_3C O HN O S—Cl O *para*-Acetamidobenzene sulphonyl chloride

***Step 2: Formation of para-acetamidobenzene sulphonamide* (sulphonylation/amination).**

H_3C O HN H O S—Cl O :NH_3 *para*-Acetamidobenzene sulphonyl chloride → H_3C O HN O Cl S NH_2—H O → H_3C O HN O S—NH_2 O *para*-Acetamidobenzene sulphonamide

***Step 3: Formation of sulphanilamide* (*deacetylation*)**

H_3C O Hydrolysis HN O S—NH_2 O *para*-Acetamidobenzene sulphonamide → H_2N O S—NH_2 O Sulphanilamide

Procedure:

Step 1: Preparation of para-acetamidobenzenesulphonyl chloride

Chemicals Required: Acetanilide, Chlorosulphonic acid

1. Transfer acetanilide (1.35 g, 10 mmol) into a two necked round bottom flask (fitted with dropping funnel and reflux condenser).
2. Add chlorosulphonic acid (3.4 mL, 51 mmol) in small portions with the help of dropping funnel fitted with calcium guard tube.
3. Shake the flask occasionally to ensure the mixing.
4. Heat the reaction mixture by placing on a water bath for 1 h.

5. Cool the contents and pour the oily mixture in a thin stream with stirring into a beaker containing crushed ice.
6. Rinse the flask with cold water and transfer into the beaker.
7. Stir vigorously to dissolve the lumps formed and obtain white solid suspension.
8. Filter the suspension and dry the residue.

Precaution:

- Chlorosulphonic acid reacts with water and produces harmful vapours, hence the addition must be slow.
- Chlorosulphonic acid is highly corrosive and may cause serious burns, hence wear gloves when handling and exercise extreme care.

Step 2: Preparation of para-acetamidobenzenesulphonamide

Chemicals Required: *para*-Acetamidobenzenesulphonyl chloride, Ammonia, Dilute sulphuric acid.

1. Mix the crude *para*-acetamidobenzenesulphonyl chloride with ammonia (3 mL, 23.8 mmol) and water (3 mL).
2. Heat the mixture for 15 min with occasional swirling.
3. Cool the suspension in an ice-bath and acidify with dilute sulphuric acid.
4. Filter the precipitate and wash with cold water.

Step 3: Preparation of sulphanilamide (deacetylation)

Chemicals Required: *para*-Acetamidobenzenesulphonamide, Hydrochloric acid, Charcoal, Sodium bicarbonate.

1. Transfer the *para*-acetamido benzenesulphanilamide to round bottom flask.
2. Add hydrochloric acid (0.7 mL) and water (2.1 mL).
3. Attach reflux condenser to the flask and reflux the mixture for 45 min.
4. Cool the solution and boil with charcoal.
5. Filter and add sodium bicarbonate (1.08 g, 19 mmol) to the filtrate to neutralize the hydrochloric acid.
6. Cool to room temperature and filter the precipitate formed.
7. Dry and recrystallize from water.
8. The melting range of pure sulphanilamide is 161 to 163 ºC.

35.2 Preparation of Sulphaguanidine

IUPAC Name: 4-Amino-N-(amino(imino))methylbenzene sulphonamide

Mol wt: 161.03 g/mol

Principle: Sulphaguanidine can be prepared from sulphanilamide by the reaction with guanidine nitrate in basic medium. Sulphanilamide can be synthesised from acetanilide through chlorosulphonation using chlorosulphonic acid and sulphonylation with ammonia followed by hydrolysis.

Sulphanilamide + Guanidine → Sulphaguanidine + NH_3

Procedure:

Chemicals Required: Sulphanilamide, Guanidine nitrate, Sodium hydroxide, Methanol, Cyclohexanol, Dilute hydrochloric acid.

1. Dissolve guanidine nitrate (1 g) in the solution of sodium hydroxide (2.4 g) in methanol (12.5 mL).
2. Stir the reaction mixture, maintaining the temperature at 50-60 °C for 15 min.
3. Cool the reaction mixture to 20 °C.
4. Filter to remove nitrite and wash the residue with two portions of methanol (3 mL).
5. Transfer the combined methanolic extract into 3-necked flask and add sulphanilamide (0.5 g, 60 mmol).
6. Stir the reaction mixture for 15 min at 50-55 °C into distil the methanol.
7. Add cyclohexanol (2.1 mL) and elevate the temperature to 180-190 °C and continue the distillation.
8. Maintain the temperature of reaction mixture between 150-160 °C for 2 h and pour into dilute hydrochloric acid (50 mL).
9. Stir, alkalinify by adding sodium hydroxide slowly with stirring.
10. Cool the mixture, filter the separated sulphaguanidine and wash with cold water.
11. Purify the sulphaguanidine by recrystallization with hot water.
12. The melting range of the pure compound is 189 to 190 °C.

KEY POINTS

- The research team of Pasteur Institute discovered the sulphanilamide from the dye prontosil.
- Chlorosulphonylation, amination with desired reactant followed by hydrolysis produces the sulphonamide of interest.
- Sulphonamides are useful in the treatment of urinary tract infection, tonsilitis, burns, conjunctivitis, peptic ulcer and bacillary dysentry.
- Chlorosulphonic acid is highly corrosive and may cause serious burns, hence wear gloves when handling and exercise extreme care.

36

Sulphonate Ester Synthesis (Nucleophilic Substitution Reaction, S_N1)

Sulphonate esters can be prepared by the reaction between sulphonyl chlorides and alcohols (alkyl or aryl alcohols). The most useful sulphonyl chlorides are methane sulphonyl chloride (mesyl chloride), benzene sulphonyl chloride, and toluene sulphonyl chloride (tosyl chloride). The chemical conversion proceeds in the presence of base and produces mesylates, tosylates, brosylates and similar sulphonate esters. Pyridine is the most preferred base, it functions as nucleophilic catalyst and solvent.

$$\underset{\text{Alcohol}}{R{-}OH} + \underset{\text{Sulphonyl chloride}}{R_1\text{-}SO_2Cl} \xrightarrow{\text{Base}} \underset{\text{Sulphonate ester}}{R{-}O{-}SO_2R_1}$$

Alcohols react most rapidly and the reactivity of primary alcohols is higher. Primary alcohols can be selectively sulphonated in the molecules containing secondary and tertiary alcoholic groups.

Reaction Mechanism

The replacement of a halogen (leaving group) by a nucleophile (incoming group) is known as nucleophilic substitution reaction (S_N1). The chloride of sulphonyl chloride is leaving group and the oxygen of alcohol is nuclophile in this reaction. The oxygen of the alcohol displaces the chloride of sulphonyl chloride.

Generation of nucleophile: Pyridine abstracts the hydrogen from alcohol and generates nucleophile (RO^-).

$$\underset{\text{Alcohol}}{R{-}OH} + \underset{\text{Pyridine}}{C_5H_5N} \longrightarrow \underset{\text{Alkoxide (nucleophile)}}{R{-}O^-} + C_5H_5N^+{-}H$$

Formation of sulphonic ester: The nucleophile attacks the sulphur of sulphonyl chloride and forms sulphonic esters. The pyridine base combines with liberated chlorine and forms pyridinium chloride (neutralization of hydrochloric acid released).

R–O⁻ (Alkoxide (nucleophile)) + R_1–SO_2–Cl ⟶ R–O–S(O⁻)(=O)(Cl)–R_1 —(pyridine)→ R–O–SO_2–R_1 (Sulphonate ester) + pyridinium chloride

36.1 Preparation of Busulphan

IUPAC Name: Butane-1,4-diol dimethanesulfonate **Mol wt**: 246.30 g/mol

Principle: Butane-1,4-diol reacts with methanesulfonyl chloride in the presence of pyridine and generates busulphan (anti-cancer drug). Pyridine acts a nucleophilic catalyst, solvent and neutralizes the liberated hydrochloric acid.

$$\begin{matrix} H_2C-CH_2-OH \\ H_2C-CH_2-OH \end{matrix} + H_3C-SO_2Cl \xrightarrow{\text{Pyridine}} \begin{matrix} H_2C-CH_2-O-SO_2-CH_3 \\ H_2C-CH_2-O-SO_2-CH_3 \end{matrix}$$

Butane-1,4-diol; Methane sulfonyl chloride; Busulphan

Pyridine abstracts the hydrogen from butane-1,4-diol and generates alkoxide nucleophile. The nucleophile attacks the sulphur of methanesulfonyl chloride and forms busulphan (sulphonic ester). The pyridine base combines with liberated chlorine and forms pyridinium chloride.

Reaction Mechanism

Generation of Nucleophile

$$\begin{matrix} H_2C-CH_2-OH \\ H_2C-CH_2-OH \end{matrix} + \text{Pyridine} \longrightarrow \begin{matrix} H_2C-CH_2-O^- \\ H_2C-CH_2-O^- \end{matrix} + \text{Pyridinium } (N^+H)$$

Butane-1,4-diol; Pyridine; Alkoxide (nucleophile)

Formation of sulphonic ester

$$\begin{matrix} H_2C-CH_2-O^- \\ H_2C-CH_2-O^- \end{matrix} + H_3C-SO_2-Cl \longrightarrow \begin{matrix} H_2C-CH_2-O-S(O^-)(=O)(Cl)-CH_3 \\ H_2C-CH_2-O^- \end{matrix} \xrightarrow{\text{pyridine}} \begin{matrix} H_2C-CH_2O-O-SO_2-CH_3 \\ H_2C-CH_2O^- \end{matrix} + H_3C-SO_2-Cl \longrightarrow$$

Alkoxide (nucleophile); pyridinium chloride (N^+H Cl^-)

$H_2C\text{-}CH_2O{-}SO_2\text{-}CH_3$

$H_2C\text{-}CH_2O{-}S(=O)(O^-){-}CH_3$ + Cl

Pyridinium ($\overset{+}{N}H$) → Pyridinium chloride ($\overset{+}{N}H\ Cl^-$)

$H_2C\text{-}CH_2SO_2CH_3$
$H_2C\text{-}CH_2SO_2CH_3$

Busulphan

Procedure:

Chemicals Required: Butane-1,4-diol, Methanesulfonyl chloride, Pyridine, Ethanol.

1. Transfer butane-1,4-diol (3.6 mL, 40 mmol) into the flask containing pyridine (10 mL) and dissolve it by mixing well.
2. Place the mixture (butane-1,4-diol in pyridine) in an ice-bath to reduce the temperature below 20 °C.
3. Add methanesulfonyl chloride (6 mL, 80 mmol) dropwise to the flask and maintain the temperature 18 ± 2 °C.
4. Allow the reaction mixture to stand at room temperature for 30 min (exothermic).
5. Cool the mixture by placing in an ice-bath and add ice-cold water (30 mL).
6. Stir the reaction mixture with glass rod to obtain white crystalline solid.
7. Isolate the solid through vacuum filtration, wash with ice-cold water and dry.
8. The crude product can be purified by recrystallization with ethanol.
9. The melting point of pure busulphan is 110 °C.

***Precautions*:**

(a) Methanesulfonyl chloride is highly toxic, corrosive and lachrymator. Hence, necessary precautions (use of PPEs) are required.

(b) Conduct the reaction in fume cupboard to avoid lachrymatory and other CNS disturbances.

KEY POINTS

- Nucleophilic substitution (S_N1) of alcohols with sulfonyl chlorides generates sulphonic ester.
- Methanesulfonyl chloride is highly toxic, corrosive and lachrymator. Hence, necessary precautions (use of PPEs) are required.
- The anticancer drug, busulphan belongs to sulphonic ester category.

37

Uracil Synthesis

Uracil is the pyrimidine nucleobase of ribonucleic acid (RNA). The methylated uracil is called as thymine, a component of deoxy ribonucleic acid (DNA) which maintains the repair and protection mechanisms of DNA replication. Ascoli (1900) isolated the uracil from yeast nucleic acid. Fisher and Roeder (1901) demonstrated the practical synthesis of uracil by condensing urea with ethylhydroxymethyleneacetate. Wheeler *et al* also proposed the method for the uracil synthesis using urea derivatives.

Brown (1994) reported simplest chemical synthesis of uracil by condensing the maleic acid with urea using fuming sulphuric acid. He also described the conversion of thiouracil into uracil through desulfuration reaction using chloroacetic acid. Malic acid also can be used in place of maleic acid.

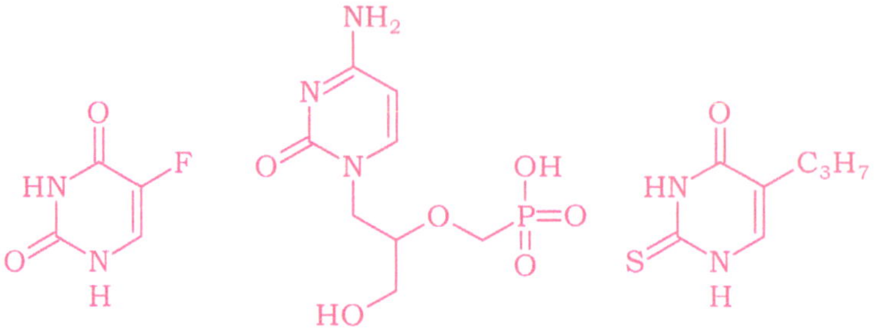

5-Fluorouracil   Cidofovir   Propylthiouracil

Pharmaceutical Applications

1) Uracil is the central core in several therapeutic molecules, such as anticancer (5-flurouracil), antithyroid (propylthiouracil) and antiherpes (cidofovir) agents.

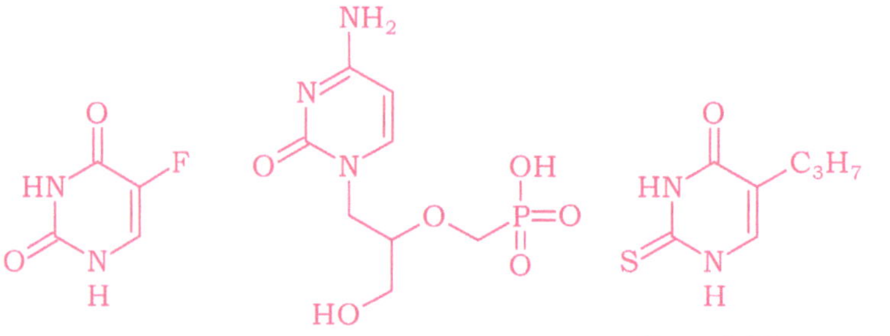

5-Fluorouracil   Cidofovir   Propylthiouracil

2) Uracil plays major role in the biosynthesis of polysaccharides and serves as a coenzyme for many biochemical reactions.
3) Preparation of antithyroid drugs (methyluracil and propylthiouracil)

Thiourea + Alkylaceto acetate → Alkylthiouracil

	R
Methylthiouracil	CH_3
Propylthiouracil	C_3H_7

37.1 Preparation of 6-Methyluracil (Method 1)

IUPAC Name: 6-Methylpyrimidine-2,4-(1H,3H)-dione

Mol wt: 126.11 g/mol

Principle: The condensation of thiourea with ethyl acetoacetate produces 6-methyluracil. At the first step, the condensation reaction generates 6-methylthiouracil. The desulphuration reaction with chloroacetic acid in alcoholic potassium hydroxide converts 6-methylthiouracil into 6-methyluracil.

Thiourea + Ethyl acetoacetate $\xrightarrow[KOH]{C_2H_5OH}$ 6-Methylthiouracil $\xrightarrow[\Delta]{Cl\ CH_2COOH}$ 6-Methyluracil

Reaction Mechanism

Generation of nucleophile: In ethyl acetoacetate, inductive effect of two carbonyl groups weakens the -C-H bonds of active methylene group and generates stable anion. Hence ethyl acetoacetate exists in *keto* and *enol* forms (tautomeric). The base abstracts proton (H^+) from thiourea and generates nucleophile.

Thiourea + $^-OC_2H_5O$ Ethoxide (base) → Nucleophile (thiourea)

Nucleophilic attack on ethyl acetoacetate: The nucleophile attacks electrophilic center of ethyl acetoacetate and upon cyclization produces 6-methylthiouracil.

H_5C_2O O O CH_3 *keto* form ⇌ Ethyl acetoacetate ⇌ H_5C_2O O HO CH_3 *enol* form

Nucleophile (thiourea) + Ethyl acetoacetate → ... → 6-Methylthiouracil ($-C_2H_5OH$)

Preparation of 6-methyluracil (desulfuration): The sulfhydryl group reacts with chloroacetic acid and forms thio ether complex, which upon hydrolysis (desulfuration) forms the 6-methyluracil.

6-Methylthiouracil $\xrightarrow[\Delta]{ClCH_2COOH}$ $HOOC\cdot H_2C-S$ ... $\xrightarrow{\text{Hydrolysis, Desulfuration}}$ 6-Methyluracil

Procedure:

Chemicals Required:Ethyl acetoacetate, Thiourea, Ethanol, Potassium hydroxide, Hydrochloric acid.

Step 1: Preparation of 6-methylthiouracil

1. Mix thiourea (1 g, 13 mmol) and ethyl acetoacetate (2 mL, 16 mmol) with ethanol (7 mL).
2. Transfer the mixture into a round bottom flask.
3. Add a solution of potassium hydroxide (0.8 g, 13 mmol) in water (3 mL)).
4. Attach condenser and reflux the mixture for 2 h.
5. Acidify the mixture with hydrochloric acid to neutralize the potassium hydroxide.

6. Cool the reaction mixture to room temperature.
7. Isolate the product through filtration and dry the product.

Step 2: Preparation of 6-methyluracil

Chemicals Required: 6-Methylthiouracil, Chloroacetic acid, Ethanol.

1. Place 6-methylthiouracil (1 g, 7 mmol) and solution of chloroacetic acid (1.4 g, 15 mmol) in water (35 mL) into a round bottom flask.
2. Heat the mixture for 2 h in fume cupboard.
3. Filter the hot solution and allow the product to crystallize.
4. Dry and recrystallize the product from hot ethanol.
5. The melting point of pure 6-methyluracil is 318 °C.

37.2 Preparation of 6-Methyluracil (Method 2)

IUPAC Name: 6-Methylpyrimidine-2,4-(1H,3H)-dione **Mol wt**: 126.11 g/mol

Principle: The acid catalysed condensation of urea with ethyl acetoacetate in ethanolic medium produces 6-methyluracil. Concentrated hydrochloric acid is the effective acid catalyst. Initially the condensation reaction generates β-uraminocrotonic ester. This ester product upon cyclization under acidic environment forms 6-methyluracil.

Urea + Ethyl acetoacetate $\xrightarrow[KOH]{C_2H_5OH}$ β-Uramino crotonic ester $\xrightarrow{HCl}$ 6-Methyluracil

Reaction Mechanism

Generation of nucleophile: In ethyl acetoacetate, inductive effect of two carbonyl groups weakens the -C-H bonds of active methylene group and generates stable anion. Hence ethyl acetoacetate exist in *keto* and *enol* forms (tautomeric). The base abstracts proton (H^+) from urea and generates nucleophile.

Urea (H_2N–CO–NH–H) + $^-OC_2H_5$ Ethoxide (base) $\longrightarrow$ H_2N–CO–NH^- Nucleophile (urea) + C_2H_5OH

Nucleophilic attack on ethyl acetoacetate: The nucleophile attacks electrophilic center of ethyl acetoacetate and generates β-uraminocrotonic ester.

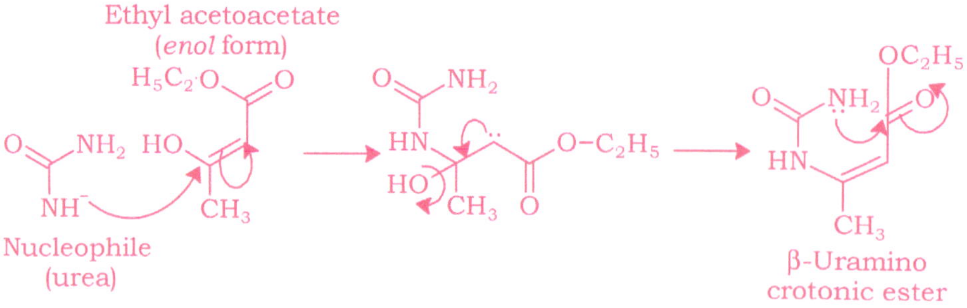

Ethyl acetoacetate (*enol* form)

Nucleophile (urea)

β-Uramino crotonic ester

Preparation of 6-methyluracil (desulfuration): The β-uraminocrotonic ester upon acid catalysed cyclization forms the 6-methyluracil.

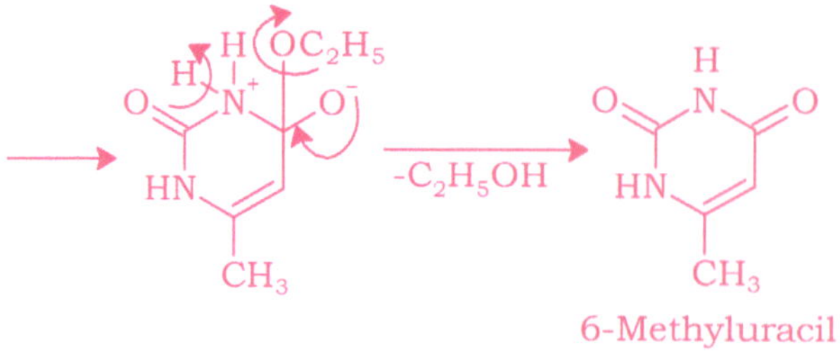

$-C_2H_5OH$

6-Methyluracil

Procedure:

Chemicals Required:Ethyl acetoacetate, Urea, Ethanol, Sodium hydroxide, Hydrochloric acid, Ether.

Step 1: Preparation of β-uraminocrotonic ester

1. Mix powdered urea (80 g, 1.33 mol), ethyl acetoacetate (155 mL, 1.23 mol) with absolute ethanol (25 mL).
2. Transfer the mixture into a beaker.
3. Add ten drops of concentrated sulphuric acid mix well and cover with watch glass.
4. Place the beaker in vacuum desiccators for 7 days to produce β-uraminocrotonic ester.

Step 2: Preparation of 6-methyluracil

1. Stir β-uraminocrotonic ester with a solution of sodium hydroxide (80 g, 2 mol) in water (1.2 L).
2. Cool the clear solution to 65 °C, and acidify slowly with concentrated hydrochloric acid.
3. The 6-methyluracil separates and isolate the product by filtration.
4. Wash the product with cold water, alcohol, ether and dry the product.
5. The melting point of pure 6-methyluracil is 318 °C.

KEY POINTS

- Fisher and Roeder (1901) demonstrated the practical synthesis of uracil by condensing urea with ethylhydroxymethyleneacetate.
- Uracil is the central core in several therapeutic molecules such as anticancer (5-flurouracil), antithyroid (propylthiouracil) and antiherpes (cidofovir) agents.

38

Vilsmeier-Haack Reaction

Anton Vilsmeir (German chemist) together with Albrecht Haack discovered the formylation reaction and is widely accepted for the aldehyde synthesis. This reaction is known as Vilsmeier-Haack reaction. N,N-Dimethylformamide (DMF) and phosphorous oxychloride ($POCl_3$) reacts to produce N,N-dimethylchloroiminium ion (Vilsmeier-Haack /formylating reagent). Phosphorous oxychloride can be replaced with oxalyl chloride and thionyl chloride. Similarly, *N*-methylformanilide can be used in place of DMF. The electrophilic substitution of electron rich aromatic ring by N,N-dimethylchloroiminium ion introduces aldehyde group (formylation). This reaction is special type of Friedel-Crafts reaction.

EDG–C6H5 —(DMF, $POCl_3$)→ EDG–C6H4–CHO

$(H_3C)_2N$–CHO + Cl–P(Cl)(Cl)=O —($-POCl_2$)→ [$(H_3C)_2N$–$\overset{+}{C}H$–Cl ⟶ $(H_3C)_2\overset{+}{N}$=CH-Cl]

N,N-Dimethyl formamide; Phosphorous oxychloride; N,N-Dimethylchloroiminium ion

Reaction Mechanism

Formation of formylating agent

Phosphorous oxychloride

N,N-Dimethyl formamide

$-Cl^-$

Cl^-

N,N-Dimethyl chloroiminium ion (formylating reagent) $(H_3C)_2\overset{+}{N}$=CH-Cl

Formylation

EDG
H_3C
$\overset{+}{N}$=CH-Cl
H_3C
N,N-Dimethyl chloroiminium ion (formylating reagent)
H Cl
CH_3
N
CH_3
EDG
Cl
CH_3
N
CH_3
EDG
CH_3
N
CH_3
EDG
Hydrolysis
CHO
EDG
Formylated product (Aldehyde)

EDG: electron withdrawing group

Pharmaceutical Applications

1. Preparation of isoflavones.

O
HO OH
2-Phenyl-2',4'-dihydroxy acetophenone
DMF
$POCl_3$
O
HO O
Isoflavones

2. Preparation of pyrans.

O O
1,3,5-triphenylpentane-1,5-dione
DMF
$POCl_3$
O
2,4,6-triphenyl tetrahydropyran

3. Preparation of furans.

H_3C CH_3
O O
Acetonyl acetone
DMF
$POCl_3$
OHC
H_3C O CH_3
2,5-dimethylfuran-3-carbaldehyde

4. Preparation of lamellarin-R (anticancer).

38.1 Preparation of 2-Phenylindole-3-carbaldehyde

IUPAC Name: 2-Phenyl-1H-indole-3-carbladehyde **Mol wt**: 221.25 g/mol

Principle: The formylation of indole ring with Vilsmeier-Haack reagent produces 2-phenylindole-3-carbaldehyde. N,N-Dimethylformamide and phosphorous oxychloride are useful in generating Vilsmeier-Haack reagent (N,N-dimethylchloroiminium ion). Pyrrole ring of indole (electron rich) attacks the reagent (electrophile) and forms schiff base. The Schiff base upon hydrolysis by aqueous sodium acetate yields, indole-3-carbaldehyde.

Reaction Mechanism

Formation of formylating agent

Formylation

N,N-Dimethyl chloroiminium ion

2-Phenylindole

CH_3COONa

Hydrolysis

2-Phenylindole-3-carbaldehyde

Procedure:

Chemicals Required: 2-Phenylindole, Phosphorous oxychloride, Dimethyl formamide, Sodium acetate.

1. Place distilled dimethylformamide (2.9 mL, 374 mmol) in three necked flask.
2. Attach reflux condenser which in turn fitted with calcium guard tube to the flask.
3. Cool the contents by placing in an ice-salt bath for about 30 min and slowly add distilled phosphorous oxychloride (0.86 mL, 9.4 mmol) with stirring.

   (*progress of formylation reaction develops pinkish colour*).
4. Slowly add the solution of 2-phenylindole (1 g, 8.5 mmol) in dimethyl formamide (1 mL, 13 mmol) to the reaction mixture and maintain the temperature below 10 °C.
5. Elevate the temperature to 35 °C, after the addition of 2-phenylindole solution.
6. Stirr the syrup formed until yellow solution turns into opaque canary yellow paste (~1 h).
7. Add crushed ice (3 g) to the paste with stirring, which turns the paste into cherry-red solution.

   (*Cool the paste in an ice-bath before adding the ice to it, because non-aqueous paste on treatment with ice generates heat (exothermic)*)

8. Transfer the solution into a three necked flask containing crushed ice (2 g) provided with mechanical stirrer and dropping funnel containing a solution of sodium hydroxide (3.8 g in 100 mL of water).
9. Add one third of the sodium hydroxide drop-wise with stirring and remaining rapidly with stirring.

   (*after red colour changes to greenish blue or greenish yellow*)
10. Add water (10 mL) to break the cake formed and to ease the stirring.
11. Boil the suspension (develops yellow-orange solution), cool to room temperature and place it in the refrigerator overnight.
12. Collect the precipitate on a filter paper and resuspend in water (100 mL), filter, wash with three 30 mL portions of water and dry.
13. Purify the product by recrystallization with ethanol.
14. The melting range of pure 2-phenylindole-3-carbaldehyde is 196 to 197 °C.

KEY POINTS

- Formylation of aromatic compounds (aldehyde synthesis) is known as Vilsmeier-Haack reaction.
- Vilsmeier-Haack reaction is a special type of Friedel-Crafts reaction.
- Lamellarin-R (anticancer agent) synthesis involves Vilsmeier-Haack formylation reaction.

39

VON Baeyer Synthesis

Albert von Baeyer (German Chemist) isolated the barbituric acid from uric acid investigations. Baeyer reported the chemical synthesis of first barbiturate from malonic acid in the year 1864. The condensation of urea and malonic acid in presence of absolute ethanol and sodium metal rendered barbiturate. It had no therapeutic effect, but served as lead for the development of therapeutically active barbiturates such as phenobarbitone. The substitution of alkyl, cycloalkyl and aryl groups to C_5 position produced therapeutically significant molecules.

$$\text{Urea} + \text{Malonic acid} \xrightarrow[\Delta]{C_2H_5OH,\ Na} \text{Barbituric acid}$$

The use of melonic ester in place of malonic acid favoured the condensation reaction.

Barbiturate therapeutics

Fisher and von Mering (1903), synthesized the therapeutically significant barbiturates attaching two ethyl groups to the C_5 position of barbiturate. This compound is known as barbital. Barbiturates posses sedative, hypnotic, anti-psychotic and anti-depressant effects. Phenobarbital was the first marketed barbiturate.

1. Synthesis of sedative and hypnotics drug- pentobarbitone: The condensation of 2-ethyl-2-pentyl diethylmalonate in presence of absolute ethanol and sodium metal produces pentobarbitone.

$$\text{Urea} + \text{2-Ethyl-2-pentyl diethylmalonate} \xrightarrow[\Delta]{C_2H_5OH,\ Na} \text{Pentobarbitone}$$

2. Synthesis of anti-convulsant - phenobarbitone: The condensation of 2-ethyl-2-phenyl diethylmalonate in presence of absolute ethanol and sodium metal produces phenobarbitone.

Urea + 2-Ethyl-2-phenyl diethylmalonate $\xrightarrow[\Delta]{C_2H_5OH,\ Na}$ Phenobarbitone

3. Synthesis of general anaesthetic drug methohexital: The condensation of 2-hexynyl-2-propenyl diethylmalonate in presence of absolute ethanol and sodium metal produces methohexital.

N-Methylurea + 2-Hexynyl,2-propenyl diethylmalonate $\xrightarrow[\Delta]{C_2H_5OH,\ Na}$ Methohexital

39.1 Preparation of Barbital

IUPAC Name: 5,5-Diethyl-1,3-diazine-2,4,6-trione **Mol wt**: 184.19 g/mol

Principle: Barbital can be synthesized by condensing urea and 2,2'-diethyl diethylmalonate in presence of absolute ethanol and sodium metal. The condensation can be effected by replacing the sodium ethoxide with phosphorous oxychloride effectively.

Urea + 2,2'-Diethyl diethyl malonate $\longrightarrow$ Barbital

Reaction Mechanism

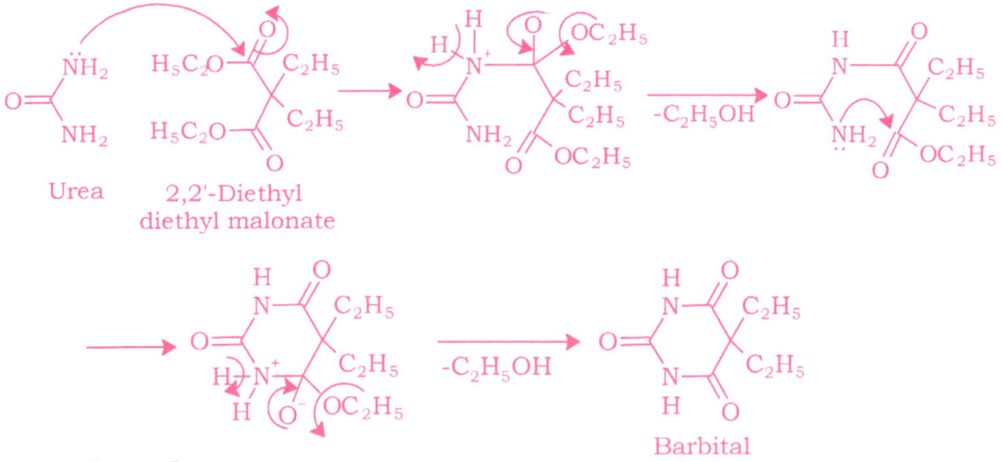

Urea

2,2'-Diethyl diethyl malonate

$-C_2H_5OH$

$-C_2H_5OH$

Barbital

Procedure:

Method 1

Chemicals Required: Urea, Sodium metal, Diethyl diethyl malonate, Ethanol and Hydrochloric acid.

Experimental steps

1. Place absolute ethanol (4 mL) and sodium metal (0.32 g, 14 mmol) into the round bottom flask.
2. Cool the mixture by placing in an ice-bath (if mixture becomes vigorous).
3. Add diethyl diethyl malonate (2 mL, 14 mmol) and solution of urea (0.84 g, 14 mmol) in hot absolute ethanol (4 mL) to the flask.
4. Shake the flask rapidly to precipitate the white solid.
5. Attach reflux condenser to the flask (fitted with calcium guard tube) and reflux the mixture for 7 h at 110 ºC.
6. Add hot water (8 mL, 50 ºC) and hydrochloric acid to acidify the mixture.
7. Cool the reaction mixture overnight in refrigerator.
8. Collect the separated barbital by vacuum filtration and wash with cold water (5 mL).
9. The melting range of the pure barbital is 188 to 192 ºC.

Method 2

Chemicals Required: Urea, Sodium metal, Diethyl diethyl malonate, Ethanol, and Hydrochloric acid.

1. Place diethyl diethylmalonate (2 mL, 14 mmol) and solution of urea (0.84 g, 14 mmol) in hot absolute ethanol (4 mL) into the round bottom flask.
2. Add phosphorous oxychloride (3 mL) to the flask.
3. Attach reflux condenser to the flask (fitted with calcium guard tube) and reflux the mixture for 7 h at 110 ºC.

4. Add hot water (8 mL, 50 ºC) and hydrochloric acid to acidify the mixture.
5. Cool the reaction mixture overnight in refrigerator.
6. Collect the separated barbital by vacuum filtration and wash with cold water (5 mL).
7. The melting range of the pure barbital is 188 to 192 ºC.

KEY POINTS

- The condensation of urea and diethyl diethyl malonate acid in presence of absolute ethanol and sodium metal produces barbiturate and the reaction is known as Von Baeyer synthesis.
- Barbiturates produce sedative, hypnotic, anti-psychotic and anti-depressant effects.
- Phenobarbitone and methohexital are the important centrally acting barbiturates.

40

Williamson's Ether Synthesis (Nucleophilic Substitution of alkaliode/ aryloxide S_N2)

The nucleophilic substitution of an alkoxide (alkali oxide) on an alkylating agent (haloalkane) generates an ether. This reaction is known as Williamson's ether synthesis. This reaction is also known as Williamson's etherification and Williamson reaction. The reaction establishes a new bond between a carbon of alkylating agent and nucleophile. This reaction also cleaves the bond between carbon and leaving group (carbon-halogen bond).

$$\underset{\text{Alcohol}}{\text{R-OH}} \xrightarrow[]{\text{Na, } C_2H_5OH} \underset{\text{Sodium salt of alkoxide}}{\text{R-ONa}} \xrightarrow{R^1\text{-X}} \underset{\text{Ether}}{\text{R-O-R}^1} + \text{Na-X}$$

The reaction produces both symmetrical and unsymmetrical ethers.

- Reaction between one alcohol and alkylating agent produces symmetrical ether.
- Reaction between different alcohols and alkylating agents produce asymmetrical ethers.

Haloalkanes are the most common alkylating agensts. Dialkyl sulphates, alkyl mesylates, tosylates, ethers of weak acids, dialkyl ethers, alkyl aryl ethers, and epoxides are useful in selective reactions. The reaction of alkoxide ion with 1° haloalkanes offers good yields. But, 2° and 3° haloalkanes (bulkier) are not suitable. The steric hindrance blocks the nucleophilic effect.

General Reaction Mechanism

Alkali alkoxide offers alkoxide, which is nucleophile in this reaction. This nucleophilic substitution follows S_N2 mechanism. The reaction mechanism can be explained in the following steps.

Step 1: Generation of alkoxide

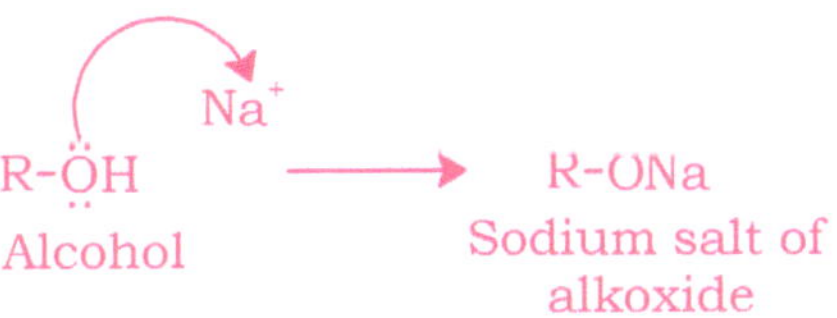

Sodium ethoxide removes the hydrogen from the hydroxyl group of substrate and generates alkoxide ion.

Step 2: Formation of ether (nucleophilic substitution, S_N2)

R-ÖNa (Sodium salt of alkoxide) + R^1-X ⟶ R-O-R^1 (Ether) + Na–X

The negative charge on alkoxide oxygen is unstable, which favours the alkyl halide to attach alkyl group to the oxygen and forms ether product.

Characteristics of Reactants

- The nucleophile must be small and should bear high electron density.
- The carbon (sp3) center must be unhindered.
- The leaving group must be weaker than the incoming nucleophile.
- Polar aprotic solvent is the choice, S_N2 reactions are well promoted in polar aprotic solvents.
- The amount of free alkoxide depends on the size of alkali cation and the polarity of the solvent.

Pharmaceutical Applications

1. Synthesis of anisole.

Phenol + CH_3I $\xrightarrow{NaOH}$ Anisole (C_6H_5-O-CH_3) + NaI + H_2O

2. Synthesis of phenetole.

Phenol + CH_3-CH_2–I $\xrightarrow{NaOH}$ Phenetole (C_6H_5-O-CH_2-CH_3) + NaI + H_2O

3. Synthesis of phenacetin.

Paracetamol (OH, $NHCOCH_3$) + CH_3CH_2I $\xrightarrow{NaOH}$ Phenacetin (OCH_2CH_3, $NHCOCH_3$) + NaI + H_2O

40.1 Preparation of Phenetole

Traditional Name: Ethylphenylether

IUPAC Name: Ethoxy benzene **Mol wt**: 122.16 g/mol

Principle: Phenetole (phenolic ethyl ether) can be prepared through Williamson's ether synthesis. The nucleophilic reaction between the phenol (phenoxide form) and ethyl iodide (alkylating agent) in presence of sodium hydroxide produces phenetole. Sodium hydroxide converts the phenol into phenoxide. The phenetole, product of Williamson ether synthesis is unsymmetrical ether.

Phenol (OH) + CH_3-CH_2-I $\xrightarrow{NaOH}$ Phenetole (O-CH_2-CH_3) + NaI + H_2O

General Reaction Mechanism

Step 1: Generation of alkoxide

Phenol (OH) $\xrightarrow{NaOH}$ Sodium phenoxide (ONa) + NaI + H_2O

The base (sodium hydroxide) removes the hydrogen from the hydroxyl group of phenol and generates sodium phenoxide ion.

Step 2: Formation of ether (nucleophilic substitution, S_N2)

Sodium salt of phenoxide (:ÖNa) + CH_3-CH_2-I $\xrightarrow{-Na^+}$ CH_3-CH_2-O^+(I) $\xrightarrow{-NaI}$ Phenetole (O-CH_2-CH_3)

The negative charge on sodium phenoxide is unstable, which favours the ethyl iodide to attach ethyl group to the phenoxide and forms ether product (phenetole).

Procedure:

Chemicals Required: Phenol, Sodium hydroxide, Ethyl iodide, Sodium chloride, Diethyl ether.

Experimental steps

1. Place phenol (4.9 g, 52 mmol) to the flask charged with solution of sodium hydroxide (2.4 g in 12 mL of water).
2. Stir the mixture to make a homogeneous solution.
3. Add ethyl iodide (4 mL, 500 mmol) dropwise with vigorous stirring (maintain the temperature below 65 °C).
4. Attach reflux condenser to the flask and heat the contents for 3 h.
5. Transfer the contents of flask to a separating funnel and mix it with saturated sodium chloride solution (3 mL).
6. Drain the lower aqueous phase and extract the remaining mixture with diethyl ether (5 mL).

   (aqueous soluble contents, such as unreacted phenol, sodium iodide can be removed)
7. Distil the ether layer at 38-40 °C and collect phenetole.
8. The boiling range of phenetole is 169 to 170 °C.

40.2 Preparation of Phenacetin

IUPAC Name: N(4-Ethoxyphenyl) acetamide **Mol wt**: 179.22 g/mol

Principle: Phenacetin, a non-steroidal anti-inflammatory drug can be prepared through Williamson ether synthesis. The nucleophilic reaction between the paracetamol (phenoxide form) and ethyl iodide (alkylating agent) in presence of sodium ethoxide produces phenacetin. Dry sodium in absolute ethanol generates sodium ethoxide *in situ*. This product is unsymmetrical in nature.

OH ... $NHCOCH_3$ Paracetamol + CH_3CH_2I $\xrightarrow[Na]{C_2H_5OH}$ OCH_2CH_3 ... $NHCOCH_3$ Phenacetin + NaI

General Reaction Mechanism

Step 1: Generation of alkoxide

OH ... $NHCOCH_3$ Paracetamol $\xrightarrow[Na^+]{C_2H_5OH}$ ONa ... $NHCOCH_3$ Sodium salt of phenoxide + NaI

The sodium ethoxide removes the hydrogen from the phenolic hydroxyl group and generates phenoxide ion.

Step 2: Formation of ether (nucleophilic substitution, S_N2)

$:\ddot{O}Na$ CH_3-CH_2-I → ($-Na^+$) → $CH_3\cdot CH_2-O^+-I$ → ($-NaI$) → OCH_2CH_3

$NHCOCH_3$ $NHCOCH_3$ $NHCOCH_3$

Sodium salt of phenoxide

Phenacetin

The negative charge on sodium phenoxide is unstable, which favours the ethyl iodide to attach ethyl group to the phenoxide and forms ether product (phenacetin).

Procedure:

Chemicals Required: Paracetamol, Sodium metal, Ethanol, Ethyl iodide.

Experimental steps

1. Place sodium metal pieces (155 mg, 6.8 mmol) to the flask containing absolute ethanol (4 mL).
2. Attach condenser and warm the flask (if necessary) to dissolve sodium completely.
3. Cool the mixture and add paracetamol (1 g, 6.6 mmol) slowly followed by ethyl iodide (0.8 mL, 10 mmol), slowly through condenser.
4. Reflux the mixture for 1 h.
5. Pour 10 mL of water through the condenser to prevent product crystallization (if crystals do separate, reflux the mixture until they dissolve).
6. Cool the flask by placing in an ice-bath, collect the phenacetin through vacuum filtration and wash with cold water.
7. Dissolve the crude phenacetin with 8 mL of ethanol (treat with charcoal boil and filter, if the solution appears colour).
8. Pour the clear solution obtained into beaker containing hot water (15 mL).
9. Allow it to cool and collect the solid product of pure phenacetin through filtration.
10. The melting range of pure phenacetin is 135 to 137 °C.

Note: Ref 3.2 (page 51) for the preparation of paracetamol.

KEY POINTS

- The nucleophilic substitution (S_N2) of an alkoxide (or alkali oxide) with an alkylating agent (haloalkane) generates an ether and the reaction is known as Williamson's ether synthesis.
- Analgesic and antipyretic molecule phenacetin can be synthesised adopting Williamson ether synthesis.
- Sodium metal-precautions: Sodium reacts with water vigorously, hence utmost care should be taken while handling sodium metal.

41

Wohl-Ziegler Reaction

Wohl-Ziegler reaction involves the free radical-based bromination of hydorocarbons (allylic or benzyllic) using an *N*-bromosuccinamide (NBS). Alfred Wohler (German Chemist, 1919), reported the bromination of 2,3-dimethyl-2-butene using NBS in diethyl ether. He observed that the bromination occurred at allylic position without affecting the double bond of butane. The free radical environment requires the stable solvent and anhydrous carbon tetrachloride (CCl_4) is identified as the suitable one. Acetonitrile, ionic liquids and solvent free (net) reactions are also effective. Succinamide formed after the bromination is insoluble in carbon tetrachloride or chloroform, hence it can be removed by filtration.

CH_3 H_3C–C=C–CH_3 CH_3 —NBS, CCl_4→ CH_3 H_3C–C=C–CH_2Br CH_3

2,3-Dimethyl-2-butene   1-Bromo-2,3-dimethyl-2-butene

The radical initiators, namely azobisisobutyronitrile (AIBN), benzoyl peroxide and UV radiation favor the homolytic cleavage of bromine bond and generate bromine radical. Conjugated olefins and 1,4-dienes does not undergo Wohl-Ziegler reaction as they are inhibitors of the reaction.

Reaction Mechanism

In order to achieve the region specific bromination, NBS is very much useful. NBS releases bromine *in situ* and offers the controlled bromination.

Bloomfield's mechanism

I· Radical initiator + Br–N (N-Bromo succinamide) —-HBr→ ·N (N-Bromosuccinamide radical)

N-Bromo succinamide   N-Bromosuccinamide radical

CH_3 H_3C C C CH_2–H CH_3 ·N O O → CH_3 H_3C C C $\dot{C}H_2$ CH_3 + HN O O

2,3-Dimethyl-2-butene — 2,3-Dimethyl-2-butene radical — Succinamide

CH_3 H_3C C C $\dot{C}H_2$ CH_3 Br–N O O —CCl_4→ CH_3 H_3C C C CH_2Br CH_3

2,3-Dimethyl-2-butene radical — N-Bromo succinamide — 1-Bromo-2,3-dimethyl-2-butene

Pharmaceutical Applications

NBS is convenient source of cationic bromine, used in radical substitution and electrophilic addition reactions.

1. Synthesis of carbamazepine (anti-convulsant drug).

10,11-Dihydro-5H-dibenzoazepine —NBS→ (Br) N H ⟶⟶ N O NH_2 Carbamazepine

2. Synthesis of oseltamivir (anti-influenza drug).

tert-Butyl 7-oxo-6-azabicyclo [3.2.1]oct-3-ene-6-carboxylate —NBS, CCl_4→ Br ... ⟶⟶ Oseltamivir phosphate (H_3C, CH_3, O, H, N, H_3C, O, H_3N^+, OC_2H_5, O, $H_2PO_4^-$)

3. Preparation of anastrazole (anti-breast cancer, aromatase inhibitor).

3,5-bis(2-cyanoprop-2-yl) toluene $\xrightarrow[CCl_4]{NBS}$ (bromomethyl intermediate) $\xrightarrow[DMF]{\text{1,2,4-triazole}}$ Anastrazole

41.1 Preparation of 3-Bromocyclohexene

IUPAC Name: 3-Bromocyclohex-1-ene **Mol wt**: 161.03 g/mol

Principle: Free radical-based bromination of cyclohexene at allylic carbon using with *N*-bromosuccinamide produces 3-bromocyclohexene. This is a typical example of Wohl-Ziegler reaction. The bromination reaction proceeds effectively using carbon tetrachloride as a solvent and benzoyl peroxide as a free radical initiator.

Cyclohexene $\xrightarrow[CCl_4]{NBS}$ 3-Bromocyclohexene

Reaction Mechanism

The free radical initiator (benzoyl peroxide) abstracts bromide from NBS and generates free radical. The NBS radical abstracts the allylic proton from cyclohexene to produce cyclohexene free radical. The cyclohexene radical undergoes bromination by NBS and generates 3-bromocyclohexene.

Benzoyl peroxide radical + N-Bromo succinamide $\xrightarrow{-HBr}$ Free radical

Cyclohexene → Cyclohexene radical + Succinamide

Cyclohexene radical + N-Bromo succinamide → 3-Bromocyclohexene

Procedure:

Chemicals Required: Cyclohexene, *N*-Bromosuccinamide, Carbon tetrachloride, Benzoyl peroxide.

1. Transfer *N*-bromosuccinamide (0.98 g, 5 mmol), redistilled cyclohexene (1.23 g, 15 mmol), carbon tetrachloride (4 mL) and benzoyl peroxide (12.5 mg) in a round bottom flask.

   (*benzoyl peroxide must be previously dried by pressing between filter papers*).
2. Attach double surface condenser to the flask and allow it to stand at room temperature for 10 min.

   (*yellowish N-bromosuccinamide becomes colourless and gets suspended in the flask*).
3. Heat the contents of the flask for 2 h by placing on the steam bath.
4. Cool the flask, filter under suction (vaccum) and wash the residue with carbon tetrachloride.
5. Distill the filtrate to remove carbon tetrachloride (b.p. 77 °C) and unreacted cyclohexene (b.p. 83 °C).
6. Distil the residue under reduced pressure to collect 3-bromocyclohexene at 72 to 77 °C.

   (*carbon tetrachloride and cyclohexane will come in first fraction*).
7. The following fraction goes brown on standing, subsequent distillation gives colourless 3-bromocyclohexene.

Starch-iodide paper test*:* The completion of the reaction may be confirmed by treating starch-iodide paper with a drop of the reaction mixture. The appearance of no colour in starch iodide paper indicates the completion of the reaction.

Precautions:

1. NBS decomposes over time giving off bromine, hence it should be stored in a refrigerator.
2. Reactions involving NBS are exothermic; hence precautions are required, in particular for large scale preparations.
3. The use of redistilled cyclohexene is advised for the effective completion of the reaction.

KEY POINTS

- The bromination at allylic position using the N-bromosuccinamide is known as Wohl-Ziegler reaction.
- This bromination occurs without affecting the double bond.
- Carbamazepine (anticonvulsant), Oseltamivir (anti-viral), anastrazole (anti-cancer) synthesis requires bromination and can be effected using Wohl-Ziegler reaction.
- Reactions involving NBS are exothermic; hence precautions are required, in particular for large scale preparations.

42

Semi Quantitative Analysis

Limit Test

Any material present in medicinal preparations, besides the active ingredient / excipient is considered as an impurity. Impurities include starting materials, by-products, interaction products, intermediates, penultimate intermediates, degradation products, reagents, ligands, catalysts and residual solvents. All the medicinal substances should be free from dangerous and/or objectionable impurities. The presence of sodium bromide in potassium bromide (hypnotic and sedative) will not produce any harm, but in large proportion reduces the medicinal value of potassium bromide. The impurities remain in active pharmaceutical ingredients (APIs) are inevitable, and even in trace amount they may influence the efficacy and safety of APIs. They may produce teratogenic, carcinogenic and mutagenic effects. The pharmaceutical industry is heavily regulated and led to the mandatory examination of all substances from starting materials to finished products. Regulation generally includes:

- Proof of product stability.
- Drug-release profiles.
- Active Pharmaceutical Ingredient (API) authentification.
- Product safety including sterility.
- Foreign materials including heavy-metals.

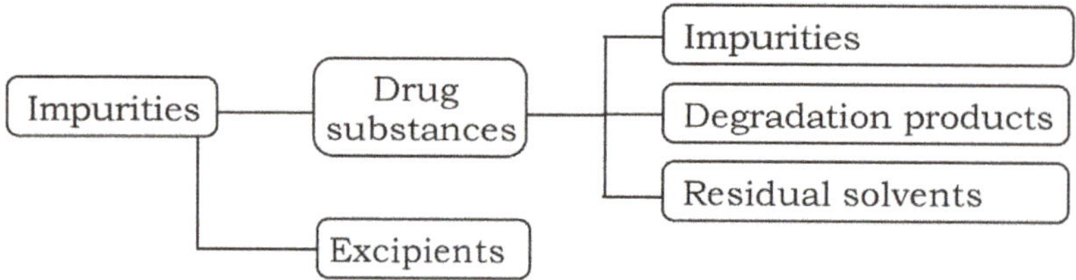

Different types of impurities known are:

1. ***Specified impurities***: An impurity that is individually listed and limited with a specific acceptance criterion in the specification.
2. ***Unspecified impurities***: An impurity that is limited by a general acceptance criterion, but not individually listed with its own specific acceptance criterion in the specification.

3. ***Identified impurities***: An impurity for which structural characterization has been achieved.
4. ***Unidentified impurities***: An impurity for which structural characterization has not been achieved and that is defined solely by qualitative analytical properties.

Limit test

One of the most common product safety-related analytical test is Limit Test. It is one of the quantification method of inorganics and/or heavy metals present in pharmaceuticals. Most of the heavy metals have significant health risks from organ failure to death. Lead, mercury, bismuth, arsenic, antimony, tin, cadmium, silver, copper, and molybdenum are the important heavy metals. Their presence in pharmaceuticals should be limited. Limit test involves the simple comparison of opalescence, turbidity and colour intensity of the samples with fixed standards.

In general, all the limit tests are carried out with an aqueous solution of the substance. But special methods are applied for selective cases.

- An alkaline substance has to be neutralized with nitric acid or hydrochloric acid.
- Water insoluble substance has to be dissolved in acid (alternatively aqueous extract can be used).

42.1 Limit Test for Chlorides

Limit test for chlorides

Principle

The chloride limit test determines the permissible limit of chloride content in the pharmaceuticals. The principle involved in the limit test for chlorides can be explained through the following steps.

- ***Chemical interaction***: Limit test for chlorides depends upon the interaction of chloride impurities present in the sample with silver nitrate in presence of dilute nitric acid.

  Importance of nitric acid: The use of hydrochloric acid instead of nitric acid produces interference in the visualization. Hydrochloric acid forms silver carbonates and oxides. Use of nitric acid prevents the formation of silver carbonates and oxides.
- ***Formation of opalescence***: Chloride content of the test (or standard) sample reacts with silver nitrate and forms fine precipitate of silver chloride. The

$$\underset{\text{Chloride ion}}{Cl^-} + \underset{\text{Silver nitrate}}{AgNO_3} \xrightarrow{\text{dilute } HNO_3} \underset{\text{Silver chloride}}{AgCl\downarrow} + NO_3^-$$

silver chloride precipitate produces opalescence.

- ***Comparison of opalescence***: The comparison of opalescence produced by the test sample with the opalescence produced by the standard under uniform conditions is basis for the conclusions.

Procedure

S. No.	Standard Nessler Cylinder	Test Nessler Cylinder
1	Transfer 1 mL of standard solution of sodium chloride (25 ppm) into a Nessler cylinder.	Transfer specified quantity (or 1 g) of test sample into a Nessler cylinder.
2	Dilute with 10 mL of distilled water.	Dissolve with 10 mL of distilled water.
3	Add 10 mL of dilute nitric acid.	Add 10 mL of dilute nitric acid.
4	Dilute to 50 mL with distilled water.	Dilute to 50 mL with distilled water.
5	Add 1 mL of silver nitrate (0.1 M) reagent.	Add 1 mL of silver nitrate (0.1 M) reagent.
6	Stir it immediately with a glass rod.	Stir it immediately with a glass rod.
7	Allow it to stand for 5 min (protect from sunlight).	Allow it to stand for 5 min (protect from sunlight).

Observation: The Nessler cylinders (standard and test) should be viewed transversely (vertically) through liquid against black background. Compare the opalescence produced by the test sample with the opalescence produced by the standard.

Table 42.1 The list of inorganic compounds and permissible limit of chloride.

Inorganic compound	Quantity	Water Solubility	Pre-treatment	Limits (in ppm)*
Dextrose	20 mL; 10% w/v	Soluble	NA	125
Sodium bicarbonate	1.25 g	Soluble	NA	200
Calcium gluconate	1 g	Soluble	NA	250
Potassium permanganate	1.5 g	Soluble	Given below in the box	250
Calamine	0.33 g	Insoluble	Acid washings of calamine	750

* as per IP 2022; NA: not available

Purple colour of potassium permanganate interferes with the limit test results.

- Boiling potassium permanganate with ethanol overcomes this problem. Potassium permanganate oxidizes the ethanol into acetaldehyde and gets reduced into insoluble manganese dioxide (brown precipitate), which can be removed by filtration. The clear filtrate can be subjected for the limit test.

$$\underset{\text{Potassium permanganate}}{2\,KMnO_4} + \underset{\text{Ethanol}}{3\,C_2H_5OH} \longrightarrow \underset{\text{Manganase dioxide}}{2\,MnO_2\downarrow} + \underset{\text{Potassium hydroxide}}{2\,KOH} + \underset{\text{Acetaldehyde}}{3\,CH_3CHO} + 2\,H_2O$$

- Boiling potassium permanganate with hydrogen peroxide and sulphuric acid also overcomes the solubility problem.

$$\underset{\text{Potassium permanganate}}{2\,KMnO_4} + \underset{\text{Hydrogen peroxide}}{5\,H_2O_2} + 3\,H_2SO_4 \longrightarrow \underset{\text{Potassium sulphate}}{K_2SO_4} + \underset{\text{Manganse sulphate}}{MnSO_4} + 8\,H_2O + 5\,O_2\uparrow$$

42.2 Limit Test for Sulphates

Principle

The sulphate limit test determines the permissible limit of sulphate content in the pharmaceuticals. The principle involved in the sulphate limit test can be explained through the following steps.

- ***Chemical interaction:*** Limit test for sulphate depends upon the interaction of soluble sulphate with barium chloride in presence of acetic acid and ethanolic standard sulphate solution.
  - o The ethanolic sulphate standard solution acts as seeding agent and increases the sensitivity of the turbidity formation.
  - o Ethanol prevents the super saturation.
  - o Acetic acid provides acidic environment and facilitates the turbidity formation.
- ***Formation of turbidity:*** Sulphate content of the test (or standard) sample reacts with barium chloride and forms turbidity. A very fine dispersed precipitate of barium sulphate produces the turbidity.

$$\underset{\text{Sulphate ion}}{SO_4^{2-}} + \underset{\text{Barium chloride}}{BaCl_2} \xrightarrow[\text{(5 M)}]{CH_3COOH} \underset{\text{Barium sulphate}}{BaSO_4\downarrow} + 2Cl^-$$

- ***Comparison of turbidity***: The comparison of turbidity produced by the test sample with the turbidity produced by the standard under uniform conditions is basis for the conclusions.

In this method, the hydrochloric acid is replaced with the acetic acid (5 M). Hydrochloric acid is useful in dissolving the barium carbonate precipitate, if any. But the hydrochloric acid is strongly acidic, hence also may dissolve the barium sulphate precipitate (turbidity). This demanded for the weak acid, hence acetic acid is substituted for hydrochloric acid. Similarly, the barium sulphate reagent is replaced with barium chloride solution. The sequential addition of ethanolic sulphate standard solution both in test and standard Nessler cylinders is useful in visualizing the distinct turbidity produced.

Procedure

S. No.	Standard Nessler Cylinder	Test Nessler Cylinder
1	Transfer 1 mL of 25% w/v solution of barium chloride into a Nessler cylinder.	Transfer 1 mL of a 25% w/v solution of barium chloride into a Nessler cylinder.
2	Add 1.5 mL of ethanolic sulphate standard solution (10 ppm).	Add 1.5 mL of ethanolic sulphate standard solution (10 ppm).

Table *Contd...*

S. No.	Standard Nessler Cylinder	Test Nessler Cylinder
3	Add 15 mL of the standard sulphate solution (10 ppm).	Add 15 mL of the test sample solution prepared as per the monograph into a Nessler cylinder (alternatively, solution of specified quantity of the test sample in 15 mL of water can be used).
4	Add 3 drops of acetic acid (5 M).	Add 3 drops of acetic acid (5 M).
5	Add sufficient distilled water to produce 50 mL.	Add sufficient distilled water to produce 50 mL.
6	Stir immediately with a glass rod.	Stir it immediately with a glass rod.
7	Allow it to stand for 5 min.	Allow it to stand for 5 min.

Observation: The Nessler cylinders (standard and test) should be viewed transversely (vertically) through liquid against black background. Compare the turbidity produced by the test sample with the turbidity produced by the standard.

Table 42.2 The list of inorganic compounds and permissible limit of sulphate.

Inorganic compound	Quantity	Water Solubility	Pre-treatment	Limits (in ppm)*
Dextrose	7.5 mL (10% w/v)	Soluble	NA	200
Sodium bicarbonate	1 g	Soluble	NA	150
Calcium gluconate	1 g	Soluble	NA	150
Ammonium chloride	1 g	Soluble	NA	150
Potassium permanganate	10 mL (pre-treatment solution)	Soluble	Required	600
Calamine	0.25 g	Insoluble	Required	0.6%

* as per IP 2022; NA: not applicable

Purple colour of potassium permanganate interferes with the limit test results.

- Boiling potassium permanganate with ethanol overcomes this problem. Potassium permanganate oxidizes the ethanol into acetaldehyde and gets reduced into insoluble manganese dioxide (brown precipitate), which can be removed by filtration. The clear filtrate can be subjected for the limit test.

$$2\,KMnO_4 + 3\,C_2H_5OH \longrightarrow 2\,MnO_2\downarrow + 2\,KOH + 3\,CH_3CHO + 2\,H_2O$$

Potassium permanganate, Ethanol, Manganase dioxide, Potassium hydroxide, Acetaldehyde

- Boiling potassium permanganate with hydrogen peroxide and sulphuric acid also overcomes the solubility problem.

$$2\,KMnO_4 + 5\,H_2O_2 + 3\,H_2SO_4 \longrightarrow K_2SO_4 + MnSO_4 + 8\,H_2O + 5\,O_2\uparrow$$

Potassium permanganate, Hydrogen peroxide, Potassium sulphate, Manganse sulphate

42.3 Limit Test for Iron

Principle

The iron limit test determines the permissible limit of iron content in the pharmaceuticals.The principle involved in the limit test for iron can be explained through the following steps.

- ***Chemical interaction:*** Limit test for iron is based upon the interaction of iron with thioglycolic acid in presence of iron-free ammonia and iron-free citric acid. Thioglycolic acid also reduces ferric (Fe^{3+}, if any ferric impurities are present) to ferrous (Fe^{2+}).

$$\underset{\text{Ferric ion}}{Fe^{3+}} + \underset{\text{Thioglycolic acid}}{2\,HS{-}CH_2{-}COOH} \longrightarrow \underset{\text{Ferrous ion}}{Fe^{2+}} + \underset{\text{Dithioglycolic acid}}{\begin{matrix} S{-}CH_2{\cdot}COOH \\ | \\ S{-}CH_2{\cdot}COOH \end{matrix}}$$

- ***Formation of purple colour:*** The reaction between ferrous and thioglycolic acid generates ferrous thioglycolate complex. This complex produces a pale pink to deep reddish purple colour in ammonia medium. The purple colour disappears upon oxidation by atmospheric oxygen, hence it should be protected.
  - o Iron-free citric acid produces ammonium citrate buffer. This buffer stabilizes the ferrous thioglycolate complex and the colour.
  - o Iron-free citric acid (20%) forms complex with other metal ions (if any) and eliminates their interference.
  - o Iron-free ammonia solution provides alkaline medium. Ferrous thioglycolate complex develops purple colour only in alkaline medium.

$$\underset{\text{Ferrous ion}}{Fe^{2+}} + \underset{\text{Thioglycolic acid}}{2HS{-}CH_2{\cdot}COOH} \xrightarrow[\text{Iron-free ammonia}]{\text{Iron-free citric acid}} \underset{\text{(purple coloured complex)}}{\underset{\text{Ferrous thioglycolate complex}}{[\text{Fe chelate: } H_2C{-}S(H){\to}Fe{\leftarrow}S(H){-}CH_2,\ C(=O){-}O{-}Fe{-}O{-}C(=O)]}} + 2H^+$$

- ***Comparison of purple colour*:** The comparison of purple colour (ferrous thioglycollate complex) produced by the test sample with the purple colour produced by the standard under uniform conditions is basis for the conclusions.

Procedure

S. No.	Standard Nessler Cylinder	Test Nessler Cylinder
1	Transfer 2 mL of iron standard solution (20 ppm of Fe) into a Nessler cylinder.	Transfer specified quantity of the test sample (or 1 g) into a Nessler cylinder.
2	Dilute with 5 mL of distilled water.	Dissolve with 5 mL of distilled water.
3	Add 2 mL of 20% iron-free citric acid.	Add 2 mL of 20% iron-free citric acid.
4	Add 2 drops of thioglycolic acid.	Add 2 drops of thioglycolic acid.
5	Make the mixture alkaline with iron-free ammonia.	Make the mixture alkaline with iron-free ammonia.
6	Dilute to 50 mL with distilled water.	Dilute to 50 mL with distilled water.
7	Stir immediately with a glass rod.	Stir it immediately with a glass rod.
8	Allow it to stand for 5 min.	Allow it to stand for 5 min.

Observation: The Nessler cylinders (standard and test) should be viewed transversely (vertically) through liquid, against a white colour background (white tile can be used).

Table 42.3 The list of inorganic compounds and permissible limit of iron.

Inorganic compound	Quantity	Water Solubility	Limits (in ppm)*
Sodium bicarbonate	2 g	Soluble	20
Ammonium chloride	2 g	Soluble	20

* as per IP 2022

42.4 Limit Test for Heavy Metals (Method A)

Principle

The principle involved in the heavy metal limit test (method A) can be explained through the following steps.

- ***Chemical interaction:*** The principle involved in the limit test of heavy metals is the reaction of metallic impurities (e.g., lead) with hydrogen sulphide solution. Dilute acetic acid or ammonia is useful in maintaining the pH (3 to 4) of the mixture.
- ***Formation of colour:*** Heavy metal content of the test (or standard) sample reacts with hydrogen sulphide and forms lead sulphide. A very fine dispersed precipitate of lead sulphide produces brown colour to the solution.

$$\underset{\text{Lead ion}}{Pb^{2+}} + \underset{\text{Hydrogen sulphide}}{H_2S} \xrightarrow[]{\text{Dilute } CH_3COOH\ /NH_3} \underset{\text{Lead sulphide}}{PbS\downarrow} + 2H^+$$

- ***Comparison of brown colour***: The comparison of brown colour produced by the test sample with the brown colour produced by the standard under uniform conditions is basis for the conclusions.

Procedure

S. No.	Standard Nessler Cylinder	Test Nessler Cylinder
1	Transfer 1 mL of standard lead solution (20 ppm, Pb) into a Nessler cylinder. Dilute the solution with distilled water 25 mL.	Transfer 25 mL of the sample solution prepared as per monograph into a Nessler cylinder. (alternatively specified quantity of the test sample can be dissolved in 25 mL of water)
2	Adjust the pH between 3.0 to 4.0 using dilute acetic acid or ammonia.	Adjust the pH between 3.0 to 4.0 using dilute acetic acid or ammonia.
3	Dilute with ~35 mL of distilled water and mix well with glass rod.	Dilute with ~35 mL of distilled water and mix well with glass rod.
4	Add 10 mL of freshly prepared hydrogen sulphide solution.	Add 10 mL of freshly prepared hydrogen sulphide solution.
5	Make up the volume upto 50 mL with distilled water.	Make up the volume upto 50 mL with distilled water.
6	Stir it immediately with a glass rod.	Stir it immediately with a glass rod.
7	Allow it to stand for 5 min.	Allow it to stand for 5 min.

Observation: The Nessler cylinders (standard and test) should be viewed transversely (vertically) through a liquid, against a white colour background (white tile can be used). Compare the brown colour produced by the test sample with the brown colour produced by the standard.

42.5 Limit Test for Heavy Metals (Method B, Substances which do not produce clear solution)

Principle

The principle involved in the heavy metal limit test (method B) can be explained through the following steps.

- ***Chemical interaction:*** The principle involved in the limit test of heavy metals is the reaction of metallic impurities (e.g., lead) with hydrogen sulphide solution. Dilute acetic acid or ammonia is useful in maintaining the pH (3 to 4) of the mixture.
- ***Formation of colour:*** Heavy metal content of the test (or standard) sample reacts with hydrogen sulphide and forms lead sulphide. A very fine dispersed precipitate of lead sulphide produces brown colour to the solution.

$$\underset{\text{Lead ion}}{Pb^{2+}} + \underset{\text{Hydrogen sulphide}}{H_2S} \xrightarrow[]{\text{Dilute } CH_3COOH\ /NH_3} \underset{\text{Lead sulphide}}{PbS\downarrow} + 2H^+$$

- ***Comparison of brown colour*:** The comparison of brown colour produced by the test sample with the brown colour produced by the standard under uniform conditions is basis for the conclusions.

Procedure

Test sample pre-treatment:

1. Weigh specified quantity of the sample as per monograph and transfer into a crucible.
2. Add sufficient sulphuric acid to dissolve the contents and ignite at low temperature (until the sample gets charred thoroughly).
3. Add 2 mL of nitric acid and 5 drops of sulphuric acid to the charred mass.
4. Heat gently until no white fumes evolves.
5. Ignite at 500 to 600 °C (use Muffle furnace).
6. Cool, add 4 mL of hydrochloric acid, cover and digest for 15 min.
7. Moisten the residue with 1 drop of hydrochloric acid, add 10 mL of hot water and digest for 2 min.
8. Add ammonia solution dropwise, until the solution becomes alkaline (litmus paper test).
9. Dilute with distilled water (25 mL) and acidify with dilute acetic acid to adjust the pH between 3.0 to 4.0 (filter if necessary).
10. Rinse the crucible and filter with 10 mL of distilled water.
11. Collect the filtrate and washings in a Nessler cylinder.
12. Dilute with distilled water to produce 35 mL with distilled water.

S. No.	Standard Nessler Cylinder	Test Nessler Cylinder
1	Transfer 1 mL of standard lead solution (20 ppm, Pb) into a Nessler cylinder. Dilute the solution with distilled water 25 mL.	Transfer 25 mL of the sample solution prepared as per monograph into a Nessler cylinder. (alternatively specified quantity of the test sample can be dissolved in 25 mL of water)
2	Adjust the pH between 3.0 to 4.0 using dilute acetic acid or ammonia.	Adjust the pH between 3.0 to 4.0 using dilute acetic acid or ammonia.
3	Dilute with ~35 mL of distilled water and mix well with glass rod.	Dilute with ~35 mL of distilled water and mix well with glass rod.
4	Add 10 mL of freshly prepared hydrogen sulphide solution.	Add 10 mL of freshly prepared hydrogen sulphide solution.
5	Make up the volume upto 50 mL with distilled water.	Make up the volume upto 50 mL with distilled water.
6	Stir it immediately with a glass rod.	Stir it immediately with a glass rod.
7	Allow it to stand for 5 min.	Allow it to stand for 5 min.

Observation: The Nessler cylinders (standard and test) should be viewed transversely (vertically) through liquid, against a white colour background (white tile can be used). Compare the brown colour produced by the test sample with the brown colour produced by the standard.

42.6 Limit Test for Heavy Metals (Method C, for the substances which give clear solution in sodium hydroxide)

Principle

The principle involved in the heavy metal limit test (method C) can be explained through the following steps.

- ***Chemical interaction:*** The principle involved in the limit test of heavy metals is the reaction of metallic impurities (e.g., lead) with sodium sulphide solution. Dilute acetic acid or ammonia is useful in maintaining the pH (3 to 4) of the mixture.
- ***Formation of colour:*** Heavy metal content of the test (or standard) sample reacts with sodium sulphide and forms lead sulphide. A very fine dispersed precipitate of lead sulphide produces brown colour to the solution.

$$\underset{\text{Lead ion}}{Pb^{2+}} + \underset{\text{Sodium sulphide}}{Na_2S} \xrightarrow{NaOH} \underset{\text{Lead sulphide}}{PbS\downarrow} + 2Na^+$$

- ***Comparison of brown colour*****:** The comparison of brown colour produced by the test sample with the brown colour produced by the standard under uniform conditions is basis for the conclusions.

Procedure

S. No.	Standard Nessler Cylinder	Test Nessler Cylinder
1	Transfer 1 mL of standard lead solution (20 ppm, Pb) into a Nessler cylinder. Dilute the solution with distilled water 25 mL.	Transfer 25 mL of the sample solution prepared as per monograph into a Nessler cylinder. (alternatively specified quantity of the test sample can be dissolved in 25 mL of water)
2	Add 5 mL of sodium hydroxide.	Add 5 mL of sodium hydroxide.
3	Dilute to 50 mL of distilled water and mix well with glass rod.	Dilute to 50 mL of distilled water and mix well with glass rod.
4	Add 5 drops of freshly prepared sodium sulphide solution.	Add 10 mL of freshly prepared sodium sulphide solution.
5	Stir it immediately with a glass rod.	Stir it immediately with a glass rod.
6	Allow it to stand for 5 min.	Allow it to stand for 5 min.

Observation: The Nessler cylinders (standard and test) should be viewed transversely (vertically) through liquid, against a white colour background (white tile can be used). Compare the brown colour produced by the test sample with the brown colour produced by the standard.

42.7 Limit Test for Heavy Metals (Method D)

Principle

The principle involved in the heavy metal limit test (method D) can be explained through the following steps.

- ***Chemical interaction:*** The principle involved in the limit test of heavy metals is the reaction of metallic impurities (e.g., lead) with thioacetamide in the presence of acetate buffer.
- ***Formation of colour:*** Heavy metal content of the test (or standard) sample reacts with thioacetamide and forms lead sulphide. A very fine dispersed precipitate of lead sulphide produces the brown colour to a solution.

$$\underset{\text{Lead ion}}{Pb^{2+}} + \underset{\text{Thioacetamide}}{H_3C\text{-}\overset{\overset{\displaystyle S}{\|}}{C}\text{-}NH_2} + H_2O \xrightarrow{\text{Acetate buffer}} \underset{\text{Lead sulphide}}{PbS\downarrow} + \underset{\text{Acetamide}}{H_3C\text{-}\overset{\overset{\displaystyle O}{\|}}{C}\text{-}NH_2} + 2H^+$$

- ***Comparison of brown colour*****:** The comparison of brown colour produced by the test sample with the brown colour produced by the standard under uniform conditions is basis for the conclusions.

Procedure

S. No.	Standard Nessler Cylinder	Test Nessler Cylinder
1	Transfer 10 mL of standard lead solution (1 or 2 ppm, Pb) into a Nessler cylinder.	Transfer 2 mL of the sample solution prepared as per monograph into a Nessler cylinder.
2	Dilute the solution with 25 mL of distilled water.	
3	Add 2 mL of acetate buffer solution (pH 3.5) and mix well with glass rod.	Add 2 mL of acetate buffer solution (pH 3.5) and mix well with glass rod.
4	Add 1.2 mL of thioacetamide reagent.	Add 1.2 mL of thioacetamide reagent.
5	Dilute the solution to 50 mL with distilled water.	Dilute the solution to 50 mL with distilled water.
6	Stir immediately with a glass rod.	Stir it immediately with a glass rod.
7	Allow it to stand for 5 min.	Allow it to stand for 5 min.

Observation: The Nessler cylinders (standard and test) should be viewed transversely (vertically) through liquid, against a white colour background (white tile can be used). Compare the brown colour produced by the test sample with the brown colour produced by the standard.

Table 42.4 The list of inorganic compounds and permissible limit of heavy metals.

Inorganic compound	Method	Quantity	Solubility	Limits (in ppm)* as per IP 2018
Dextrose	A	4 g	Water	5
Calcium gluconate	A	1 g	Water	20
Ammonium chloride	A	2 g	Water	10
Sodium bicarbonate	A	4 g	Water	5
Bentonite	D	5 g	Acetic acid	50
Barium sulphate	A	4 g	Acetic acid	10

* as per IP 2022

42.8 Limit Test for Lead

Principle

The lead limit test determines the permissible limit of lead content in the pharmaceuticals. The limit test for lead is indicated in the individual monograph in terms of ppm, i.e., parts of lead per million parts of the substance under examination. The more obvious source of lead in chemicals are sulphuric acid used in the manufacture and the use of lead apparatus. The principle involved in the limit test for lead is extraction of lead by solutions of dithizone.

- ***Chemical interaction:*** Limit test for lead is based upon the chemical reaction with dithizone and lead in presence of ammonia. This forms lead dithizonate complex.

- ***Formation of brown colour:*** The lead dithizonate complex is brown in colour.
- ***Comparison of brown colour***: The brown colour (lead dithizonate complex) produced by test is compared with the brown colour produced by the standard.

Procedure

S. No.	Standard Nessler Cylinder	Test Nessler Cylinder
1	Transfer lead standard solution equivalent to 1 ppm into a separating funnel (transfer volume of lead standard solution equivalent to the permitted limit of lead in the sample).	Transfer specified quantity of the test sample (as per monograph) into a separating funnel.
2	Add 6 mL of ammonium citrate solution Sp and 2 mL of hydroxylamine hydrochloride solution Sp.	Add 6 mL of ammonium citrate solution Sp and 2 mL of hydroxylamine hydrochloride solution Sp.
3	Add 2 drops of phenol red solution.	Add 2 drops of phenol red solution.
4	Add strong ammonia to bring the pH to alkaline (red colour).	Add strong ammonia to bring the pH to alkaline (red colour).
5	Cool and add 2 mL of potassium cyanide solution Sp.	Cool and add 2 mL of potassium cyanide solution Sp.
6	Extract with dithizone extraction solution (5 mL; several times) into another separating funnel. (extraction should be continued until the solution shows stable green colour)	Extract with dithizone extraction solution (5 mL; several times) into another separating funnel. (extraction should be continued until the solution shows stable green colour)

Table *Contd...*

S. No.	Standard Nessler Cylinder	Test Nessler Cylinder
7	Shake the combined extracts with 30 mL of 1%v/v nitric acid solution for 30 sec.	Shake the combined extracts with 30 mL of 1%v/v nitric acid solution for 30 sec.
8	Discard the chloroform layer.	Discard the chloroform layer.
9	Add 5 mL of dithizone standard solution to acidic layer (aqueous layer) and shake for 30 sec.	Add 5 mL of dithizone standard solution to acidic layer (aqueous layer) and shake for 30 sec.

Ammonium citrate, potassium cyanide, hydroxylamine hydrochloride are used to make pH optimum so interference and influence of other impurities have been eliminated. Phenol red is used as indicator to develop the color at the end of process. Lead present as an impurity in the substance gets separated by extracting an alkaline solution with a dithizone extraction solution.

Note: For the determination of lead in iron salts (e.g., $FeSO_4$), use ammonium citrate solution.

Observation: The Nessler cylinders (standard and test) should be viewed transversely (vertically) through liquid, against a white colour background (white tile can be used). Compare the brown colour produced by the test sample with the brown colour produced by the standard.

Table 42.5 The list of inorganic compounds and permissible limit of lead.

Inorganic compound	Quantity	Limits (in ppm)*
Ferrous sulphate	8 g	50 ppm
Calamine	2 g	

* as per IP 2018

42.9 Limit Test for Arsenic

Principle

The arsenic limit test determines the arsenic content in the pharmaceuticals. The limit is expressed with reference to the arsenic trioxide (As_2O_3). The limit test for arsenic is indicated in the individual monographs in terms of parts per million (ppm). The principle involved in the limit test for arsenic can be explained through the following steps.

- ***Reduction of arsenic:*** The hydrochloric acid reduces arsenic present in the sample into arsenious acid (if arsenic is trivalent) or arsenic acid (if arsenic is pentavalent). The combined effect of hydrochloric acid, stannous chloride and potassium iodide reduces arsenic acid (if any) into arsenious acid. The nascent hydrogen produced by the reaction of zinc and hydrochloric acid reduces arsenious acid into arsine gas (AsH_3, arsenious hydride).

Action of hydrochloric acid

$$\underset{\text{Arsenic (trivalent)}}{As^{3+}} \xrightarrow{H^+} \underset{\text{Arsenious acid}}{H_3AsO_3}$$

$$\underset{\text{Arsenic (pentavalent)}}{As^{5+}} \xrightarrow{H^+} \underset{\text{Arsenic acid}}{H_3AsO_4}$$

Reduction of arsenic acid into arsenious acid

$$\underset{\text{Arsenic acid}}{H_3AsO_4} \xrightarrow[\text{HCl, SnCl}_2]{\text{KI}} \underset{\text{Arsenious acid}}{H_3AsO_3}$$

Generation of arsine

$$\underset{\text{Arsenious acid}}{H_3AsO_3} \xrightarrow[\text{Nascent hydrogen}]{\overset{Zn + HCl}{\downarrow} \; 6H} \underset{\text{Arsine}}{AsH_3} \uparrow + 3H_2O$$

- ***Stain formation***: The nascent hydrogen carries the arsine into mercuric chloride paper present in the tube and stains the paper yellow (or brown). The intensity of the colour depends upon the quantity of arsenic impurity present. This chemical reaction is known as 'Modified Gutzeit test'. The cotton wool moistened with lead acetate present in the tube traps hydrogen sulphide, if any formed. Otherwise hydrogen sulphide produces yellow stain with mercuric chloride paper (instead of AsH_3) and leads to erroneous conclusions.

$$\underset{\text{Arsine}}{AsH_3} + \underset{\text{Mercuric chloride}}{HgCl_2} \longrightarrow \underset{\text{Yellow stain}}{Hg(AsH_2)_2} + 2\,HCl$$

  In original Gutzeit test, the mouth of the flask is covered with filter paper and on the paper crystals of silver nitrate is placed. The liberated arsine gas reacts with silver nitrate and produce silver arsenide (yellow colour). It turns into black colour.

- ***Comparison of yellow stain***: The intensity of the stain produced by sample under test is compared with intensity of the stain produced by the standard.

The presence of a small quantity of stannous chloride in the hydrochloric acid ensures rapid reaction between the acid and the zinc and steady evolution of hydrogen.

Apparatus

The arsenic limit test apparatus consists of the following parts:

1. ***Generator bottle***: It holds sample and reactants including reducing agents.

2. ***Glass tube***: Tube with 20 cm length and 5 mm diameter.

   Lower part of tube is drawn to an internal diameter of 1 mm and 15 mm from its tip is a later orifice of 2 to 3 mm diameter. The lower tube is inserted with 50 to 60 mg of lead acetate impregnated cotton.

   The orifice should be at least 3 mm below the lower surface of stopper.

   A second glass tube with 30 mm long and 5 mm internal diameter above the first tube using spiral springs.
3. ***Rubber or ground glass stopper (bung)***: It provides space for inserting the glass tube and seals the container.
4. ***Spiral springs (clip)***: This is useful in fixing the mercuric chloride paper.

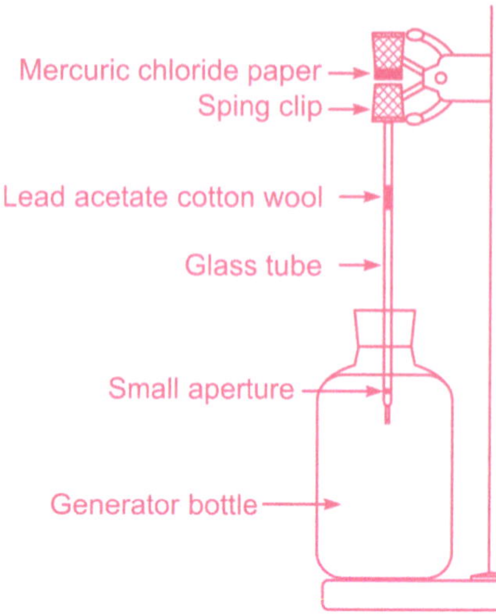

Preparation of Reagents

- **Standard arsenic solution (10 ppm)**: Dissolve 0.33 g of arsenic trioxide in 5 mL of 2 M sodium hydroxide. Dilute to 250 mL with water. Dilute 1 mL of this solution to 100 mL with water.
- **Stannous chloride solution**:

  Method 1: Weigh 330 g stannous chloride and dissolve with 100 mL of hydrochloric acid. Add sufficient water to produce 1000 mL.

  Method 2: Dilute 60 mL of hydrochloric acid with 20 mL of water. Add 2 g of tin. Heat the mixture gently, until no more gas evolves. Add sufficient water to produce 100 mL. Store over a little of the undissolved tin remaining in the solution and protected from light.
- **Stannated-Hydrochloric acid:** Dilute 1 mL of stannous chloride solution AsT to 100 mL with hydrochloric acid.
- **Potassium iodide:** Dissolve 16.6 g of potassium iodide in sufficient water to produce 100 mL.
- **Lead acetate cotton wool**: Moisten the cotton wool with lead acetate solution.

- **Mercuric chloride paper**: Soak 25 mm width white paper in a saturated mercuric chloride solution. Dry the paper at 60 °C.

Procedure

S. No.	Standard Nessler Cylinder	Test Nessler Cylinder
1	Transfer 1 mL of standard arsenic solution (10 ppm) into a Gutzeit apparatus.	Dissolve 1 g sample with distilled water (or use solution prepared as per monograph).
2	Dilute with 10 mL of distilled water.	
3	Dilute with distilled water to 50 mL.	Dilute with distilled water to 50 mL.
4	Add 10 mL of stannated-hydrochloric acid.	Add 10 mL of stannated-hydrochloric acid.
5	Add 5 mL of potassium iodide (1 M) and mix well.	Add 5 mL of potassium iodide (1 M) and mix well.
6	Add 10 g of zinc to the cylinder.	Add 10 g of zinc to the cylinder.
7	Immediately assemble the apparatus and immerse in a water-bath.	Immediately assemble the apparatus and immerse in a water-bath.
8	Allow it to stand for 40 min at constant temperature.	Allow it to stand for 40 min at constant temperature.

Observation: The yellow stain produced on the mercuric chloride papers (test and standard) should be compared.

Marsh's test: The yellow stain produced by the Gutzeit method, is inferior in terms of accuracy and results. The stain is light sensitive and gets affected by foreign gases and moisture. Hence, an alternative method called 'Marsh's test' is developed. Extremely small quantities of arsenic can be detected by this method. The apparatus consists of drying tube loaded with lead acetate wool followed by calcium chloride to dry the evolved gas. The hard glass exit tube is connected to the tube, the exit tube is heated at one point using micro burner. The evolved arsine forms the mirror of arsenic beyond the heated part of the tube.

Fleitmann's test: The arsine gas can be detected by using filter paper moistened with silver nitrate solution. The formation of greyish-black stain of metallic silver on the paper indicates the presence of arsenic. The stain disappears upon treatment with dilute acid.

Table 42.6 The list of inorganic compounds and permissible limit of arsenic.

Inorganic compound	Quantity	Solubility	Pre-treatment	Limits (in ppm)*
Dextrose	10 g	Soluble	NA	1
Sodium bicarbonate	5 g	Soluble	NA	2
Calcium gluconate	5 g	Soluble	NA	2
Ammonium chloride	2.5 g	Soluble	NA	4
Calamine	1.25 g	Insoluble	Required	8

* as per IP 2022; NA: not applicable

KEY POINTS

- Any material present in medicinal preparations, besides the active ingredient / excipient is considered as an impurity.
- Limit Test is useful in the quantification of inorganics and/or heavy metals present in pharmaceuticals.
- The use of nitric acid in the limit test for chlorides prevents the formation of silver carbonates and oxides.
- The ethanolic sulphate standard solution acts as seeding agent and increases the sensitivity of the turbidity formation in the limit test for sulphae.
- The reaction between ferrous and thioglycolic acid generates a reddish purple coloured ferrous thioglycolate complex.
- The arsine gas reacts with mercuric chloride paper and stains the paper yellow to brown.

Qualitative Analysis

Qualitative chemical analysis is a branch of chemistry that deals with the systematic identification of elements or grouping of elements present in a sample. It is a process of identifying a chemical substance. Qualitative test results are basis for the limit tests. The qualitative analysis of inorganic compounds includes the identification of acidic radicals and basic radicals.

They are based on the systematic elimination of compounds by observing reactions of the sample with various known compounds to form precipitates or substances with known properties (colour, odour, etc). By observing the products of such reactions, the correct ion present in the sample can be identified.

43

Analysis of Inorganic Compounds

The analysis of inorganic compounds is generally attempted in two steps: identification of cations and identification of anions. Cations and anions are divided into several groups based on their ability to react with a common reagent or similar group ions may exhibit similar end products. After identifying the group, independent tests are conducted to further differentiate the right ion in the group.

Grouping of anionic radicals

Group I	Carbonates, Bicarbonates, Sulphides, Acetates and Nitrates
Group II	Chlorides, Bromides, Iodides and Nitrites
Group III	Sulphates, Phosphates
Others	Gluconates

Grouping of basic radicals

Based on the reaction with the group categorizing reagents, the basic radicals are classified into the following categories.

Group I	Mercurous, Lead, Gold, Silver
Group II	Mercuric, Copper, Lead, Bismuth, Cadmium, Arsenic, Strontium, Stannous
Group III	
Group IIIa	Aluminium, Ferric, Ferrous, Chromium
Group IIIb	Zinc, Manganese, Cobalt, Nickel
Group IV	Calcium, Barium, Strontium
Group V	Magnesium
Group VI	Ammonium
Group VII	Sodium, Potassium

43.1 Systematic Analysis of Inorganic Compunds

Preliminary tests

S No	Experiment	Observation	Inference
1	**Physical nature**	Amorphous	Calcium carbonate.
		Crystalline	Magnesium sulphate
		Deliquescent	Ammonium carbonate
		Efflorescent	Copper sulphate.
2	***Colour:*** Observe the colour of the given inorganic compound.	Blue or green	Copper or Nickel salt
		Bluish green	Lead
		Light green	Ferrous salts
		Dark green	Chromium salts
		Dark brown	Ferric salts
		Light pink	Manganese salts
3	**Heat test:** Heat the given sample in a dry test tube.	Decrepitation (cracking noise).	May be Sodium, Potassium, Lead.
		Smell of ammonia.	Ammonium salts
		Yellow colour changes to brown on cooling.	May be Copper.
		Colourless gas turns lime water milky.	May be Carbonates and Bicarbonates.
		Violet vapour turns starch iodide paper blue.	May be Iodine.
		Fusion accompanied by condensation of water drops on the sides of the test tube.	Hygroscopic salts (e.g., Magnesium sulphate).
4	**Dilute sulphuric acid test:** Place 50 mg of sample into a dry test tube. Add 1 mL of dilute sulphuric acid to the test tube. Heat gently.	White fumes turn blue litmus red.	May be Chlorides
		Colourless gas with vinegar smell.	May be Acetates
		Evolution of carbon dioxide with brisk effervescence, which turns lime water milky.	May be Carbonates and Bicarbonates
		Evolution of hydrogen sulphide (rotten egg smell) gas. The gas turns lead acetate paper black.	May be Sulphides
		Brown gas turns ferrous sulphate solution slowly	May be Nitrites.
5	**Concentrated sulphuric acid test:** Place 50 mg of the sample in a dry test tube. Add 1 mL of concentrated sulphuric acid. Heat gently.	Colourless gas with pungent odour	May be Chlorides.
		Reddish fumes with pungent odour	May be Bromides.
		Violet vapour turns moist iodide paper dark blue. Sublimes solid on the sides of the test tube.	May be Iodides.
		Brown gas turns ferrous sulphate solution in to black.	May be Nitrates.

Table *Contd...*

S No	Experiment	Observation	Inference
6	**Manganese dioxide test:** Place 50 mg of sample, into a test tube. Add manganese dioxide and 2 mL of concentrated sulphuric acid to the test tube. Heat gently.	A greenish yellow fume evolves. The fumes turn blue litmus into red.	May be Chlorides.
		A brown fume evolves. It turns starch iodide paper into blue and starch paper into yellow.	May be Bromides.
		A violet vapour evolves. It turns starch paper into bluish black.	May be Iodides.
7	**Flame test:** Prepare the sample paste with concentrated hydro-chloric acid. Introduce the paste into the non-luminous flame with the help of glass rod.	Persistent golden yellow	Sodium
		Pale violet	Potassium
		Brick red or orange	Calcium
		Yellowish-grassy green	Barium
		Bluish-green or blue	Copper

43.2 Detection of Acid Radicals

***Preparation of extract of acid radicals*:** Place 1 g of the sample, 3 g of sodium carbonate and 15 mL of water into a small beaker. Boil the contents for 5 min, cool and filter. The filtrate is known as sodium carbonate extract. Neutralize the extract by adding dilute nitric acid (slightly acidic; litmus paper test). Add ammonia to turn slightly alkaline to litmus. Boil the solution to expel off ammonia and cool.

The extract is useful in the determination acid radical through the following chemical tests.

S No	Experiment	Observation	Inference
1	**Silver nitrate test:** Transfer 1 mL of neutralized extract into a test tube. Add 1 mL of silver nitrate solution.	Formation of white precipitate ($AgCl$, soluble in ammonia).	Indicates the presence of Chlorides.
		Formation of pale yellow precipitate ($AgBr$, soluble in ammonia).	Indicates the presence of Bromides.
		Formation of yellow precipitate (AgI, soluble in excess of ammonia)	Indicates the presence of Iodides.
		Formation of white or brown precipitate (Ag_2CO_3, soluble in nitric acid).	Indicates the presence of Carbonates.
		Formation of white precipitate (AgO_4, insoluble in nitric acid).	Indicates the presence of Sulphates.
		Formation of black precipitate (AgS).	Indicates the presence of Sulphides.
		No precipitate.	Indicates the presence of Nitrates.

Table *Contd...*

S No	Experiment	Observation	Inference
2	**Barium nitrate test:** Transfer 1 mL of the neutralized extract into a test tube. Add 1 mL of barium nitrate reagent.	Formation of white precipitate ($BaSO_4$, insoluble in nitric acid).	Indicates the presence of Sulphates.
		Soluble in dilute acids with effervescence, due to the formation of $BaCO_3$.	Indicates the presence of Carbonates.
3	**Ferrous sulphate test:** Transfer 1 mL of the neutralized extract into a test tube and neutralize with acetic acid. Add 1 mL of freshly prepared ferrous sulphate solution.	Formation of brown colour.	Indicates the presence of Nitrates.
4	**Lead acetate test:** To 1 mL of neutralized extract add lead acetate solution.	White precipitate (soluble in hot water).	Indicates the presence of Chlorides and /Bromides.
		White precipitate (insoluble in dilute acids; soluble in ammonium acetate).	Indicates the presence of Sulphates.
		Yellow precipitate (soluble in boiling water, and on cooling separates golden yellow crystals).	Indicates the presence of Iodides.
		Black precipitate.	Indicates the presence of Sulphides.

43.3 Confirmatory Tests for Acid Radicals

GROUP I acid radicals

Confirmatory Tests for Carbonates and Bicarbonates

S No	Experiment	Observation	Inference
1	Place 1 mL of the sample into a test tube. Add 1 mL of dilute sulphuric acid.	Brisk effervescence of carbon dioxide.	Indicates the presence of Carbonates.
	Pass the fumes into a test tube containing lime water.	It turns the lime water milky white.	Confirms the presence of Carbonates and Bicarbonates.
	$CO_3^{2-} + H_2SO_4 \longrightarrow CO_2\uparrow$; CO_2 + Lime water $\longrightarrow$ Milky white		
2	**Barium nitrate test**: Place 1 mL of the sample into a test tube. Add 1 mL of barium nitrate solution to the test tube.	Formation of white precipitate. It is soluble in dilute acids with effervescence.	Confirms the presence of Carbonates and Bicarbonates.
	$CO_3^{2-} + Ba(NO_3)_2 \longrightarrow BaCO_3\downarrow + 2NO_3^-$		

Table ***Contd...***

S No	Experiment	Observation	Inference
3	**Distinct test for carbonates and bicarbonates:** Transfer 1 mL of aqueous solution of the sample into a test tube. Add magnesium sulphate solution to the test tube.	Formation of white precipitate.	Confirms the presence of Carbonates.
	$CO_3^{2-} + MgSO_4 \longrightarrow MgCO_3 \downarrow + SO_4^{2-}$		
		Observation of clear solution.	Confirms the presence of Bicarbonates
	$2\ HCO_3^- + MgSO_4 \longrightarrow Mg(HCO_3)_2 \downarrow + SO_4^{2-}$		

Confirmatory Test for Sulphides

S No	Experiment	Observation	Inference
1	**Sodium nitroprusside test:** Transfer 1 mL of sample into a test tube. Add 1 mL of sodium nitroprusside solution.	Appearance of violet colour.	Confirms the presence of Sulphides.
	$Na_2[Fe(CN)_5NO] + S^- \longrightarrow Na_4[Fe(CN)_5NOS]$ Sodium nitroprusside + Sulphide → Sodium nitroprusside sulphide complex		

Confirmatory Tests for Nitrates

S No	Experiment	Observation	Inference
1	**Brown ring test:** Transfer 1 mL of sample into a test tube. Add 1 mL of sulphuric acid, cool and add ferrous sulphate solution from the sides of the test tube.	Development of brown ring at the junction of two layers.	Confirms the presence of Nitrates.

GROUP II acid radicals

Confirmatory Tests for Chlorides

S No	Experiment	Observation	Inference
1	**Chromyl chloride test:** Place 1 mL of the sample solution into a test tube. Add 50 mg of potassium dichromate and 5 mL sulphuric acid into a test tube. Heat the contents gently. Pass the vapours to the test tube containing lead acetate solution.	Formation of yellow precipitate of lead chromate.	Confirms the presence of Chloride.
	$4\ Cl^- + K_2Cr_2O_7 + 3\ H_2SO_4 + Pb(CH_3COO)_2 \longrightarrow PbCrO_4 \downarrow$		
2	**Manganese dioxide test:** Place 1 mL of the sample solution into a test tube. Add 50 mg of manganese dioxide and 1 mL of dilute sulphuric acid. Heat the contents gently.	Liberates the greenish yellow vapour. It turns blue litmus red.	Confirms the presence of Chloride.
	$2\ Cl + MnO_2 + 3\ H_2SO_4 \longrightarrow Cl_2 \uparrow$ Cl_2 ↓ Blue litmus ⟶ Red		

Confirmatory Test for Bromides

S No	Experiment	Observation	Inference
1	**Manganese dioxide test:** Place 1 mL of the sample solution into a test tube. Add 50 mg of manganese dioxide and 1 mL of dilute sulphuric acid. Heat the contents gently.	Liberates brownish vapour. It turns starch iodide paper blue and starch paper yellow.	Confirms the presence of Bromides.
	$2 Br^- + MnO_2 + 3 H_2SO_4 \longrightarrow Br_2\uparrow$ $\downarrow$ Starch iodide paper $\longrightarrow$ Blue Starch paper $\longrightarrow$ Yellow		

Confirmatory Tests for Iodides

S No	Experiment	Observation	Inference
1	**Manganese dioxide test:** Place 1 mL of the sample solution into a test tube. Add 50 mg of manganese dioxide and 1 mL of dilute sulphuric acid. Heat the contents gently.	Liberates violet vapour. It turns starch paper blue.	Confirms the presence of Iodide.
	$2 I^- + MnO_2 + 3 H_2SO_4 \longrightarrow I_2\uparrow$ $\downarrow$ Starch iodide paper $\longrightarrow$ Blue		
2	**Mercuric chloride test:** Place 1 mL of the sample solution into a test tube. Add 1 mL of mercuric chloride solution.	Red precipitate of mercuric iodide formed.	Confirms the presence of Iodides.
	$2 I^- + HgCl_2 \longrightarrow HgI_2\downarrow$		

GROUP III acid radicals

Confirmatory Test for Sulphates

S No	Experiment	Observation	Inference
1	**Barium chloride test**: Transfer 1 mL of extract into a test tube. Add 1 mL of barium chloride solution.	Formation of white precipitate. It is insoluble in hydrochloric acid and nitric acid.	Confirms the presence of Sulphates.
	$SO_4^{2-} + BaCl_2 \longrightarrow BaSO_4\downarrow + 2 Cl^-$		

Confirmatory Test for Phosphates

S No	Experiment	Observation	Inference
1	**Ammonium molybdate test**: Transfer 1 ml of sample into a test tube. Acidify with concentrated nitric acid. Add ammonium molybdate solution and boil the mixture.	Formation of canary yellow precipitate.	Confirms the presence of Phosphate.
	$PO_4^- + 3(NH_4)_2MoO_4 + 2HNO_3 + 6H_2O \longrightarrow (NH_4)_3PO_4.12MoO_3.6H_2O\downarrow$ Ammonium molybdate (for $(NH_4)_2MoO_4$) Ammonium phosphate molybdate (canary yellow precipitate) (for $(NH_4)_3PO_4.12MoO_3.6H_2O$)		

43.4 Detection of Basic Radicals

Preparation of the sample solution

1. **Solution in water:** Transfer 50 mg of sample into the test tube. Add 2 mL of water and boil. The aqueous solution is useful for group analysis.

For water insoluble compounds

2. **Solution in dilute hydrochloric acid:** Transfer 50 mg of sample into the test tube. Add 10 mL of dilute hydrochloric acid and boil to remove the gases (CO_2 and H_2S) completely, if they evolve.

   The solution is useful for analysis from group II elements onwards.

3. **Solution in concentrated hydrochloric acid:** Transfer 50 mg of sample into the test tube. Add 10 mL of concentrated hydrochloric acid and boil to remove the gases. Cool the acidic solution and dilute with water. The acidic solution is useful for the group analysis.

For water insoluble and mineral acid insoluble compounds

4. **Solution in Aqua regia:** Transfer 50 mg of sample into the test tube. Add 3 mL of aqua regia and boil. Cool the acidic mixture and dilute with water. The acidic solution is useful for the group analysis.

   ***Aqua regia*:** The mixture of 3 parts of concentrated hydrochloric acid and 1 parts of concentrated nitric acid.

   Filter to remove the insoluble compounds, if any present.

S No	Experiment	Observation	Inference
Test for Group I: Mercurous, Lead, Silver			
1	Place 1 mL of the aqueous solution of the sample into a test tube. Add 1 mL of dilute hydrochloric acid.	Formation of white precipitate (chlorides of Group I elements) The precipitate is insoluble in water.	Indicates the presence of Group I basic radicals.
Test for Group II: Copper, Lead, Bismuth, Mercuric (Mercury II),			
2	Place 1 mL of the sample solution into a test tube. Add 1 mL of dilute hydrochloric acid and pass hydrogen sulphide gas.	Formation of black precipitate (sulphides of Group II elements). The precipitate is insoluble in dilute acid.	Indicates the presence of Group II basic radicals.
Test for Group III			
Group IIIa: Aluminium, Ferric, Ferrous, Chromium			
3	Place 1 mL of the sample solution into a test tube. Neutralize with ammonium hydroxide. Add excess of ammonium chloride and ammonium hydroxide solutions into a test tube.	Formation of white precipitate ($Al(OH)_3$).	Indicates the presence of Aluminum.
		Formation of reddish brown precipitate ($Fe(OH)_3$).	Indicates the presence of Ferric.
		Formation of dirty-green precipitate ($Fe(OH)_2$).	Indicates the presence of Ferrous.
	Hydroxides insoluble in presence of ammonium chloride and ammonium hydroxide.		

Table ***Contd...***

S No	Experiment	Observation	Inference
Group IIIb: Zinc, Manganese, Cobalt, Nickel			
4	Place 1 mL of the sample solution into a test tube. Neutralize with ammonium hydroxide. Add excess of ammonium chloride, ammonium hydroxide and sodium or hydrogen sulphide solutions into a test tube.	Formation of white precipitate (ZnS).	Indicates the presence of Zinc.
		Formation of pinkish precipitate (MnS).	Indicates the presence of Manganese.
		Formation of black precipitate (CoS/NiS).	Indicates the presence of Cobalt/Nickel.
	Sulphides insoluble in presence of ammonium chloride and ammonium hydroxide.		
Test for Group IV: Calcium, Barium, Strontium			
5	Place 1 mL of the sample solution into a test tube. Add excess of ammonium chloride, ammonium hydroxide and ammonium carbonate solutions to the test tube.	Formation of white precipitate ($CaCO_3$, $BaCO_3$, $SrCO_3$). Carbonate precipitates are insoluble in presence of ammonium chloride and ammonium hydroxide.	Indicates the presence of Calcium / Barium / Strontium.
Test for Group V: Magnesium			
6	Place 1 mL of the sample solution into a test tube. Add excess of ammonium chloride, ammonium hydroxide and disodium hydrogen phosphate solutions to the test tube.	Formation of white precipitate ($MgNH_4PO_4$). (Insoluble in the presence of ammonium chloride and ammonium hydroxide)	Indicates the presence of Magnesium.
Test for Group VI and VII			
7	No characteristic reactions of above mentioned reactions, indicates that the sample contains either of Group VI (Ammonium) and Group VII (Sodium, Potassium).		

43.5 Confirmatory Tests for Basic Radicals

Confirmatory Tests to differentiate Group I radicals

General: Place 50 mg of the sample into a test tube. Dissolve the sample with 2 mL of dilute hydrochloric acid. Wash the precipitate with water several times. Add 10 mL of ammonium hydroxide to dissolve the precipitate and collect the filtrate.

Confirmatory tests for Silver (Group I)

S No	Experiment	Observation	Inference
1	Place 1 mL of filtrate into a test tube. Acidify the filtrate with dilute nitric acid (blue litmus paper test).	Formation of white precipitate. It turns into grey colour upon exposure to sun light. $Ag^+ + HNO_3 \longrightarrow AgNO_3 \downarrow$	Confirms the presence of Silver.
2	Place 1 mL of sample solution into a test tube. Add ammonia or sodium hydroxide.	Formation of brown precipitate. $2\,Ag^+ + HO^- \longrightarrow Ag_2O \downarrow$	Confirms the presence of Silver.
3	**Potassium iodide test**: Place 1 mL of filtrate into a test tube. Add 1 mL of potassium iodide solution into the test tube.	Formation of pale yellow precipitate. $Ag^+ + I^- \longrightarrow AgI \downarrow$	Confirms the presence of Silver.

Confirmatory tests for Lead (Group I)

S No	Experiment	Observation	Inference
1	Place 1 mL of sample solution into a test tube. Add 1 mL of dilute hydrochloric acid / dilute sulphuric acid (2 M).	Formation of white crystals (insoluble in excess of acid).	Indicates the presence of Lead.
2	**Potassium iodide test**: Place 1 mL of filtrate into a test tube. Add 1 mL of potassium iodate solution into the test tube.	Formation of yellow precipitate (dissolves in boiling water). $Pb^{2+} + 2I^- \longrightarrow PbI_2\downarrow$	Confirms the presence of Lead.
3	**Potassium chromate test**: Place of 1 mL of filtrate into a test tube. Add 1 mL of potassium chromate solution into the test tube.	Formation of brilliant yellow precipitate (dissolves in sodium hydroxide).	Confirms the presence of Lead.
	$Pb^{2+} + K_2Cr_2O_7 \longrightarrow PbCr_2O_7\downarrow + 2K$		
4	Place of 1 mL of sample solution into a test tube. Add 1 mL of sodium hydroxide (or ammonium hydroxide).	Formation of white precipitate (dissolves on excess of sodium hydroxide; insoluble in excessive ammonia). $Pb^{2+} + 2OH^- \longrightarrow Pb(OH)_2\downarrow$	Confirms the presence of Lead.

Confirmatory Tests for Group II

Confirmatory tests for Copper (Group II)

S No	Experiment	Observation	Inference
1	**Ferrocyanide test**: Place 1 mL of filtrate into a test tube. Add 1 mL of potassium ferrocyanide solution into the test tube.	Formation of chocolate red (or pink) precipitate.	Confirms the presence of Copper.
	$Cu^{2+} + K_4[Fe(CN)_6 \longrightarrow Cu_2[Fe(CN)_6\downarrow + 4K$		
2	Place 1 mL of the sample solution into a test tube. Add 1 mL of ammonium hydroxide into the test tube.	Formation of bluish white precipitate (copper hydroxide). It turns black on warming.	Confirms the presence of Copper.
	$Cu^{2+} + 2NH_4OH \longrightarrow Cu(OH)_2\downarrow + 2NH_4^+$		
3	**Potassium iodide test**: Place 1 mL of sample solution into a test tube. Add 1 mL of potassium iodide solution into the test tube.	Formation of brown precipitate. It turns black on warming.	Confirms the presence of Copper.
	$Cu^{2+} + 2KI \longrightarrow CuI_2\downarrow + 2K$		

Confirmatory Tests for Group III

Confirmatory tests for Aluminium (Group IIIa)

S No	Experiment	Observation	Inference
1	Place 1 mL of the filtrate (or sample solution) into a test tube. Add 1 mL of ammonia into the test tube and boil.	Formation of white gelatinous precipitate. $Al^{3+} + 3\ OH^- \longrightarrow Al(OH)_3 \downarrow$	Confirms the presence of Aluminium.
2	Place 1 mL of the filtrate (or sample solution) into a test tube. Add 1 mL of ammonium hydroxide (or sodium hydroxide) into the test tube.	Formation of white gelatinous precipitate. $Al^{3+} + 3\ OH^- \longrightarrow Al(OH)_3 \downarrow$	Confirms the presence of Aluminium.
3	**Lake test**: Place 1 mL of the filtrate (or sample solution) into a test tube. Acidify with dilute hydrochloric acid, add 2 drops of blue litmus solution and 2 drops of ammonium hydroxide, shake gently.	A crystalline blue precipitate floats.	Confirms the presence of Aluminium.
4	Place 1 mL of the filtrate (or sample solution) into a test tube. Add 1 mL of ammonium acetate into the test tube and boil.	Formation of gelatinous white precipitate (disappears on cooling).	Confirms the presence of Aluminium.
	$Al^{3+} + 3\ CH_3COONH_4 \longrightarrow Al(CH_3COO)_3 \downarrow + 3\ NH_4^+$		
5	Place 1 mL of the filtrate (or sample solution) into a test tube. Add 1 mL of disodium hydrogen phosphate into the test tube.	Formation of gelatinous white precipitate.	Confirms the presence of Aluminium.
	$2\ Al^{3+} + 3\ Na_2HPO_4 \longrightarrow Al_2(PO_4)_3 \downarrow + 6\ Na^+ + 3\ H^+$		

Confirmatory tests for Ferric (Group IIIa)

S No	Experiment	Observation	Inference
1	Place 1 mL of the filtrate (or sample solution) into a test tube. Add 1 mL of potassium ferrocyanide into the test tube.	Formation of Prussian blue precipitate (insoluble in acetic acid).	Confirms the presence of Ferric.
	$Fe^{3+} + K_4[Fe(CN)_6 \longrightarrow Fe_3[Fe(CN)_6 \downarrow$		
2	Place 1 mL of the filtrate (or sample solution) into a test tube. Add 1 mL of disodium hydrogen phosphate into the test tube.	Formation of yellowish white precipitate. $Fe^{3+} + Na_2HPO_4 \longrightarrow FePO_4 \downarrow$	Confirms the presence of Ferric.
3	Place 1 mL of the filtrate (or sample solution) into a test tube. Add 1 mL of ammonium hydroxide (or sodium hydroxide) into the test tube.	Formation of reddish-brown gelatinous precipitate. $Fe^{3+} + 3\ OH^- \longrightarrow Fe(OH)_3 \downarrow$	Confirms the presence of Ferric.

Table *Contd...*

S No	Experiment	Observation	Inference
4	Place 1 mL of the filtrate (or sample solution) into a test tube. Add 1 mL of sodium acetate into the test tube.	Formation of reddish-brown colouration.	Confirms the presence of Ferric.
	$3\ Fe^{3+} + 6\ CH_3COONa \longrightarrow Fe_3(OH)\ (CH_3COO)_6 \downarrow + 6\ Na^+$		

Confirmatory tests for Ferrous (Group IIIa)

S No	Experiment	Observation	Inference
1	Place 1 mL of the filtrate (or sample solution) into a test tube. Add 1 mL of potassium ferricyanide into the test tube.	Formation of deep blue Turn's Bull blue (ferrous ferro cyanide).	Confirms the presence of Ferrous.
	$Fe^{2+} + K_3[Fe(CN)_6] \longrightarrow Fe_3[Fe(CN)_6]_2 \downarrow$		
2	Place 1 mL of the filtrate (or sample solution) into a test tube. Add 1 mL of ammonium hydroxide into the test tube.	Formation of green gelatinous precipitate. $Fe^{2+} + NH_4OH \longrightarrow Fe(OH)_2 \downarrow$	Confirms the presence of Ferrous.
	$Fe^{2+} + 2\ NH_4OH \longrightarrow Fe(OH)_2 \downarrow + 2\ NH_4^+$		
3	Place 1 mL of the filtrate (or sample solution) into a test tube. Add 1 mL of sodium hydroxide into the test tube.	Formation of white precipitate.	Confirms the presence of Ferrous.
	$Fe^{2+} + 2\ NaOH \longrightarrow Fe(OH)_2 \downarrow + 2\ Na^+$		
4	Place 1 mL of the filtrate (or sample solution) into a test tube. Add 1 mL of 1,10-phenanthroline into the test tube.	Formation of red coloration.	Confirms the presence of Ferrous.

Distinct tests for Ferric and Ferrous

S No	Experiment	Observation	Inference
1	Place 1 mL of the filtrate (or sample solution) into a test tube. Add 1 mL of ammonium thiocyanate into the test tube.	Formation of deep-red color.	Confirms the presence of Ferric.
	$Fe^{3+} + 3\ NH_4SCN \longrightarrow Fe(SCN)_3 + 3\ NH_4^+$		

Confirmatory tests for Manganese (Group IIIb)

S No	Experiment	Observation	Inference
1	Place 1 mL of the sample solution into a test tube. Add 1 mL of sodium hydroxide into the test tube.	Formation of white precipitate (insoluble in excess sodium hydroxide).	Confirms the presence of Manganese.
	$Mn^{2+} + 2\ NaOH \longrightarrow Mn(OH)_2 \downarrow$		

Table ***Contd...***

S No	Experiment	Observation	Inference
2	Place 1 mL of the filtrate (or sample solution) into a test tube. Add 1 mL of disodium hydrogen phosphate into the test tube.	Formation of white precipitate.	Confirms the presence of Manganese.
	$3\ Mn^{2+} + 2\ Na_2HPO_4 \longrightarrow Mn_3(PO_4)_2\downarrow + 4\ Na^+ + 2\ H^+$		
3	Place 1 mL of the filtrate (or sample solution) into a test tube. Add 1 mL of concentrated hydrochloric acid and 0.5 mL of sodium bismuthate into the test tube. Shake and allow it stand.	Formation of pink (or purple) colour. $Mn^{2+} + NaBiO_3 \longrightarrow MnO_2^-$	Confirms the presence of Manganese.

Confirmatory tests for Zinc (Group IIIb)

S No	Experiment	Observation	Inference
1	Place 1 mL of the sample solution into a test tube. Add 1 mL of ammonium hydroxide into the test tube.	Formation of white (or bluish-white) precipitate (insoluble in excess of ammonium hydroxide).	Confirms the presence of Zinc.
	$Zn^{2+} + 2\ NH_4OH \longrightarrow Zn(OH)_2\downarrow + 2\ NH_4^+$		
2	Place 1 mL of the filtrate (or sample solution) into a test tube. Add 1 mL of disodium hydrogen phosphate into the test tube.	Formation of white precipitate.	Confirms the presence of Zinc.
	$3\ Zn^{2+} + 2\ Na_2HPO_4 \longrightarrow Zn_3(PO_4)_2\downarrow + 4\ Na^+ + 2\ H^+$		
3	**Ferro cyanide test:** Place 1 mL of the filtrate (or sample solution) into a test tube. Acidify with hydrochloric acid and add 1 mL of potassium ferro cyanide solution.	Formation of white (or bluish-white) precipitate.	Confirms the presence of Zinc.
	$Zn^{2+} + K_4[Fe(CN)_6 \longrightarrow Zn_2[Fe(CN)_6]\downarrow + 4\ K^+$		

Confirmatory Tests for Group IV

Confirmatory tests for Calcium (Group IV)

S No	Experiment	Observation	Inference
1	**Flame test:** Introduce the glass rod dipped in paste of sample made with hydrochloric acid into the non-luminous flame.	Appearance of brick red flame.	Indicates the presence of Calcium.
2	Place 1 mL of the sample solution into a test tube. Add 1 mL of ammonium carbonate solution into the test tube.	Formation of white precipitate.	Confirms the presence of Calcium.
	$Ca^{2+} + (NH_4)_2CO_3 \longrightarrow CaCO_3\downarrow + 2\ NH_4^+$		

Table ***Contd...***

S No	Experiment	Observation	Inference
3	Place 1 mL of the sample solution into a test tube. Add 1 mL of ammonium oxalate solution into the test tube.	Formation of white precipitate. (soluble in hydrochloric acid and sparingly soluble in dilute acetic acid)	Confirms the presence of Calcium.
	$Ca^{2+} + (COONH_4)_2 \longrightarrow Ca(COO)_2 \downarrow + 2\ NH_4^+$		
4	**Ferro cyanide test:** Place 1 mL of the filtrate (or sample solution) into a test tube. Acidify with glacial acetic acid and add 1 mL of potassium ferrro cyanide solution.	Formation of white precipitate.	Confirms the presence of Calcium.
	$Ca^{2+} + K_4[Fe(CN)_6 \longrightarrow Ca[Fe(CN)_6] \downarrow + 4\ K^+$		

Confirmatory tests for Barium (Group IV)

S No	Experiment	Observation	Inference
1	**Flame test:** Introduce the glass rod dipped in paste of sample made with hydrochloric acid into the non-luminous flame.	Appearance of pale green flame.	Indicates the presence of Barium.
2	Place 1 mL of the filtrate (or sample solution) into a test tube. Add 1 mL of dilute hydrochloric acid (or 1 mL of dilute sulphuric acid).	Formation of white precipitate.	Confirms the presence of Barium.
	$Ba^{2+} + 2\ HCl \longrightarrow BaCl_2 \downarrow + 2\ H^+$		
3	Place 1 mL of the sample solution into a test tube. Add 1 mL of ammonium carbonate solution into the test tube.	Formation of white precipitate.	Confirms the presence of Barium.
	$Ba^{2+} + (NH_4)_2CO_3 \longrightarrow BaCO_3 \downarrow + 2\ NH_4^+$		
4	**Potassium chromate test**: Place 1 mL of filtrate into a test tube. Add 1 mL of potassium chromate solution into the test tube.	Formation of yellow precipitate (insoluble in water and dilute acetic acid).	Confirms the presence of Barium.
	$Ba^{2+} + K_2Cr_2O_7 \longrightarrow BaCr_2O_7 \downarrow + 2\ K^+$		
5	Place 1 mL of the sample solution into a test tube. Add 1 mL of ammonium oxalate solution into the test tube.	Formation of white precipitate (sparingly soluble in dilute acetic acid and soluble in hydrochloric acid).	Confirms the presence of Barium.
	$Ba^{2+} + (COONH_4)_2 \longrightarrow Ba(COO)_2 \downarrow + 2\ NH_4^+$		
6	Place 1 mL of the filtrate (or sample solution) into a test tube. Add 1 mL of disodium hydrogen phosphate into the test tube.	Formation of white precipitate.	Confirms the presence of Barium.
	$Ba^{2+} + Na_2HPO_4 \longrightarrow Ba(PO_4)_2 \downarrow + 2\ Na^+$		

Confirmatory Tests for Group V

Confirmatory tests for Magnesium (Group V)

S No	Experiment	Observation	Inference
1	**Filter paper ash test:** Place 1 mL of sample solution into a test tube. Add drop of cobalt nitrate solution and dip a filter paper in it. Hold the paper in a flame until it burns away and leaves ash.	Formation of pink colour ash.	Confirms the presence of Magnesium.
2	**Magneson test:** Place 1 mL of the filtrate (or sample solution) into a test tube. Add 1 mL of dilute hydrochloric acid and 2 drops of Magneson reagent and 2 mL of sodium hydroxide (2 M).	Formation of flocculent blue precipitate.	Confirms the presence of Magnesium.
	Magneson reagent: (4-(4-Nitrophenylazo)-resorcinol)		
3	Place 1 mL of the sample solution into a test tube. Add 1 mL of sodium hydroxide into the test tube.	Formation of white precipitate.	Confirms the presence of Magnesium.
	$Mg^{2+} + 2\ NaOH \longrightarrow Mg(OH)_2\downarrow + 2\ Na^+$		
4	Place 1 mL of the sample solution into a test tube. Add 1 mL of ammonium hydroxide into the test tube.	Formation of white gelatinous precipitate (soluble in excess of ammonium chloride).	Confirms the presence of Magnesium.
	$Mg^{2+} + 2\ NH_4OH \longrightarrow Mg(OH)_2\downarrow + 2\ NH_4^+$		
5	Place 1 mL of the filtrate (or sample solution) into a test tube. Add 1 mL of disodium hydrogen phosphate and 1 mL of ammonium chloride solution into the test tube.	Formation of white crystalline precipitate.	Confirms the presence of Magnesium.
	$Mg^{2+} + Na_2HPO_4 + NH_4Cl \longrightarrow Mg(NH_4)PO_4\downarrow + 2\ Na^+ + H^+$		

Confirmatory Tests for Group VI

Confirmatory tests for Ammonium (Group VI)

S No	Experiment	Observation	Inference
1	Place 1 mL of the sample solution into a test tube. Add 1 mL of picric acid into the test tube.	Formation of yellow precipitate.	Indicates the presence of Ammonium.
2	**Nesslers test:** Place 1 mL of the sample solution into a test tube. Add 1 mL of sodium hydroxide into the test tube. Boil the mixture and pass the evolving ammonia gas.	Formation of reddish-brown precipitate.	Confirms the presence of Ammonium.
	$4\ NH_3 + NaOH + 2\ K_2HgI_4 \longrightarrow 8\ NH_4HgOHgI\downarrow + Na^+ + 4\ K^+$		

Confirmatory Tests for Group VII

Confirmatory tests for Potassium (Group VII)

S No	Experiment	Observation	Inference
1	**Flame test:** Introduce the glass rod dipped in paste of sample made with hydrochloric acid into the non-luminous flame.	Appearance of violet flame.	Indicates the presence of Potassium.
2	Place 1 mL of the sample solution into a test tube. Add 1 mL of picric acid into the test tube.	Formation of yellow precipitate.	Indicates the presence of Potassium.
3	Place 1 mL of the sample solution into a test tube. Add 1 mL of perchloric acid into the test tube.	Formation of white crystalline precipitate.	Confirms the presence of Potassium.
	$K^+ + HClO_4 \longrightarrow KClO_4 \downarrow + H^+$		
4	Place 1 mL of the sample solution into a test tube. Add 1 mL of sodium cobalt nitrite solution into the test tube.	Formation of yellow precipitate.	Confirms the presence of Potassium.
5	Place 1 mL of the sample solution into a test tube. Add 1 mL of tartaric acid (buffered with sodium acetate) into the test tube.	Formation of white crystalline precipitate.	Confirms the presence of Potassium.

Confirmatory tests for Sodium

S No	Experiment	Observation	Inference
1	**Flame test:** Transfer the pinch of sample into a test tube. Add 1ml of con. hydrochloric acid. Stir and introduce the paste into the non-luminous flame with the help of glass rod.	Appearance of persistent golden yellow.	Indicates the presence of sodium.
2	**Magnesium uranylacetate test:** Transfer 0.1 g sample into a test tube. Add 2 ml of water. Acidify with acetic acid. Add magnesium uranylacetate solution.	Formation of yellow crystalline precipitate.	Confirms the presence of sodium.
	$Na^+ + \underset{\text{Uranylacetate}}{UO_2(CH_3COO)_2} + \underset{\text{Magnesiumacetate}}{Mg(CH_3COO)_2} \longrightarrow \underset{\text{Sodium-magnesium uranylacetate}}{NaMg(UO_2)_3(CH_3COO)_2}$		
3	**Potassium pyroantimonate test:** Transfer 0.1 g of the sample into a test tube. Add 2 ml of water and 2 ml of 15% potassium carbonate solution. Heat to boil. • Add 4 ml freshly prepared dil. potassium pyroantimonate solution. Heat to boil. • Cool and scratch the sides of the test tube.	Formation of dense white precipitate.	Confirms the presence of sodium.
	$Na^+ + \underset{\text{Potassium pyroantimonate}}{KH_2SbO_4} \longrightarrow \underset{\text{Sodium pyroantimonate}}{NaH_2SbO_4} + K^+$		

44

Analysis of Organic Compounds

Qualitative analysis of organic compounds involves series of chemical tests to establish the identity of the unknown organic compound. The unknown organic compound identity can be established through the following parameters.

1. Physical appearance
   - Colour: Blue, dull white
   - Physical nature: Crystalline, amorphous
   - Physical form: Solid, liquid
   - Solubility: Water soluble, organic solvent soluble
2. Melting point or boiling point.
3. Solubility tests
4. Saturation state: saturated, unsaturated
5. Nature of carbon chain: Aliphatic, aromatic
6. Special elements: Nitrogen, sulphur, halogen
7. Functional groups: Carboxylic acids, amines, carbonyls, alcohols, esters, amides, etc.
8. Chemical derivatization

Practical tips

1. Sample size:

   For functionality detection

   Solid: 0.1 g

   Liquid: 2 to 3 drops

   For chemical derivatization

   Solid: 1 g

   Liquid: 1 mL
2. Tests with authentic samples (control): The comparison of results of a test sample and the authentic compound provides effective conclusion.

Organic compounds	Aliphatic	Aromatic
Carboxylic acids	Formic acid, Acetic acid	Benzoic acid, Salicylic acid
Phenols	Thioalcohols	Phenol, Resorcinol, Thiophenol
Amines	Methylamine	Aniline
Aldehydes	Formaldehyde, Acetaldehyde	Benzaldehyde, Salicylaldehyde
Ketones	Acetone, Cyclohexanone	Acetophenone
Alcohols	Methanol, Ethanol, Propyl alcohol	Benzyl alcohol
Amides	Acetamide	Benzamide
Anhydrides	Acetic anhydride	Phthalic anhydride
Carbohydrates	Glucose, Fructose, Sucrose	-

44.1 Preliminary Tests

S. No.	Experiment	Observation	Inference
1	**Physical state** Solid / Liquid	Solid	It may be phenols, acids, amides
		Liquid	It may be alcohols, aldehydes, ketones, esters, acids, anhydrides
2	**Colour** Solids	Pale yellow	Nitro compounds, iodoform
		Orange to red	Nitro anilines, azo compounds
		Pink	Naphthols
		Brown	Aromatic amines, amino phenols
		Green	*p*-Nitrosophenol
		Colourless	Aldehydes, ketones, carbohydrates, alcohols
	Colour Liquids	Reddish brown	Amines
		Orange to red	Nitro compounds
3	**Odour**	Pleasant	Ethers, aliphatic alcohols, chloroform
		Bitter almonds	Benzaldehyde, nitro benzene
		Fishy	Amines
		Pungent	Acetic acid, acetic anhydride, formic acid
		Rotten egg	Sulphur compounds
		Fruity smell	Esters

44.2 Solubility Tests

S. No.	Experiment	Observation	Inference
General Procedure: Dissolve the sample (solid (0.1 g) / liquid (0.2 mL)) with the solvent (3 mL).			
1	**Test with water** If the sample is water souble, then test the aqueous solution with litmus paper. **Note**: High molecular weight alcohols, aldehydes and ketones do not dissolve in water.	Turns blue litmus red	Acids and phenols
		Add sodium bicarbonate solution (10%) to the sample solution.	• Evolution of carbon dioxide by effervescence indicates the presence of carboxylic acids and nitro phenols. • No evolution of carbon dioxide indicates the presence of phenols.
		• Turns red litmus blue	Amines, alcohols, aldehydes, carbohydrates
		• Neutral to litmus	Esters, ethers, amides, nitriles

Table *Contd...*

S. No.	Experiment	Observation	Inference
2.	Test with sodium hydroxide (5%)	• Completely soluble (reappears by the addition of hydrochloric acid)	Acids, phenols, oximes, thiophenols, thiols, sulphonic acids, sulphonamides, β-ketoesters
		• Soluble in hot condition and turns into brown colour	Carbohydrates
		• Soluble and produces alcohol odour.	Esters
3.	Test with hydrochloric acid (5%). Add sodium hydroxide solution.	Completely soluble Precipitates the dissolved sample.	Amines and hydrazines.
4.	Test with cold sulphuric acid.	Completely soluble	Aromatic nitro compounds, ethers, esters, alcohols, aldehydes, ketones, unsaturated hydrocarbons and anhydrides.

44.3 Tests for Saturation

S. No.	Experiment	Observation	Inference
1.	**Baeyer test:** Dissolve 0.2 g (or 0.2 mL) of the sample with suitable solvent (2 mL). Add sodium carbonate (10 mL) and potassium permanganate (2%) drop-wise.	Decolourisation of potassium permanganate.	Indicates the presence of Unsaturated compound.
		No decolourisation of potassium permanganate.	Indicates the presence of Saturated compound.
	Alkene + $KMnO_4$ $\xrightarrow{Na_2CO_3}$ HO–C–C–OH (diol)		
2.	**Bromine test:** Dissolve 0.2 g (or 0.2 mL) of the sample with carbon tetrachloride (2 mL). Add this solution (drop wise) to test tube containing bromine solution (2 mL, 2%) in carbon tetrachloride and shake well.	Disappearance of the bromine colour (yellow).	Indicates the presence of Unsaturated compound.
		No decolourisation.	Indicates the presence of Saturated compound.
	Alkene + Br_2 $\xrightarrow{CCl_4}$ Br–C–C–Br		
	Note: Bromine reagent is very dangerous, hence protect skin, eyes and nose.		

44.4 Tests for Aromaticity

S. No.	Experiment	Observation	Inference
1.	**Ignition test**: Ignite the sample using metal spatula.	Burns with non-smoky (or less smoky) flame.	Indicates the aliphatic nature of the compound.
		Burns with very smoky flame.	Indicates the aromatic nature of the compound.

Table *Contd...*

S. No.	Experiment	Observation	Inference
2.	**Nitration test:** Place the sample to a beaker containing mixture of concentrated sulphuric acid and nitric acid (1:1). Heat the mixture and pour into a beaker containing water.	Development of yellowish solution (or precipitate).	Indicates the aromatic nature of the compound.
3.	**Fuming sulphuric acid test:** Dissolve the sample (0.2 g or 0.2 mL) in fuming sulphuric acid (2 mL, 20%).	Aromatic hydrocarbon dissolves and evolves heat.	Indicates the aromatic nature of the compound.
	Warm gently and pour into beaker containing crushed ice.	Aromatic compounds produce homogenous solution.	

44.5 Tests for the Special Elements

Lassaigne's Sodium Fusion Test

The detection of elements namely oxygen, nitrogen, sulphur, chlorine, bromine, fluorine and iodine is essential. The ionic tests convert these elements into water-soluble ionic compounds (NaX, NaCN, Na_2S and NaCNS).

***Preparation of sodium fusion extract*:**

1. Place a piece of sodium metal into a fusion tube and melt the sodium.
2. Add the sample (50 mg or 3 drops) portion-wise on to the molten sodium. Heat the bottom of the tube to redness for about 2 min.
3. Place the tube into a porcelain dish containing cold distilled water (15 mL) and crush the tube.
4. Boil for 15 min and remove the glass splinters by filtration.
5. The clear filtrate is known as *sodium fusion extract*. The extract can be used for the specific tests described below.

   ***Caution*:** The residual sodium metal (if any) reacts with water vigorously and leads to explosion. Hence, personal protective equipment (PPE) and operation in fume cupboard is advisable.

Lassaigne's Test for Nitrogen

S. No.	Experiment	Observation	Inference
1	***Prussian blue test:*** Transfer 2 mL of extract into a test tube. Add pinch of powdered ferrous sulphate crystals and 1 mL of sodium hydroxide solution. Heat the mixture gently with shaking. Cool and 2 drops of ferric chloride solution. Acidify the solution with dilute sulphuric acid.	Formation of a Prussian blue (bluish-green) precipitate.	Confirms the presence of Nitrogen.
		Formation of pale yellow colour.	Confirms the absence of Nitrogen.
	$NaCN + FeCl_3 + Fe_2(SO_4)_3 \longrightarrow Fe_4[Fe(CN)_6]_3 \downarrow$ Ferric ferrocyanide (Prussian blue)		

Table ***Contd...***

Lassaigne's Test for Sulphur

S. No.	Experiment	Observation	Inference
2	**Lead acetate test:** Acidify 1 mL of the extract with acetic acid and add 2 drops of lead acetate solution.	Formation of black precipitate	Confirms the presence Sulphur.
	$Na_2S + (CH_3COO)_2Pb \xrightarrow{CH_3COOH} PbS\downarrow$		
3	**Sodium nitroprusside test:** Transfer 2 mL of extract into a test tube. Add 2 drops of dilute sodium hydroxide and 4 drops of cold sodium nitroprusside solution (freshly prepared).	Development of deep red or purple colour	Confirms the presence of Sulphur (strong positive results are significant).
	$\underset{\text{Sodium nitroprusside}}{Na_4[Fe(CN)_6]NO} + \underset{\text{Sodium sulphide}}{Na_2S} \longrightarrow Na_4[Fe(CN)_5]NOS$		

Lassaigne's Test for Nitrogen and Sulphur

S. No.	Experiment	Observation	Inference
4	Transfer 1 mL of the extract into a test tube. Add 2 drops of ferric chloride solution.	Formation of blood red colour.	Confirms the presence of Nitrogen and Sulphur.
5	Transfer 1 mL of the extract into a test tube. Add 2 mL of ethanol and 2 drops of cobalt nitrate solution.	Formation of blue colour.	Confirms the presence of Nitrogen and Sulphur.

Lassaigne's Test for Halogens

S. No.	Experiment	Observation	Inference
6	Transfer 2 mL of the extract into a test tube and acidify with 2 drops of dilute nitric acid. (Boil for 2 min to expel hydrogen sulphide and or hydrogen cyanide, (if any present). Their presence causes interference with the results.) Add 2 mL of aqueous silver nitrate solution.	Formation of white precipitate. It is soluble in ammonium hydroxide.	Confirms the presence of Chlorides.
		$NaCl + AgNO_3 \xrightarrow{HNO_3} AgCl\downarrow$	
		Formation of pale yellow precipitate. It is soluble in excess of ammonium hydroxide.	Confirms the presence of Bromides.
		$NaBr + AgNO_3 \xrightarrow{HNO_3} AgBr\downarrow$	
		Formation of yellow precipitate. It is insoluble in ammonium hydroxide.	Confirms the presence of Iodides.
		$NaI + AgNO_3 \xrightarrow{HNO_3} AgI\downarrow$	

44.6 Functional group Identification

Tests for Carboxylic Acids

S. No.	Experiment	Observation	Inference
1	**Litmus test:** Place drop of sample solution on blue litmus paper.	Blue litmus turns into red colour.	Indicates the presence of Carboxylic acid or Phenols.
2	Transfer 1 mL of sample solution into a test tube. Add 2 mL of potassium iodide (5%) and 2 mL of potassium iodate. Boil for 2 min and add drop of starch solution.	Appearance of blue colour.	Indicates the presence of Carboxylic acid and or Phenols.
3	**Distinction test for carboxylic acids:**		
	Transfer 1 mL of sample solution into a test tube. Add 1 mL of aqueous sodium bicarbonate solution (5%).	Brisk effervescence of carbon-dioxide.	Indicates the presence of Carboxylic acids (phenols do not respond to this test).
	$\underset{\text{Carboxylic acid}}{\text{R-COOH}} + \underset{\text{Sodium bicarbonate}}{\text{NaHCO}_3} \longrightarrow \underset{\text{Sodium salt of carboxylic acid}}{\text{R-COONa}}$		

Distinction tests for different carboxylic acids

S. No.	Experiment	Observation	Inference
	Distinction tests between aliphatic and aromatic acids		
4	**Soda lime test:** Transfer sample solution and sodalime (1:2) into a test tube. Heat the contents of the test tube.	A gas with smoky flame.	Indicates the presence of Aromatic acids (distinction from aliphatic acids).
	$\text{R-COOH} + \text{NaHCO}_3 \longrightarrow \text{R-COONa}$		
5	***Esterification test*:** Transfer the sample and absolute ethanol (1:2) into a test tube. Add 1 part of concentrated sulphuric acid into a test tube. Warm the mixture for 2 min. Cool and pour the hot mixture into beaker containing aqueous sodium hydroxide solution.	Fruity (sweet) odour.	Confirms the presence of Carboxylic acid.
		$\underset{\text{Carboxylic acid}}{\text{R-COOH}} + \underset{\text{Alcohol}}{\text{R}^1\text{-OH}} \xrightarrow[\text{NaOH}]{\text{H}^+} \underset{\text{Ester}}{\text{R-CO-O-R}^1}$	
		Gum like odour	Formic acid
		Apple-fruity and or Banana odour	Acetic acid
		Mint odour	Benzoic acid
		Balmy odour	Salicylic acid
6	Dissolve the sample (0.5 g) with water and add dilute sodium hydroxide (*until it becomes alkaline*). Acidify with dilute hydrochloric acid and add dilute nitric acid (1 mL). Boil the solution to remove the excess of ammonia (litmus paper test). Add 3 drops of ferric chloride solution to the neutralized solution (boil if necessary).	Development of reddish brown precipitate.	Indicates the presence of Acetic acid.
		Development of faint yellow colour.	Indicates the presence of Oxalic acid.
		Development of buff coloured precipitate.	Indicates the presence of Benzoic acid or Cinnamic acid.
		Development of violet colour.	Indicates the presence of Salicylic acid.

Table *Contd...*

S. No.	Experiment	Observation	Inference
	Test for dicarboxylic acids		
7	***Fluorescein test***: Transfer the sample and resorcinol (1:2) into a test tube and mix well. Add 4 drops of concentrated sulphuric acid and heat till deep red solution is obtained (~5 min). Pour the red solution into a beaker containing dilute sodium hydroxide.	Appearance of intense greenish-yellow fluorescence.	Confirms the presence of *di*-carboxylic acid.
	Phthalic acid (dicarboxylic acid) + Resorcinol $\xrightarrow[NaOH]{H_2SO_4}$ Fluorescein		

Test for Alcohols

S. No.	Experiment	Observation	Inference
8	Transfer 1 mL of the sample solution into a test tube. Add piece of dry sodium metal. Heat the mixture by placing on a water bath.	Brisk effervescence of hydrogen gas evolves.	Indicates the presence of Alcohols.
	$R\text{-}OH + Na \longrightarrow H_2\uparrow + R\text{-}ONa$		
9	***Ceric ammonium nitrate test***: Transfer 1 mL of the sample solution into a test tube. Add 2 drops of cerric ammonium nitrate solution.	Development of red colour.	Indicates the presence of Alcohol.
		Development of green colour.	Indicates the presence of Phenols.
	$R\text{-}OH + (NH_4)_2Ce(NO_3)_6 \longrightarrow (NH_4)_2Ce(OR)(NO_3)_5 + HNO_3$ Alcohol; Cerric ammonium nitrate (yellow); Cerric ammonium nitrate alcohol complex (red)		
10	***Esterification test***: Transfer the sample and acetic acid (2:1) into a test tube. Add 1 part of concentrated sulphuric acid into a test tube. Warm the mixture for 2 min. Cool and pour the hot mixture into beaker containing aqueous sodium hydroxide solution.	Fruity (sweet) odour.	Confirms the presence of Alcohol.
	$R\text{-}COOH + R^1\text{-}OH \xrightarrow[NaOH]{H^+} R\text{-}CO\text{-}O\text{-}R^1$ Carboxylic acid; Alcohol; Ester		
11	***Xanthate test (carbon disulphide test):*** Transfer the sample solution into a test tube. Add sodium hydroxide pellets, dissolve and cool. Add 5 drops of carbon disulphide and shake.	Formation of yellow precipitate of thioxanthate.	Confirms the presence of Alcohol.
	$R\text{-}OH + CS_2 \xrightarrow[-H_2O]{NaOH} R{-}O{-}C({=}S){-}SK$ Alcohol; Xanthate (yellow)		

Table *Contd...*

S. No.	Experiment	Observation	Inference
12	***Oxidation test***: Heat copper wire in a non luminous flame and introduce into the solution of sample present in fusion tube 3 times. Divide this solution into 2 parts.	Crystalline yellow precipitate	Confirms the presence of Alcohol.
	1) To one part add few drops of Schiff reagent.	Formation of purple colour.	Indicates the presence of Methyl and Ethyl alcohol.
	2) To the another part add few drops of 2,4-dinitrophenylhydrazine.	Odour of oil of bitter almond.	Indicates the presence of Benzyl alcohol.

Differentiation between 1°, 2° and 3° alcohols

S. No.	Experiment	Observation	Inference
13	***Lucas test***: Transfer 1 mL of sample solution into a test tube. Add 2 mL of Lucas reagent and shake the mixture. Keep it aside for 5 min. ***Lucas reagent***: Mixture of anhydrous zinc chloride and concentrated hydrochloric acid.	Solution remains clear.	Primary alcohols.
		$R\text{-}CH_2OH \longrightarrow$ Clear solution	
		Cloudy (becomes two phase after 5 min to 1 h).	Secondary alcohols.
		$R\text{—}CH(R)\text{-}OH \xrightarrow{ZnCl_2\text{-}HCl} R\text{—}CH(R)\text{-}Cl$ Cloudy	
		Immediate separation into two phases.	Tertiary alcohols.
		$R\text{—}C(R)_2\text{—}OH \xrightarrow{ZnCl_2\text{-}HCl} R\text{—}C(R)_2\text{—}Cl$ Two phases	
14	***Jones test***: Transfer 1 mL of sample solution in acetone into a test tube. Add one drop of Jones reagent and shake to mix the contents. **Jones Reagent:** Potassium chromate and concentrated sulphuric acid.	Formation of a green or blue-green precipitate (or emulsion).	Confirms the presence of Primary and Secondary alcohols.
		$R\text{-}CH_2OH \xrightarrow{(O)} R\text{-}CHO \xrightarrow{(O)} R\text{-}COOH$ $R\text{—}CH(R)\text{-}OH \xrightarrow{(O)} R\text{—}C(R){=}O$	
		Tertiary alcohols do not react.	

Tests for Phenols

S. No.	Experiment	Observation	Inference
15	**Litmus test:** Place drop of sample solution on blue litmus paper.	Blue litmus turns into red colour.	Indicates the presence of acidic compound (Carboxylic acid or Phenols produce positive results).
16	Transfer 1 mL of the sample solution into a test tube. Add 5 mL of sodium hydroxide solution.	Formation of clear solution (sodium hydroxide dissolves the sample).	Indicates the presence of Carboxylic acid or Phenols.

Table *Contd...*

S. No.	Experiment	Observation	Inference
17	Transfer 1 mL of the sample solution into a test tube. Add 5 mL of sodium bicarbonate solution.	Evolution of no carbon dioxide gas. (carboxylic acids releases carbon dioxide)	Indicates the presence of phenols.
18	***Neutral ferric chloride test*:** Transfer 1 mL of aqueous (or alcoholic) solution into a test tube. Add 1 drop of neutral (1% w/v) ferric chloride solution. Add another drop neutral (1% w/v) ferric chloride after 3 sec.	Development of green or blue or purple colour.	Indicates the presence of Phenols.
		Development of white to violet precipitate.	Indicates the presence of α-Naphthol.
		Development of green to white precipitate.	Indicates the presence of β-Naphthol.
		Development of bluish white precipitate.	Indicates the presence of Resorcinol.
		Development of greenish black or blue precipitate.	Indicates the presence of Hydroquinone.
		Development of red precipitate.	Indicates the presence of Pyrogallol. (presence of enol)
19	***Bromine water test*:** Transfer 1 mL aqueous solution of the sample into a test tube. Add bromine water drop wise until the colour persists after shaking (slow decolourization).	Development of white precipitate.	Indicates the presence Phenol or Resorcinol.
		Development of yellowish needle like crystals.	Indicates the presence of α-Naphthol.
	Phenol (OH) + Br_2 → Tribromo phenol (OH, Br, Br, Br)		
20	***Ceric ammonium nitrate test*:** Transfer 1 mL of the sample solution into a test tube. Add 2 drops of ceric ammonium nitrate solution to the test tube.	Development of green colour.	Indicates the presence of Phenols.
21	***Liebermann's nitroso test*:** Transfer sample (0.2 g or 1 mL) and sulfuric acid (1 mL) into a test tube. Add crystals of sodium nitrite into a test tube and heat gently.	Formation of black colour precipitate.	Indicates the presence of β-Naphthol.
	Add the sample and 1 mL of concentrated sulphuric acid to the orange-red colour solution.	Green to blue-green-brown colouration. • Dilution with water turns red. • Basification gives original colour.	Confirms the presence of Phenols.
	Phenol (–OH) —$NaNO_2$/H_2SO_4→ HO–N(H)–C₆H₄=O —Phenol→ HO–C₆H₄–N=C₆H₄=O (Indo phenol) —NaOH→ NaO–C₆H₄–N=C₆H₄=O (Indo phenol sodium salt)		

Table ***Contd...***

S. No.	Experiment	Observation	Inference
22	***Phthalein test***: Transfer the equal weight of sample and phthalic anhydride into a dry test tube. Mix the contents. Add 1 drop of concentrated sulphuric acid. Heat the contents for 4 min. Cool and add to a beaker containing sodium hydroxide solution (10%).	Green to blue-green-brown colouration.	Confirms the presence of Phenols.
		• Red colouration	• Phenol/*o*-Cresol
		• Blue colouration	• *m*-Cresol/Pyrogallol
		• Yellowish red with green fluroscence	• Resorcinol
		• Green colouration	• *α*-Naphthol
		• Faint green with fluroscence	• *β*-Naphthol
	Phthalic anydride + Phenol $\xrightarrow[H_2O]{H^+}$ (phenolphthalein, HO…OH) $\xrightarrow{NaOH}$ (quinonoid form with COONa)		

Tests for Carbonyl Compounds

S. No.	Experiment	Observation	Inference
23	***Brady's reagent: 2,4-Dinitrophenylhydrazine test***: Transfer small amount (0.1 g or 0.2 mL) of sample into a test tube. Add 3 mL of 2,4-diphenylhydrazine and shake. Allow to stand for 10 min.	Oily precipitate turns into yellow to reddish crystalline precipitate.	Confirms presence of Carbonyl compounds.
	$RR_1C{=}O$ (Carbonyl compound) + $H_2N{-}HN{-}C_6H_3(NO_2)_2$ (2,4-Dinitrophenylhydrazine) $\longrightarrow$ $RR_1C{=}N{-}HN{-}C_6H_3(NO_2)_2$ (Hydrazone)		

Tests for Carbonyl Compounds: Aldehydes

S. No.	Experiment	Observation	Inference
24	***Tollen's reagent test (silver mirror test)***: Place 2 mL of Tollen's reagent and 5 drops of sample solution into a test tube. Boil for 5 min and cool. ***Tollen's reagent***: Ammoniacal silver nitrate solution.	Appearance of black color or silver mirror on the sides of the test tube. *Caution:* The silver mixture is highly explosive. Hence, pour the contents into the sink and wash the test tube with dilute nitric acid.	Confirms the presence of Aldehyde. (Aldehydes reduces silver ions (Ag^+) in Tollen's reagent to silver (Ag)).
	$RHC{=}O$ (Aldehyde) + $[Ag(NH_3)_2NO_3]$ (Tollens reagent) $\xrightarrow[NaOH]{\Delta}$ $2Ag\downarrow$ (Silver mirror)		

Table *Contd...*

S. No.	Experiment	Observation	Inference
25	***Fehling's test***: Transfer small amount of sample (0.5 g or 2 drops) into a test tube. Add 3 mL of Fehling's solution A and B. Warm the solution in a water bath for 3 min.	Formation of yellowish red precipitate of cuprous oxide.	Confirms the presence of Aldehyde.
	$RCHO + Cu^{2+} \xrightarrow[NaOH]{\Delta} Cu_2O\downarrow$ Aldehyde + Fehling's reagent → Cuprous oxide (red precipitate)		
	Fehling's solution A: Copper sulphate in distilled water. **Fehling's solution B**: Sodium-potassium tartarate (Rochelle salt) in aqueous sodium hydroxide.		
26	**Benedict's test:** Transfer small amount of sample (0.5 g or 2 drops) into a test tube. Add 2 mL of Benedict's reagent and boil for few min.	Yellow to red precipitate of cuprous oxide.	Indicates the presence of Aldehyde.
	$RCHO + Cu^{2+} \xrightarrow[NaOH]{\Delta} Cu_2O\downarrow$ Aldehyde + Benedict's reagent → Cuprous oxide (red precipitate)		
	Benedict's reagent: Copper sulphate and sodium citrate in aqueous sodium carbonate solution.		
27	***Schiff's reagent test - Caro's test***: Transfer small amount of sample (0.5 g) in to a test tube, add 2 mL of Schiff's reagent and shake the mixture by keeping on ice-cold condition.	Formation of instantaneous purple colour.	Confirms the presence of aliphatic Aldehyde.
		Formation of purple colour on standing.	Confirms the presence of aromatic Aldehyde
	Schiff's reagent: p-Rosaniline hydrochloride in aqueous sulphur dioxide solution.		
28	***Jones test***: Transfer 1 mL of sample in acetone into a test tube. Add one drop of the Jones reagent and mix the contents.	Formation of a green or blue-green precipitate (or emulsion). (disappearance of orange colour of the reagent).	Confirms the presence of Aldehydes.
		$R\text{-}CHO \xrightarrow{(O)} R\text{-}COOH$	
	Jones Reagent: Potassium chromate and concentrated sulphuric acid.		

Tests for Carbonyl Compounds: Ketones

S. No.	Experiment	Observation	Inference
29	***Iodoform test***: Transfer aqueous sample solution into test tube. Add 2 mL of sodium hydroxide (5%) and iodine reagent drop-wise with shaking, until iodine persists. Allow the contents to stand for 3 min.	Formation of yellow precipitate of iodoform.	Confirms the presence of Methyl ketone. *Acetaldehyde and secondary alcohols also produces positive results.*

Table ***Contd...***

S. No.	Experiment	Observation	Inference
	Warm and add iodine reagent drop-wise, until iodine colour persist. Add dilute sodium hydroxide drop-wise with shaking (to remove excess of iodine). Dilute with equal volume of water and allow standing for 10 min.		
	$R(H_3C)C{=}O + KI\text{-}I_2 \xrightarrow{NaOH} CHI_3$ (Methyl ketone → Iodoform)		
30	***Sodium nitroprusside test***: To the sample add sodium nitroprusside solution and excess of 30% sodium hydroxide.	Orange colour changes to pink/purple colour (formation of complex).	Indicates the presence of methyl ketone.
31	***Zimmerman reaction*** (*m*-dinitrobenzene test): To the sample add powdered *m*-dinitrobenzene. Add excess of sodium hydroxide solution and shake.	• Red colour develops immediately • Light red colour on standing • Yellow turns to red on standing	• Methyl ketone • Benzophenone/Benzaldehyde • Salicyladehyde

Test for Esters and Anhydrides

S. No.	Experiment	Observation	Inference
32	***Phenolphthalein test***: To the sample, add a drop of phenolphthalein and add sodium hydroxide solution drop-wise. Heat the mixture.	Disapperance of odour and colour.	Indicates the presence of Anhydrides and Esters.
33	***Hydroxamic acid test***: To 0.2 g of the sample add 2 g of hydroxylamine hydrochloride in ethanol. Add saturated solution of ethanolic potassium hydroxide, until mixture becomes alkaline (litmus test). Boil for 2 min, cool and acidify with hydrochloric acid and add 2 drops of ferric chloride solution.	Development of violet/wine red colour.	Confirms the presence of anhydrides and esters.
	$R\text{-}CO\text{-}O\text{-}R^{1+} + NH_2OH \xrightarrow[KOH]{H^+} R\text{-}C(=O)\text{-}NHOH + R^1\text{-}OH$ (Ester + Hydroxyl amine → … + Alcohol)		
	Esters react with hydroxylamine in basic condition and forms sodium salt of the corresponding hydroxamic acid. Addition of ferric chloride produces the magenta-coloured iron (III) complex of the hydroxamic acid.		

Test for Ethers

S. No.	Experiment	Observation	Inference
34	Transfer 1 mL of iodine in carbon disulphide to a test tube. Add 0.5 mL of the substance.	Purple colour changes to tan colour.	Confirms the presence of Ethers.

Test for Polyhydric Alcohols and Carbohydrates

S. No.	Experiment	Observation	Inference
35	**Molisch's test** (General test for carbohydrates): Place 1 mL of the sample solution in a clean test tube. Add 2 drops of Molisch's reagent (alcoholic α-naphthol, 10%) and mix well. Incline the test tube and slowly add 0.5 mL of concentrated sulfuric acid in drops along the sides of the test tube.	Appearance of purple colour ring at the interface. Sulphuric acid dehydrates reducing sugars to furfural derivatives. These furfurals condense with alcoholic α-naphthol (Molisch's reagent) and forms violet colored products.	Indicates the presence of Carbohydrates.
	Glucose → HOH_2C–(furan)–CHO (5-Hydroxymethyl furfural) + 2 α-naphthol —($-H_2O$)→ Furfuryl-diphenyl methane dye		
	Note: Concentrated solution of organic compounds may give a red colour instead violet due to charring action of the sulphuric acid. In case of doubt, the experiment should be repeated on a more diluted solution of the substance to be tested.		
36	***Tollen's test (silver mirror test)*:** Place 2 mL of Tollen's reagent and 5 drops of sample solution into a test tube. Boil for 5 min and cool. ***Tollen's reagent***: Ammoniacal silver nitrate solution.	Appearance of black color or silver mirror on the sides of the test tube. *Caution:* The silver mixture is highly explosive. Hence, pour the contents into the sink and wash the test tube with dilute nitric acid.	Confirms the presence of Reducing sugar. (Aldehydes reduce silver ions (Ag^+) in Tollen's reagent to silver (Ag)).
	$R_2C{=}O$ (Aldehyde or ketone) + $[Ag(NH_3)_2NO_3]$ (Tollens reagent) $\xrightarrow[NaOH]{\Delta}$ $2Ag\downarrow$ (Silver mirror)		
37	***Fehling's test*:** Transfer small amount of sample (0.5 g or 2 drops) into a test tube. Add 3 mL of Fehling's solution A and B. Warm the solution in a water-bath for 3 min.	Formation of yellowish red precipitate of cuprous oxide.	Confirms the presence of Reducing sugar.

Table *Contd...*

S. No.	Experiment	Observation	Inference
	$RCHO$ (Aldehyde) + Cu^{2+} (Fehling's reagent) $\xrightarrow[NaOH]{\Delta}$ $Cu_2O\downarrow$ (Cuprous oxide (red precipitate))		
	Fehling's solution A: Copper sulphate solution. **Fehling's solution B**: Sodium-potassium tartarate (Rochelle salt) in aqueous sodium hydroxide.		
38	**Benedict's test:** Transfer small amount of sample (0.5 g or 2 drops) into a test tube. Add 2 mL of Benedict's reagent and boil for few min.	Yellow to red precipitate of cuprous oxide.	Confirms the presence of Reducing sugar.
	$RCHO$ (Aldehyde) + Cu^{2+} (Benedict's reagent) $\xrightarrow[NaOH]{\Delta}$ $Cu_2O\downarrow$ (Cuprous oxide (red precipitate))		
	Benedict's reagent: Copper sulphate and sodium citrate in aqueous sodium carbonate solution.		

Tests for Compounds Containing Nitrogen

Tests for Amines

S. No.	Experiment	Observation	Inference
39	***Concentrated hydrochloric acid test:*** To the sample add concentrated hydrochloric acid.	Formation of white precipitate.	Confirms the presence of Amines.
40	***Diazotization test:*** To the sample add 3 mL of concentrated hydrochloric acid, cool thoroughly to 0 - 5 °C in an ice-bath for 5 min.and add few drops cold solution (kept in ice-bath) of sodium nitrite (0.5 g sodium nitrite in 2 mL of water) from a dropper. Add the above solution to ice cold solution of 0.2 g of β-naphthol in 2 mL of sodium hydroxide with swirling keeping the test tube in ice-bath.	Formation of an orange-red azo dye.	Confirms the presence of Amines.
	1° Aromatic amines	Orange red dye	
	$Ar-NH_2$ (Aromatic primary amine) $\xrightarrow[HCl]{NaNO_2}$ $Ar-N{=}N-Cl$ (Diazonium salt)		
	1° Aliphatic amines	Orange red dye (evolves nitrogen gas)	
	2° Aromatic amines		
	2° Aliphatic amines	Yellow oily nitrosamines	

Table ***Contd...***

S. No.	Experiment	Observation	Inference
	3° Aromatic amines	No colouration, but gives blue colour with starch iodide paper (nitrous acid liberates iodine from starch iodide and produces blue colour)	
	3° Aliphatic amines	Reddish-green solid forms upon the addition of sodium hydroxide.	
41	**Hinsberg test:** Place 0.5 mL (or 0.5 g) of the sample, 10 mL of sodium hydroxide (5%) and 1 mL of benzenesulphonyl chloride in a test tube. Stopper the tube and shake until the disappearance of odour of the sulphonyl chloride.	Formation of white precipitate.	Confirms the presence of Amines (primary and secondary).
	If there is no precipitate, acidify it cautiously with concentrated hydrochloric acid.	Formation of white precipitate.	Indicates the presence of primary amines.
	$C_6H_5-SO_2-Cl$ (Benzenesulphonyl chloride) + H_2N-R (Primary amine) $\xrightarrow{NaOH}$ $C_6H_5-SO_2-NHR$ (N-Substituted sulphonamides) + NaCl + H_2O		
	Formation of white precipitate, which is insoluble in alkali and unaffected by hydrochloric acid.		Indicates the presence of secondary amines.
	$C_6H_5-SO_2-Cl$ (Benzenesulphonyl chloride) + $HN(R)-R$ (Secondary amine) $\xrightarrow{NaOH}$ $C_6H_5-SO_2-N(R)-R$ (N, N-Disubstituted sulphonamides) + NaCl + H_2O		
	The sample remains unreactive and dissolves upon acidification with hydrochloric acid.		Indicates the presence of tertiary amines.

Tests for Amides (R-CO-NH$_2$)

S. No.	Experiment	Observation	Inference
42	**Hydroxamic acid test:** Transfer sample (0.2 g/0.2 mL) to the test tube. Add 2 g of hydroxylamine hydrochloride in ethanol and 5 mL of sodium hydroxide (10%). Boil for 2 min, cool and add 2 drops of ferric chloride.	Formation of deep red colour.	Confirms the presence of Amides.
	$R-CO-NH_2$ (Amide) + $NH_2OH.HCl$ (Hydroxylamine hydrochloride) $\xrightarrow[-R-OH]{NaOH}$ $R-CO-NHOH$ $\xrightarrow[-HCl]{FeCl_3}$ $[R-CO-NHOH]_3Fe$		

Table *Contd...*

S. No.	Experiment	Observation	Inference
43	Add 1 mL of sodium hydroxide sodium hydroxide (10%) to the sample and boil.	Smell of ammonia and white fumes.	Confirms the presence of Amides.
	$R-\overset{O}{\overset{\parallel}{C}}-NH_2 + NaOH \longrightarrow R-\overset{O}{\overset{\parallel}{C}}-ONa + NH_3$ (Amide)		
44	Add 5 drops of concentrated hydrochloric acid to the above solution.	Formation of white precipitate	Confirms the presence of aromatic Amides.
45	Transfer 1 mL of ice-cold sodium nitrite solution and 1 mL of acetic acid in to a test tube. Add ice-cold sample solution to the above tube.	Brisk effervescence of nitrogen.	Confirms the presence of Amides.
46	**Biuret test:** Heat 0.2 g of the sample to melt. Cool and dissolve with sodium hydroxide (10%). Add 1 drop of 1% copper sulphate solution.	Develops violet/ purple colour	Indicates the presence of *di*-amides.
	$H_2N-\overset{O}{\overset{\parallel}{C}}-NH_2 \xrightarrow{NaOH} H_2N-\overset{O}{\overset{\parallel}{C}}-NH-\overset{O}{\overset{\parallel}{C}}-NH_2 \xrightarrow{CuSO_4}$ Cu-Biuret complex (Blue precipitate) (Urea; Biuret)		
47	**Action of hypobromide:** To a solution of the substance add sodium hypobromide solution.	Brisk effervescence.	
	$R-\overset{O}{\overset{\parallel}{C}}-NH_2 + 6\ NaOBr \longrightarrow N_2 + CO_2 + NaBr + H_2O$ (Amide)		

Tests for Anilides

S. No.	Experiment	Observation	Inference
48	**Tafel's test:** To 0.2 g of the sample add 5 mL of sulphuric acid, shake and add 0.2 g potassium dichromate solution.	Red to violet colour (changes to green colour).	Confirms the presence of Anilides.
49	**Hydrolysis test:** To 0.2 g of the sample add 5 mL of dilute hydrochloric acid. Boil, cool and add sodium nitrite solution followed by β-naphthol in sodium hydroxide.	Formation of orange-red azo dye. (due to the cleavage of anilide into aniline).	Confirms the presence of Anilides.

Tests for Thiourea

S. No.	Experiment	Observation	Inference
50	**Ferric chloride test:** Heat the sample to melt. Cool and add ferric chloride solution.	Formation of deep-red colour.	Confirms the presence of Thiourea.
51	**Potassium ferrocyanide test:** To the hot solution of substance in acetic acid add 2 mL of potassium ferrocyanide.	Green colour changes to blue.	Confirms the presence of Thiourea.

Tests for Nitro Compounds

S. No.	Experiment	Observation	Inference
52	***Mulliken Barker test:*** To 0.2 g of sample in 2 mL of ethanol add 3 drops of calcium chloride solution and pinch of zinc dust. Boil, cool and filter. *Divide the filtrate into 2 parts.*		
	To one part of the filtrate, add Tollen's reagent.	Formation of black (or gray) precipitate.	Confirms the presence of Nitro group.
	$R\text{—}NO_2 \xrightarrow[-H_2O]{Zn,\ CaCl_2} R\text{—}NH\text{—}OH$ (Nitrate → Hydroxyl amine compound)		
	To the second part add equal volumes of Fehling's solutions A and B and heat.	Red brown precipitate	Confirms the presence of Nitro group.
53	To the sample add 2 mL of Ferric ammonium sulphate (5%) and drop of dilute sulphuric acid, followed by 1 mL of methanolic potassium hydroxide. Shake vigorously.	Red brown precipitate	Confirms the presence of Nitro group
	$R\text{-}NO_2 + Fe(NH_3)_2SO_4 \longrightarrow R\text{-}NO_2 + 6\ Fe\ (OH)_3 + 2\ NH_3$ (Nitrate + Ferric ammonium sulphate)		
54	***Azo dye test:*** Heat 0.1 g compound with 0.5 mL of hydrochloric acid. Add metal tin and boil for 3-4 minutes.	Smell of aniline	Confirms the presence of Nitro group.
55	Filter the above solution and add 3 mL of aqueous sodium nitrite solution, pour into a beaker containing cold β-naphthol.	Formation of brick-orange dye.	Confirms the presence of Nitro group.

44.7 Methods for the Preparation of Derivatives

1. **Acid derivative**

   1A) ***Amides, anilides and p-toluidides:*** Place the sample (0.5 g) into the flask and thionyl chloride (3 mL). Attach condenser with cotton plug on the top and reflux the mixture for 30 min (operation under in a fume cupboard is must). Distil the excess (unreacted) thionyl chloride (b.p. 78 °C). Treat the acid chloride product with concentrated ammonia solution (5 mL) or aniline (1 mL) or *p*-toluidine (1 g). Collect the solid derivative and recrystallize from alcohol.

   Note: Phosphorous pentachloride can be used in place of thionyl chloride.

2. **Alcohol Derivative**

   2A) ***3,5-Dinitrobenzoates:***

   Heat the mixture of 3,5- dinitrobenzoic acid (1 g) and phosphorus pentachloride (1.5 g) in a dry test tube, until it liquifies (5 min). Pour off the liquid on a dry watch glass and allow it to solidify. Remove the phosphoryl chloride by pressing the solid with a spatula on a wad of filter paper. Mix the solid (3,5-dinitrobenzoyl chloride) with the alcohol (1 mL) in a loosely corked dry test tube and heat on a steam bath for about 10 min (secondary and tertiary alcohols requires ~30 min). Cool and add 10 mL of sodium bicarbonate solution and stir until the ester crystallizes out. Filter the product under vacuum, and wash with sodium carbonate solution. Recrystallize the product from hot ethanol.

Note: Work under fume hood. Fumes are irritating to the eyes and nose.

3. Phenol Derivative

3A) ***Benzoates (Schotten-Baumann method):*** Dissolve phenol (0.5 g) in 5% sodium hydroxide solution (10 mL) in a small conical flask. Add benzoyl chloride (2 mL) in small quantities, and shake the mixture vigorously with occasional cooling. Maintain the pH as alkaline and the product (benzoate) separates after 15 min. Isolate the product by filtration and recrystallize from hot ethanol.

3B) ***Acetates:*** Acetate is a suitable derivative for polyhydric and substituted phenols. Dissolve phenol (0.5 g) in 10% sodium hydroxide solution in a clean test tube. Add equal quantity of crushed ice and acetic anhydride (2 mL). Shake the mixture vigorously, until the acetate separates out. Filter the product and recrystallize from alcohol.

3C) ***Bromo derivatives:*** Suspend phenol (0.3 g) in dilute hydrochloric acid (10 mL) and add bromine water drop wise, until no more decolourisation. Filter the bromo derivative and recrystallize from alcohol.

4. Aldehydes and Ketones

4A) ***Semicarbazones:*** Dissolve semicarbazide hydrochloride (1 g) and sodium acetate (1.5 g) in water (10 mL) contained in a conical flask. Add aldehyde or ketone (0.3 mL) and shake the mixture for a few min. Cool in ice-water and filter off the crystals, Wash the crystals with cold water and recrystallize from ethanol.

4B) ***2,4-Dinitrophenylhydrazones:*** Suspend 0.3 g of 2,4-dinitrophenylhydrazine in 5 mL of methanol and add 0.5 mL of concentrated sulphuric acid. Filter the warm solution and add solution of 0.2 g of the carbonyl compound in 1 mL of methanol to the above solution. Shake well and filter the yellow precipitate. Recrystallize the derivative from ethanol.

4C) ***Oximes:*** Transfer hydroxylamine hydrochloride (0.5 g) in to a test tube containing water (2 mL). Add solution of 10% sodium hydroxide (2 mL) and the carbonyl compound (0.3 g) in alcohol (2 mL) to the above tube. Warm the mixture by placing on a water bath for 10 min and then cool in ice. Induce the crystallisation by scratching the sides of the test tube with a glass rod. Dry and recrystallize from ethanol.

5. **Amine Derivatives**

5A) ***Acetyl derivatives (acetamides):*** Suspend amine (1 g) with acetic anhydride (3 mL) in a flask. Reflux the mixture for 15 min. Cool the mixture and pour into beaker containing 20 mL of cold water. Boil the mixture to decompose excess of acetic anhydride. Cool, collect the product by filtration and recrystallize from ethanol.

5B) ***Benzoyl derivatives (benzamides):*** Suspend amine (1 g) in aqueous sodium hydroxide (20 mL, 5%) in a well-corked flask. Add benzoyl chloride (2 mL, fume hood) slowly with constant shaking. Shake the mixture vigorously for 5-10 min, until the odour of the benzoyl chloride disappears. Maintain the alkaline pH, and filter the solid derivative. Wash the product with cold water and recrystallize from ethanol.

5C) ***Benzenesulphonamides:*** Suspend amine (1 g) in aqueous sodium hydroxide (20 mL, 5%) in a well-corked flask. Add benzenesulphonyl chloride (1 mL, fume hood) and shake the mixture until the odour disappears. Maintain the alkaline pH, and filter the solid derivative. Wash the product with cold water and recrystallize from ethanol.

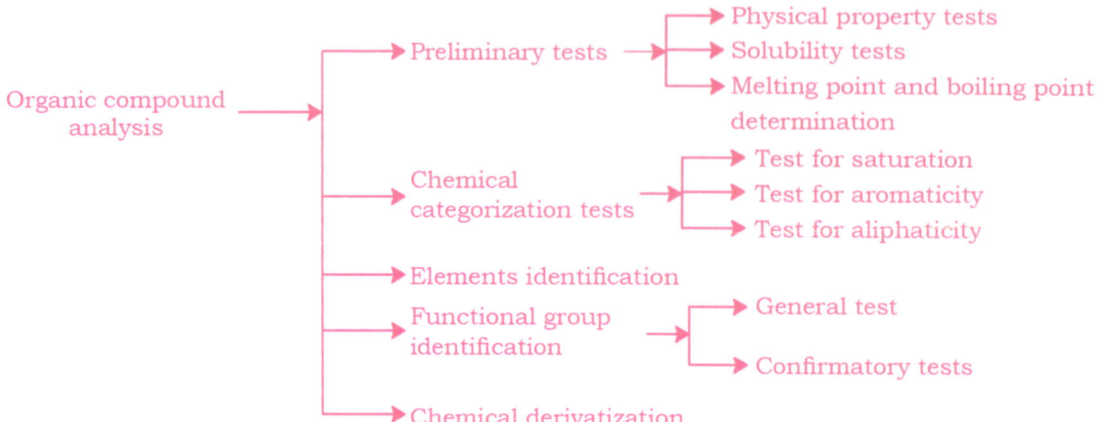

Titrimetric Analysis

In general, titration is an analytical technique for the quantification of analytes. The basic principle involved in the titration is the reaction between two solutions, one being the standard and another one is an analyte. The amount of analyte can be quantified based on the stoichiometry.

***Titrant*:** A solution used in the titration with known concentration serves as a standard and is known as titrant.

***Titrand (analyte)*:** A solution for which the quantification is required and to which the titrant is added is known as titrand.

Types of Titrations

The chemical property of analyte will be the basis for the titrimetric analysis. For example, in case of acids and bases, determination of pH is the basis. The following are the most important titrimetric analysis used in the chemical analysis.

1. Acid-base titrations
2. Non-aqueous titrations
3. Redox titrations
4. Precipitation titrations
5. Complexometric titrations

Indicators

The chemical compounds in solution form shows well-defined colour change according to the H^+ ion concentration (pH) of the mixture are known as indicators. They can be weak acids and bases and exhibit different colour in their conjugate base and acid forms (two colour). Some indicators produce no colour in either of these forms.

- In acid solution, the excess of H^+ ions depress the ionization of weakly acidic indicator. The concentration of ionized molecule of indicator will be very small and produces colour of unionized form of indicator. For example, phenolphthalein in acidic medium remains unionized and produce no colour.
- In base solution, the excess of OH^- ions promotes the ionization of weakly acidic indicator. The concentration of ionized molecule produces colour of unionized form of indicator. For example, phenolphthalein in basic medium undergoes ionization and produce pink colour.

45

Estimation of Drugs by Acid-Base Titration

Theory

Acid-base titrations involve the neutralization reaction between the analyte and titrant. The solution of sample for which quantification is intended is known as analyte (titrand). The second solution added for the neutralization is known as titrant. The neutralization of acid and base produces salt and liberates water.

Acid + Base $\longrightarrow$ Salt + Water

Principle

In acid-base titrations, either solutions of free acids or free bases are titrated against standard solutions to neutralize them.

***Acidimetry*:** Titration between solutions of free acids against standard alkali solutions is known as acidimetric titration. For example, the neutralization of hydrochloric acid by sodium hydroxide (titrant).

$$\underset{\text{Hydrochloric acid (titrand)}}{HCl} + \underset{\text{Sodium hydroxide (titrant)}}{NaOH} \longrightarrow \underset{\text{Sodium chloride}}{NaCl} + H_2O$$

***Alkalimetry*:** It is specific for the quantification of basic analyte. Titration between solutions of free bases against standard acid solutions. For example, the neutralization of sodium hydroxide by hydrochloric acid (titrant).

$$\underset{\text{Sodium hydroxide (titrand)}}{NaOH} + \underset{\text{Hydrochloric acid (titrant)}}{HCl} \longrightarrow \underset{\text{Sodium chloride}}{NaCl} + H_2O$$

Residual/ back titration: Titration of excess (residual) of neutralizing agent (acid/base) against suitable titrant is known as residual/back titration.

45.1 Estimation of Sodium Bicarbonate

Sodium bicarbonate is an antacid drug.

Principle

Sodium bicarbonate is a base and can be determined by acid-base titration. Sodium bicarbonate can be titrated against standard hydrochloric acid (alkalimetry). Methyl orange is used as an indicator and colour change from red to yellow indicates the endpoint.

$$\underset{\text{Sodium bicarbonate}}{NaHCO_3} + \underset{\text{Hydrochloric acid}}{HCl} \longrightarrow \underset{\text{Sodium chloride}}{NaCl} + CO_2\uparrow + H_2O$$

Procedure:

Chemicals required: Sodium bicarbonate, Hydrochloric acid (1 M), Methyl orange, Distilled water.

Experimental steps

1. Transfer accurately weighed sample (1.5 g) into a clean conical flask.
2. Add carbon dioxide free distilled water (50 mL) to dissolve the contents.
3. Titrate the aqueous solution of sample against standard hydrochloric acid (1 M) using methyl orange solution as an indicator (in basic pH it produces red colour).
4. The colour change from red to yellow indicates the end point.

   Each mL of 1 M hydrochloric acid is equivalent to 0.08401 g of sodium bicarbonate.

$$\text{Amount of sodium bicarbonate present in the sample} = \frac{\text{Equivalent weight factor} \times \text{Volume of hydrochloric acid (Titre value)} \times \text{Molarity of hydrochloric acid (actual)}}{\text{Weight taken} \times \text{Molarity of hydrochloric acid (standard)}}$$

45.2 Estimation of Ibuprofen Present in Tablets

Ibuprofen is a non-steroidal anti-inflammatory drug.

Principle

The amount of ibuprofen present in the sample can be quantified through acid-base titration. Ibuprofen (free acid) present in the sample can be determined by titrating against standard sodium hydroxide (acidimetry; direct titration). Phenolphthalein is used as an indicator and the appearance of pale pink colour is the endpoint.

$$\text{Ibuprofen (COOH)} \xrightarrow{NaOH} \text{Sodium salt of ibuprofen (COONa)} + HCl$$

Ibuprofen present in the tablets can be extracted with chloroform. The ethanolic solution of ibuprofen can be titrated against 0.1 M sodium hydroxide using phenolphthalein as an indicator. Sodium hydroxide (0.1 M) converts Ibuprofen into its sodium salt. The slight excess of sodium hydroxide makes the solution basic and produces pink colour (end point).

Procedure

Chemicals required: Ibuprofen tablets, Chloroform, Ethanol (95%), Sodium hydroxide (0.1 M), Phenolphthalein, Distilled water.

Experimental steps

1. Weigh and powder 20 ibuprofen tablets.
2. Weigh the ibuprofen tablet powder equivalent to 0.2 g of ibuprofen.
3. Transfer the powder into a separatory funnel and extract with 15 mL of chloroform (two times).
4. Filter and wash the residue with 5 mL of chloroform, three times.
5. Mix the chloroform layers and evaporate to dryness.
6. Dissolve the residue in 5 mL of ethanol (95%).
7. Titrate the ethanolic solution of sample with standard sodium hydroxide (0.1 M) using phenolphthalein as an indicator (**a**)
8. The appearance of pale pink colour is the end point.
9. Perform blank titration (without the substance; **b**).

   [(**a** – **b**) is the volume of sodium hydroxide consumed to neutralize the ibuprofen present in the given formulation]

   Each mL of 0.1 M sodium hydroxide is equivalent to 0.02063 g of ibuprofen

$$\text{Amount of ibuprofen present in the sample} = \frac{\text{Equivalent weight factor} \times \text{Volume of sodium hydroxide (titre value)} \times \text{Molarity of sodium hydroxide (actual)}}{\text{Weight taken} \times \text{Molarity of sodium hydroxide (standard)}}$$

45.3 Estimation of Salicylic Acid

Salicylic acid is an antibacterial drug.

Principle

The amount of salicylic acid (free acid) can be determined through acid-base titration. The titration of ethanolic solution of salicylic acid against 0.1 M sodium hydroxide is the reaction involved in the quantification. Phenol red is the indicator and the colour change from yellow to red indicates the endpoint of the titration. Sodium hydroxide converts salicylic acid into its sodium salt. The slight excess of sodium hydroxide makes the reaction mixture basic and converts yellow colour of the indicator into red (end point).

$$\text{Salicylic acid (COOH, OH)} \xrightarrow[C_2H_5OH]{NaOH} \text{Sodium salt of salicylic acid (COONa, OH)} + HCl$$

Procedure

Chemicals required: Salicylic acid, Sodium hydroxide (0.1 M), Phenol red, Distilled water.

Experimental steps

1. Transfer accurately weighed salicylic acid (0.1 g) into a clean conical flask.
2. Add 15 mL of ethanol and 7 mL of water to the flask to effect the solution.
3. Titrate the ethanolic solution of sample against sodium hydroxide (0.1 M) using phenol red as an indicator.
4. The colour change from yellow to red is the end point.

   Each mL of 0.1 M sodium hydroxide is equivalent to 0.01381 g of salicylic acid.

$$\text{Amount of salicylic acid present in the sample} = \frac{\text{Equivalent weight factor} \times \text{Volume of sodium hydroxide (Titre value)} \times \text{Molarity of sodium hydroxide (actual)}}{\text{Weight taken} \times \text{Molarity of sodium hydroxide (standard)}}$$

45.4 Estimation of Acetylsalicylic Acid Present in Tablets

Acetylsalicylic acid (aspirin) is an anti-inflammatory, analgesic and anti-platelet drug.

Principle

The amount of acetylsalicylic acid (aspirin) present in the tablets can be determined by acid-base titration. Aspirin upon boiling with sodium hydroxide undergoes hydrolysis and generates sodium salt of salicylic acid. Excess of base (sodium hydroxide) can be titrated against hydrochloric acid by residual titration (alkalimetry method). The volume of sodium hydroxide consumed by aspirin for the hydrolysis can be calculated from the volume of hydrochloric acid required to neutralize the excess of sodium hydroxide (residual). Phenol red is used as an indicator, and the colour change from red to yellow is the end point.

Aspirin (benzene ring with COOH and $OCOCH_3$) $\xrightarrow[\text{Hydrolysis}]{\text{NaOH}}$ Sodium salt of salicylic acid (benzene ring with COONa and OH) + CH_3COONa (Sodium acetate)

$$\underset{\text{(excess)}}{NaOH} + HCl \longrightarrow NaCl + H_2O$$

Procedure

Chemicals required: Aspirin tablets, Sodium hydroxide (0.5 M), Hydrochloric acid (0.5 M), Phenol red, Distilled water.

Experimental steps

1. Weigh and powder 20 aspirin tablets.
2. Weigh the tablet powder equivalent to 0.2 g of aspirin and transfer into a conical flask.
3. Add 15 mL of sodium hydroxide (0.5 M) to the flask and boil the mixture for 10 min.
4. Cool the mixture and titrate the excess sodium hydroxide against standard hydrochloric acid using phenol red as an indicator (**a**).
5. The colour change from red to yellow indicates the end point.
6. Perform the blank titration (without sample, **b**).

   Each mL of 0.5 M sodium hydroxide is equivalent to 0.04504 g of aspirin.

$$\text{Amount of aspirin present in the sample} = \frac{\text{Equivalent weight factor} \times \text{Volume of sodium hydroxide } (\mathbf{b\text{-}a}) \times \text{Molarity of sodium hydroxide (actual)}}{\text{Molarity of sodium hydroxide (standard)}}$$

45.5 Estimation of Busulphan

Busulphan is an anticancer drug.

Principle

The amount of busulphan can be estimated through acid-base titration. Busulphan upon hydrolysis produces butane-1,4-diol and methane sulphonic acid. The liberated methane sulphonic acid can be titrated against sodium hydroxide (0.1 M) using phenolphthalein as an indicator. After the complete conversion of methane sulphonic acid into its sodium salt, phenolphthalein in the slight excess of sodium hydroxide gives pale pink colour (endpoint).

$$\text{Busulphan} + H_2O \longrightarrow \underset{\text{Butane-1,4-diol}}{HO-CH_2CH_2CH_2CH_2-OH} + \underset{\text{Methane sulphonic acid}}{2H_3C-SO_2-OH}$$

$$\underset{\text{Methane sulphonic acid}}{H_3C-SO_2-OH} + NaOH \longrightarrow \underset{\text{Sodium salt of methane sulphonic acid}}{H_3C-SO_2-ONa} + H_2O$$

Procedure

Chemicals required: Busulphan, Sodium hydroxide (0.1 M), Phenolphthalein, Distilled water.

Experimental steps

1. Transfer the accurately weighed busulphan (0.25 g) into a conical flask.
2. Add 25 mL of distilled water to the flask to dissolve the contents.
3. Boil the mixture for 30 min.
4. Wash the condenser with distilled water and cool the mixture.
5. Titrate the mixture against standard sodium hydroxide using phenolphthalein as an indicator.
6. The appearance of pale pink colour indicates the end point.

   Each mL of sodium hydroxide (0.1 M) is equivalent to 0.01232 g of busulphan.

$$\text{Amount of busulphan present in the sample} = \frac{\text{Equivalent weight factor} \times \text{Volume of sodium hydroxide (titre value)} \times \text{Molarity of sodium hydroxide (actual)}}{\text{Weight taken} \times \text{Molarity of sodium hydroxide (standard)}}$$

45.6 Estimation of Codeine Phosphate Present in Syrup

Codeine phosphate is an anti-tussive and analgesic agent.

Principle

The amount of codeine phosphate present in the formulation (syrup) can be determined by acid-base titration. Codeine phosphate upon treatment with ammonium hydroxide liberates codeine (free base). The liberated codeine (base) reacts with hydrochloric acid and forms hydrochloride salt. The unreacted hydrochloric acid can be titrated against standard sodium hydroxide by acidimetry (residual titration). The volume of hydrochloric acid consumed by the codeine base is calculated from the volume of sodium hydroxide required to neutralize the acid.

H_3C H_3PO_4. 1/2 H_2O ... H_3CO ... O ... OH — Codeine phosphate $\xrightarrow{NH_3}$ Codeine base $\xrightarrow{HCl}$ Codeine hydrochloride (Cl^-)

Codeine phosphate | Codeine base | Codeine hydrochloride

Procedure

Chemical Required: Codeine phosphate syrup, Dilute ammonia, Chloroform, Ethanol (95%), Hydrochloric acid (0.05 M), Sodium hydroxide (0.05 M), Methyl red, Distilled water.

Experimental steps

1. Transfer accurately weighed codeine phosphate syrup (10 g) into a porcelain dish.
2. Add dilute ammonia until the solution turns to alkaline with litmus paper.
3. Extract the alkaline solution with chloroform (25 mL, four volumes) and collect the chloroform layer.
4. Wash each extract with 10 mL of water and combine all the extracts.
5. Evaporate the chloroform to dryness in water bath.
6. Add 5 mL of ethanol (95%) to the residue and evaporate the solvent to dryness.
7. Dissolve the residue with 5 mL of standard hydrochloric acid.
8. Titrate the excess of acid against standard sodium hydroxide solution using methyl red as an indicator **(a)**.
9. The colour change from orange red to golden yellow indicates the endpoint.
10. Perform the blank titration (without the substance being examined, **b)**.

    (b – a) is the volume of sodium hydroxide consumed for the codeine phosphate.

    Each mL of 0.05 M hydrochloric acid is equivalent to 0.02 g of codeine phosphate ($C_{18}H_{21}NO_3 .\ H_3PO_4 .\ ½\ H_2O$).

$$\text{Amount of codeine phosphate present in the sample} = \frac{\text{Equivalent weight factor} \times \text{Volume of hydrochloric acid } (\mathbf{b\text{-}a}) \times \text{Molarity of hydrochloric acid (actual)}}{\text{Weight taken} \times \text{Molarity of hydrochloric acid (standard)}}$$

45.7 Estimation of Frusemide Present in Tablets

Frusemide is a diuretic drug.

Principle

Frusemide is chemically 4-chloro-N-furfuryl-5-sulphamoyl anthranilic acid. The drug contains carboxylic acid group (acidic), hence it can be quantified by titrating against standard sodium hydroxide (acidimetry). Phenolphthalein is used as an indicator and the appearance of pale pink colour is the endpoint.

Frusemide $\xrightarrow{NaOH}$ Sodium salt frusemide

Procedure

Chemicals Required: Frusemide tablets, Sodium hydroxide (0.1 M), Dimethylformamide, Bromothymol blue, Distilled water.

Experimental steps

1. Weigh and powder 20 frusemide tablets.
2. Weigh the tablet powder equivalent to 0.2 g of frusemide and transfer into a conical flask.
3. Add 16 mL of dimethylformamide into the flask to dissolve the contents.
4. Titrate the solution against standard sodium hydroxide using bromothymol blue as indicator (**a**)
5. The appearance of pale pink colour is the end point.
6. Perform blank titration (without the substance; **b**).

   Each mL of 0.1 M sodium hydroxide is equivalent to 0.03307 g of frusemide.

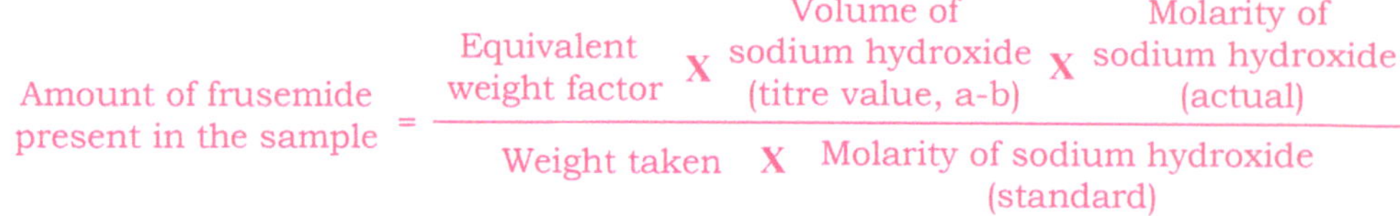

$$\text{Amount of frusemide present in the sample} = \frac{\text{Equivalent weight factor} \times \text{Volume of sodium hydroxide (titre value, a-b)} \times \text{Molarity of sodium hydroxide (actual)}}{\text{Weight taken} \times \text{Molarity of sodium hydroxide (standard)}}$$

KEY POINTS

- Acid-base titrations involve the neutralization reaction between the analyte and titrant.
- Titration of excess (residual) of neutralizing agent (acid/base) against suitable titrant is known as residual/back titration.

- Sodium bicarbonate can be titrated against standard sulphuric acid (alkalimetry).
- Ibuprofen, busulphan and frusemide can be titrated against standard sodium hydroxide (acidimetry).
- Codeine phosphate can be treated with excess of hydrochloric acid and the excess of acid is back titrated with standard base (residual titration).

46

Estimation of Drugs by Non-Aqueous Titration

Theory

The weakly acidic and weakly basic drugs does not produce sharp endpoint, hence aqueous acid-base titration is not suitable. Titrations of chemicals and drugs dissolved in solvents other than water (non-aqueous) are known as non-aqueous titrations. Non-aqueous titration is suitable for the weakly acidic (pKa > 7) and weakly basic (pKa < 7) drugs. In case of weakly acidic analyte, water acts as base and abstracts the proton (competes with the titrant).

$$H_2O + H^+ \longrightarrow H_3O^+$$

Similarly, with weakly basic analyte, water acts as an acid and donates the proton.

$$H_2O + B^- \longrightarrow BH^+ + OH^-$$

The amphoteric nature of water (acidic and basic), cause interference for the weakly acidic and basic analytes, hence it is not suitable for the titrations.

Principle

Most organic acids and bases are extremely water insoluble and it is difficult to analyze them through acid-base titrations. Also, the chemical nature of most drugs is either weakly acidic or weakly basic. The quantification of these drugs through acid-base titrations are very difficult. Hence, non-aqueous titration is the best alternative method for the quantification. Non-aqueous titration enhances the acidity and basicity of the solvent as well as analyte.

- **Acidimetric non-aqueous titrations:** For the quantification of weakly acidic compounds.

  Perchloric acid titrations: Perchloric acid in glacial acetic acid is the most common titrant for the estimation of inorganic and organic salts in non-aqueous acidic or inert solvent medium. This method is also useful for the estimation of salts of strong acids.
- **Alkalimetric non-aqueous titrations:** For the quantification of weakly basic compounds.

Sodium methoxide, potassium methoxide, lithium methoxide and tetrabutylammonium hydroxide are the most common titrants for the quantification of inorganic and organic bases.

46.1 Estimation of Amitriptyline Present in Tablets

Amitriptyline is an anti depressant drug.

Principle

Amitriptyline is a weakly basic drug and cannot be quantified through acid-base titration. It can be estimated effectively through non-aqueous titration using acetous perchloric acid as a titrant. Amitriptyline is available as a hydrochloride salt. In general, the halide ions (chloride, bromide and iodide) are weakly basic in character, and cannot react quantitatively with acetous perchloric acid. This problem can be overcome by the addition of mercuric acetate. It replaces the halide ion by an equivalent amount of acetate ion, which serves as a strong base in acetic acid medium. The end point can be determined potentiometrically. A visible end point determination using crystal violet in glacial acetic acid is also possible. Crystal violet develops blue (violet) to bluish green (or yellow) colour with basic substances in acetic acid.

Amitryptyline hydrochloride $\xrightarrow[(CH_3COO)_2Hg]{HClO_4}$ Amitryptyline perchlorate + HCl

(Amitryptyline hydrochloride: N, H, Cl^-, N^+—CH_3, CH_3; Amitryptyline perchlorate: N, H, ClO_4^-, N^+—CH_3, CH_3)

$$(CH_3COO)_2Hg + 2\,Cl^- \longrightarrow 2\,CH_3COO^- + HgCl_2$$

Mercuric acetate; Chloride ion of drug; Acetate ion of drug

$$HClO_4 \rightleftharpoons ClO_4^- + H^+$$

$$CH_3COOH + H^+ \rightleftharpoons CH_3COOH_2^+$$

$$CH_3COOH_2^+ + CH_3COO^- \rightleftharpoons 2CH_3COOH + \text{Drug}$$

Acetate ion of drug

Procedure

Chemicals required: Amitriptyline hydrochloride tablets, Glacial acetic acid, Acetone, Mercuric acetate (acetous), Crystal violet (acetous), Acetous Perchloric acid (0.1 M).

Experimental steps

1. Weigh and powder 20 amitriptyline hydrochloride tablets.
2. Weigh the powder equivalent to 50 mg of amitryptyline hydrochloride.
3. Transfer the tablet powder into a clean and dry conical flask.
4. Add 16 mL of glacial acetic acid (or acetone) and 15 mL of mercuric acetate (10 mg in 1 mL) solution into the flask.
5. Titrate the mixture with standard perchloric acid using crystal violet as an indicator (**a**).
6. The colour change from violet to green indicates the end point.
7. Perform blank titration (omitting the substance being examined; **b**).

   Each mL of 0.1 M perchloric acid is equivalent to 0.03139 g of amitriptyline hydrochloride.

$$\text{Amount of amitriptyline present in the sample} = \frac{\text{Equivalent weight factor} \times \text{Volume of perchloric acid (titre value, } \mathbf{a\text{-}b}) \times \text{Normality of perchloric acid (actual)}}{\text{Weight taken} \times \text{Normality of perchloric acid (standard)}}$$

46.2 Estimation of Chlorpromazine Present in Tablets

Chloropromazine is an anti-psychotic drug.

Principle

Chloropromazine is a weakly basic drug and cannot be quantified through acid-base titration. It can be estimated effectively through non-aqueous titration using acetous perchloric acid as a titrant. Chloropromazine is available as a hydrochloride salt. In general, the halide ions (chloride, bromide and iodide) are very weakly basic in character, and cannot react quantitatively with acetous perchloric acid. This problem can be overcome by the addition of mercuric acetate. It replaces the halide ion by an equivalent amount of acetate ion, which serves as a strong base in acetic acid medium. The end point can be determined potentiometrically. A visible end point determination using crystal violet in glacial acetic acid is also possible. Crystal violet develops blue (violet) to bluish green (or yellow) colour with basic substances in acetic acid.

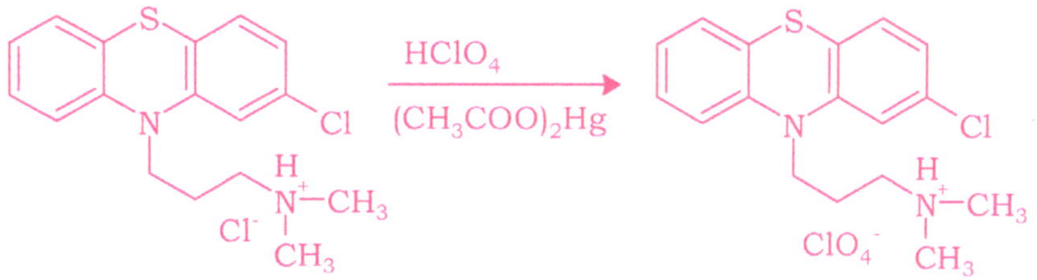

Chlorpromazine hydrochloride $\xrightarrow[(CH_3COO)_2Hg]{HClO_4}$ Chlorpromazine perchlorate

$$(CH_3COO)_2Hg + 2\,Cl^- \longrightarrow 2\,CH_3COO^- + HgCl_2$$

Mercuric acetate; Chloride ion of drug; Acetate ion of drug

$$HClO_4 \rightleftharpoons ClO_4^- + H^+$$

$$CH_3COOH + H^+ \rightleftharpoons CH_3COOH_2^+$$

$$CH_3COOH_2^+ + CH_3COO^- \rightleftharpoons 2CH_3COOH + \text{Drug}$$

Acetate ion of drug

Procedure

Chemicals required: Chlorpromazine hydrochloride tablets, Mercuric acetate (acetous), Perchloric acid (0.1 M), Glacial acetic acid , Acetone, Methyl orange (acetous), Crystal violet (acetous).

Experimental steps

1. Weigh and powder 20 chlorpromazine hydrochloride tablets.
2. Weigh the powder equivalent to 50 mg of chlorpromazine hydrochloride.
3. Transfer the tablet powder into a clean and dry conical flask.
4. Add 16 mL of glacial acetic acid (or acetone) and 15 mL of mercuric acetate (10 mg in 1 mL) solution into the flask.
5. Titrate the mixture with standard perchloric acid using saturated acetous methyl orange as an indicator (**a**)
6. The appearance of emerald green colour is the end point.
7. Perform blank titration (without the substance; **b**).

   Each ml of 0.1 M perchloric acid is equivalent to 0.03553 g of chlorpromazine hydrochloride.

$$\text{Amount of chlorpromazine present in the sample} = \frac{\text{Equivalent weight factor} \times \text{Volume of perchloric acid (titre value, } \mathbf{a}\text{-}\mathbf{b}\text{)} \times \text{Normality of perchloric acid (actual)}}{\text{Weight taken} \times \text{Normality of perchloric acid (standard)}}$$

46.3 Estimastion of Phenytoin Present in Tablets

Phenytoin is an anticonvulsant drug and is available as phenytoin sodium.

Principle

Phenytoin sodium can be estimated by non-aqueous titration using acetous perchloric acid as a titrant. In the estimation, the drug phenytoin gets converted into hydrochloride salt by the hydrochloric acid treatment. Halides (chloride, bromide and iodide) are very weakly basic, hence cannot react quantitatively with acetous perchloric acid. This problem can be overcome by the addition of mercuric acetate. It replaces the halide ion by an equivalent amount of acetate ion, which serves as a strong base in acetic acid medium. The end point can be determined potentiometrically. A visible end point determination using crystal violet in glacial acetic acid is also possible. Crystal violet develops blue (violet) to bluish green (or yellow) colour with basic substances in acetic acid.

Phenytoin sodium $\xrightarrow{HCl}$ Phenytoin hydrochloride $\xrightarrow[(CH_3COO)_2Hg]{HClO_4}$ Phenytoin perchlorate + HCl

$$(CH_3COO)_2Hg + 2\,Cl^- \longrightarrow 2\,CH_3COO^- + HgCl_2$$

Mercuric acetate; Chloride ion of drug; Acetate ion of drug

$$HClO_4 \rightleftharpoons ClO_4^- + H^+$$

$$CH_3COOH + H^+ \rightleftharpoons CH_3COOH_2^+$$

$$CH_3COOH_2^+ + CH_3COO^- \rightleftharpoons 2CH_3COOH + Drug$$

(CH_3COO^-: Acetate ion of drug)

Procedure

Chemicals: Phenytoin tablets, Sodium hydroxide, Hydrochloric acid, Acetous perchloric acid (0.1 M), Glacial acetic acid, Acetic anhydride, Ether, Acetous mercuric acetate, Acetous crystal violet.

Experimental steps

1. Weigh and powder 20 phenytoin sodium tablets.

2. Weigh the powder equivalent to 0.5 g of phenytoin sodium.
3. Transfer the tablet powder into a clean and dry conical flask.
4. Add sodium hydroxide (40 mL, 0.1 M) to the flask and shake for 5 min.
5. Add sodium hydroxide (0.1 M) to produce 50 mL.
6. Centrifuge the basic solution and acidify 25 mL of the clear solution with 10 mL of hydrochloric acid (0.1 M).
7. Extract the acidified solution with ether three times (successively, 50, 40, 25 mL).
8. Combine the ether extracts and wash with water (10 mL).
9. Evaporate the ethereal solution to dryness and dry the residue at 105 °C.
10. Dissolve the residue in glacial acetic acid (50 mL).
    (warm if necessary, to effect the solution)
11. Cool the solution and add mercuric acetate solution (10 mL).
12. Titrate the mixture with standard perchloric acid using acetous crystal violet (or 1-naphtholbenzein) as an indicator.
13. The colour change from violet to green indicates the end point (a).
14. At the end point color changes from violet to bluish-green.
15. Perform blank titration (omitting the substance being examined) (b).
    Each mL of 0.1 M perchloric acid is equivalent to 0.02743 g of phenytoin.

$$\text{Amount of phenytoin present in the sample} = \frac{\text{Equivalent weight factor} \times \text{Volume of perchloric acid (titre value, } \mathbf{a}\text{-}\mathbf{b}\text{)} \times \text{Normality of perchloric acid (actual)}}{\text{Weight taken} \times \text{Normality of perchloric acid (standard)}}$$

46.4 Estimation of Methyldopa

Methyldopa is an antihypertensive drug.

Principle

Methyldopa can be estimated by non-aqueous titration using acetous perchloric acid as titrant. The end point can be determined using crystal violet in glacial acetic acid. Crystal violet develops blue (violet) to bluish green (or yellow) colour with basic substances in acetic acid.

$$C_6H_5\text{-}CH_2\text{-}C(NH_2)(CH_3)\text{-}COOH \cdot nH_2O \xrightarrow{HClO_4} C_6H_5\text{-}CH_2\text{-}C(NH_3^+)(CH_3)\text{-}COOH \; ClO_4^-$$

Methyldopa — Methyldopa perchlorate

Procedure

Chemicals required: Methyldopa, Acetous perchloric acid (0.1 M), Glacial acetic acid, Formic acid (acetous), Dioxane, Acetous crystal violet.

Experimental steps

1. Accurately weigh 0.2 g of methyldopa and transfer into a conical flask.
2. Add anhydrous formic acid (15 mL), glacial acetic acid (30 mL) and dioxane (30 mL) to the flask to dissolve the contents.
3. Titrate the mixture with standard perchloric acid using acetous crystal violet as indicator.
4. The colour change from violet to green indicates the end point (a).
5. At the end point color changes from violet to bluish-green.
6. Perform blank titration (omitting the substance being examined) (b).

   Each mL of the acetous perchloric acid (0.1 M) is equivalent to 0.02262 g of methyldopa.

$$\text{Amount of methyldopa present in the sample} = \frac{\text{Equivalent weight factor} \times \text{Volume of perchloric acid (titre value, } \mathbf{a}\text{-}\mathbf{b}\text{)} \times \text{Normality of perchloric acid (actual)}}{\text{Weight taken} \times \text{Normality of perchloric acid (standard)}}$$

46.5 Estimation of Ethambutol Present in Tablets

Ethambutol is an antitubercular drug.

Principle

Ethambutol can be estimated by non-aqueous titration using acetous perchloric acid as a titrant. Ethambutol is available as a hydrochloride salt. In general, the halide ions (chloride, bromide and iodide) are very weakly basic in character, and cannot react quantitatively with acetous perchloric acid. This problem can be overcome by the addition of mercuric acetate. It replaces the halide ion by an equivalent amount of acetate ion, which serves as a strong base in acetic acid medium. The end point can be determined using α-naptholbenzein in glacial acetic acid. The colour change from violet to bluish green colour indicates the endpoint.

HO, HO, N—CH$_2$, H, CH$_2$—N, H, OH, OH, 2HCl $\xrightarrow[(CH_3COO)_2Hg]{HClO_4}$ HO, HO, $\overset{+}{N}$—CH$_2$, H$_2$, CH$_2$—CH$_2$—$\overset{+}{N}$, H$_2$, OH, OH, 2ClO$_4^-$

Ethambutol hydrochloride Ethambutol perchlorate

$$(CH_3COO)_2Hg + 2Cl^- \longrightarrow 2CH_3COO^- + HgCl_2$$

Mercuric acetate; Chloride ion of drug; Acetate ion of drug

$$HClO_4 \rightleftharpoons ClO_4^- + H^+$$

$$CH_3COOH + H^+ \rightleftharpoons CH_3COOH_2^+$$

$$CH_3COOH_2^+ + CH_3COO^- \rightleftharpoons 2CH_3COOH + \text{Drug}$$

Acetate ion of drug

Procedure

Chemicals Required: Ethambutol tablets, Acetous perchloric acid (0.1M), Glacial acetic acid, Acetous mercuric acetate, Acetous crystal violet.

Experimental steps

1. Weigh and powder 20 ethambutol hydrochloride tablets.
2. Weigh the powder equivalent to 0.2 g of ethambutol hydrochloride.
3. Transfer the tablet powder into a clean and dry conical flask.
4. Add glacial acetic acid (50 mL) to dissolve the contents.
5. Stir the contents for 30 min on a rotary shaker.
6. Add 5 mL of acetous mercuric acetate (5%) and 10 drops of acetous crystal violet (0.1%).
7. Titrate the mixture with 0.1 N perchloric acid.
8. The colour change from violet to bluish-green indicates the end point.
9. At the end point color changes from violet to bluish-green.
10. Perform blank titration (omitting the substance being examined).

    Each mL of the 0.1 N perchloric acid is equivalent to 0.01386 g of ethambutol.

$$\text{Amount of ethambutol present in the sample} = \frac{\text{Equivalent weight factor} \times \text{Volume of perchloric acid (titre value, } \mathbf{a}\text{-}\mathbf{b}) \times \text{Normality of perchloric acid (actual)}}{\text{Weight taken} \times \text{Normality of perchloric acid (standard)}}$$

46.6 Estimation of Phenobarbitone Present in Tablets

Phenobarbitone is sedative, hypnotic and anticonvulsant drug.

Principle

Phenobarbitone is chemically 5-phenyl, 5-ethyl barbituric acid and is a weakly basic drug. The weakly acidic and weakly basic drugs does not produce sharp endpoint, hence aqueous acid base titration is not suitable. Non-aqueous titration is suitable for the weakly acidic (pKa >7) and weakly basic (pKa < 7) drugs. Non-aqueous titration enhances the acidity and basicity of the solvent as well as analyte. Phenobarbitone like weakly basic drugs can be estimated through titration against alcoholic sodium hydroxide using crystal violet as indicator. The development of emerald green colour is the end point.

$$\text{Phenobarbitone} \xrightarrow{C_2H_5OH\text{-}NaOH} \text{Phenobarbitone sodium}$$

Phenobarbitone

Phenobarbitone sodium

Procedure

Chemicals Required: Phenobarbitone tablets, Pyridine, Thymolphthalein, Sodium hydroxide, Ethanol, Silver-nitrate-Pyridine reagent.

Experimental steps

1. Weigh and powder 20 phenobarbitone tablets.
2. Weigh accurately a quantity of powder equivalent to 0.1 g of phenobarbitone.
3. Transfer the tablet powder into a clean and dry conical flask.
4. Add 5 mL of pyridine and 10 mL of silver nitrate-pyridine reagent into the flask.
5. Titrate the resulting mixture with ethanolic sodium hydroxide using 0.25 mL of thymolphthalein as an indicator.
6. Appearance of blue colour is the end point (**a**).
7. Repeat the operation without the substance being examined (**b**).

   Each mL of 0.1 M sodium hydroxide is equivalent to 0.01161 g of phenobarbitone

$$\text{Amount of phenobarbitone present in the sample} = \frac{\text{Equivalent weight factor} \times \text{Volume of sodium hydroxide (titre value, } \mathbf{a}-\mathbf{b}) \times \text{Normality of sodium hydroxide (actual)}}{\text{Weight factor} \times \text{Normality of sodium hydroxide (standard)}}$$

KEY POINTS

- Most organic acids and bases are extremely water insoluble in nature and it is difficult to analyze them through normal acid-base titrations.

- Non-aqueous titration is suitable for the weakly acidic (pKa > 7) and weakly basic (pKa < 7) drugs.
- Mercuric acetate replaces the weakly basic halide ions (chloride, bromide and iodide) with acetate ion, which serves as a strong base in acetic acid medium.
- Phenobarbitone can be estimated through titration against alcoholic sodium hydroxide using thymolphthalein as indicator.

47

Estimation of Drugs by Diazotization Titration

Theory

Diazotization is an important chemical analysis method for the pharmaceuticals. An important pharmaceutical application of diazotization titration is the quantitative analysis of sulphonamides. Local anaesthetic drugs (benzocaine, procaine), antileprotic drugs (dapsone, solapsone) also can be quantified by this method. The primary aromatic amines present in these class of drugs undergo diazotization and produce dye (diazonium compound). Aromatic primary amino group can be quantified by measuring the volume of sodium nitrite solution required to convert them into diazonium salts.

Principle

The principle involved in the estimation is the reaction between aromatic primary amine and nitrous acid (*in situ* generated).The reaction between aromatic primary amine and nitrous acid (*in situ*) under ice-cold condition (0 to 5 °C) in presence of excess of mineral acid forms diazonium salt. This reaction is known as diazotization. In place of hydrochloric acid, other mineral acids, inorganic acids and glacial acetic acid can also be used. Sodium nitrite reacts with hydrochloric acid and generates nitrous acid (HONO) *in situ*. The unreacted nitrous acid can be detected by using starch iodide paper (or starch paste) as an external indicator. Nitrous acid reacts with indicator (HI) and liberates iodine this in turn gives blue colour with starch. This is the basic principle involved in the estimation of amine containing drugs through diazotization.

$$\underset{\text{Sodium nitrite}}{NaNO_2} + HCl \xrightarrow[\text{0 to 5 °C}]{-NaCl} HONO$$

$$\underset{\text{Arylamine}}{Ar{-}NH_2} + \underset{\text{Nitrous acid}}{HONO} \xrightarrow{\text{0 to 5 °C}} \underset{\text{Aryldiazonium salt}}{Ar{-}N_2^+Cl^-} + H_2O$$

$$\underset{\text{Potassium iodide}}{KI} + HCl \longrightarrow \underset{\text{Hydrogen iodide}}{HI} + KCl$$

$$\underset{\text{Hydrogen iodide}}{HI} + \underset{\text{Nitrous acid}}{HONO} \longrightarrow \underset{\text{Iodine}}{I_2} + 2NO + 2H_2O$$

$$I_2 + \text{Starch} \longrightarrow \underset{\text{(end point)}}{\text{Blue colour}}$$

47.1 Estimation of Sulphanilamide

Principle

Sulphanilamide can be estimated by diazotization reaction. The principle involved in the estimation is the reaction between aromatic primary amine of sulphanilamide and nitrous acid (*in situ* generated) under ice-cold condition (0 to 5 ºC). Sodium nitrite reacts with hydrochloric acid and generates nitrous acid (*in situ*). The volume of sodium nitrite required to convert the amine groups into diazonium salts is basis for the quantification. Unreacted nitrous acid remains in the solution and can be detected by using starch iodide paper or paste as external indicator. Nitrous acid reacts with indicator (HI) and liberates iodine this in turn gives blue colour with starch. Blank titration determines the nitrous acid consumed by the sulphanilamide during diazotization reaction.

$$\underset{\text{Sodium nitrite}}{NaNO_2} + HCl \xrightarrow[-NaCl]{0\ \text{to}\ 5\ °C} HONO$$

$$\underset{\text{Sulphanilamide}}{H_2N{-}C_6H_4{-}SO_2{-}NH_2} + \underset{\text{Nitrous acid}}{HONO} \xrightarrow{0\ \text{to}\ 5\ °C} \underset{\text{Sulphanilamide diazonium salt}}{Cl^-N_2^+{-}C_6H_4{-}SO_2{-}NH_2} + H_2O$$

$$\underset{\text{Potassium iodide}}{KI} + HCl \longrightarrow \underset{\text{Hydrogen iodide}}{HI} + KCl$$

$$\underset{\text{Hydrogen iodide}}{HI} + \underset{\text{Nitrous acid}}{HONO} \longrightarrow \underset{\text{Iodine}}{I_2} + 2NO + 2H_2O$$

$$I_2 + \text{Starch} \longrightarrow \underset{\text{(end point)}}{\text{Blue colour}}$$

Procedure

Chemicals Required: Sulphanilamide, Concentrated hydrochloric acid, Sodium nitrite (0.1 M), Starch iodide paper, Distilled water.

Experimental steps

1. Transfer accurately weighed sample (1 g) into a clean conical flask.
2. Add concentrated hydrochloric acid (40 mL) and distilled water (100 mL) to dissolve the contents.
3. Titrate the acidic mixture against 0.1 M sodium nitrite using starch iodide paper as an external indicator (starch paste also can be used).
4. Appearance of blue colour indicates the end point.
5. Note down the volume of sodium nitrite rundown (**a**).
6. Perform blank titration by omitting the sample. Note down the volume rundown (**b**).

   Each mL of 0.1 M sodium nitrite is equivalent to 0.01722 g of sulphanilamide.

$$\text{Amount of sulphanilamide present in the sample} = \frac{\text{Equivalent weight factor} \times \text{Volume of sodium nitrite (Titre value, } \mathbf{a\text{-}b}\text{)} \times \text{Molarity of sodium nitrite (actual)}}{\text{Weight taken} \times \text{Molarity of sodium nitrite (standard)}}$$

47.2 Estimation of Dapsone Present in Tablets

Dapsone is an antileprotic drug.

Principle

Dapsone can be estimated by diazotizaion reaction. The principle involved in the estimation is the reaction between aromatic primary amine groups of dapsone and nitrous acid (*in situ* generated) under ice-cold condition (0 to 5 ºC). Sodium nitrite reacts with hydrochloric acid and generates nitrous acid (*in situ*). The volume of sodium nitrite required to convert the amine groups into diazonium salts is basis for the quantification. Unreacted nitrous acid remains in the solution and can be detected by using starch iodide paper or paste as external indicator. Nitrous acid reacts with indicator and liberates (HI) iodine this in turn gives blue colour with starch. Blank titration determines the nitrous acid consumed by the dapsone during diazotization reaction.

$NaNO_2$ + HCl
Sodium nitrite
0 to 5 °C | -NaCl
HONO
Nitrous acid

$$H_2N-C_6H_4-SO_2-C_6H_4-NH_2 \xrightarrow[0\text{-}5\ ^\circ C,\ -H_2O]{\text{HONO (Nitrous acid)}} Cl^-N_2^+-C_6H_4-SO_2-C_6H_4-N_2^+Cl^-$$

Dapsone → Dapsone diazonium salt

$$\underset{\text{Potassium iodide}}{KI} + HCl \longrightarrow \underset{\text{Hydrogen iodide}}{HI} + KCl$$

$$\underset{\text{Hydrogen iodide}}{HI} + \underset{\text{Nitrous acid}}{HONO} \longrightarrow \underset{\text{Iodine}}{I_2} + 2NO + 2H_2O$$

$$I_2 + \text{Starch} \longrightarrow \underset{\text{(end point)}}{\text{Blue colour}}$$

Procedure

Chemicals Required: Dapsone tablets, Sodium nitrite (0.1 M), Hydrochloric acid (2 M), Starch iodide paper, Distilled water.

Experimental steps

1. Weigh and powder 20 dapsone tablets.
2. Weigh accurately a quantity of the powder equivalent to 0.2 g of dapsone.
3. Transfer the powder into a conical flask.
4. Add distilled water (15 mL) and hydrochloric acid (15 mL, 2 M) to dissolve the contents.
5. Keep the mixture in an ice bath to reduce temperature below 5 °C (0 to 5 °C).
6. Titrate the ice cold mixture with 0.1 M sodium nitrite, shaking continuously using starch iodide paper as an external indicator.
   (maintain the ice cold condition throughout the titration)
7. Appearance of blue colour instantaneously with starch iodide paper, when the drop of titrated solution is placed indicates the end point (**a**).
8. Perform a blank determination (**b**).
   Each mL of 0.1 M sodium nitrite is equivalent to 0.01242 g of dapsone.

$$\text{Amount of dapsone present in the sample} = \frac{\text{Equivalent weight factor} \times \text{Volume of sodium nitrite (Titre value, } \mathbf{a}\text{-}\mathbf{b}) \times \text{Molarity of sodium nitrite (actual)}}{\text{Weight taken} \times \text{Molarity of sodium nitrite (standard)}}$$

47.3 Estimation of Metronidazole Present in Tablets

Metronidazole is an antiprotozoal drug.

Principle

Metronidazole can be estimated by diazotizaion reaction. The first step in the quantification is the reduction of nitro group of metronidazole into amino through Clemmenson reduction. The reaction between aromatic amine group and nitrous acid (*in situ* generated) under ice-cold condition (0 to 5 ºC) is basis for the estimation. Sodium nitrite reacts with hydrochloric acid and generates nitrous acid ((*in situ*). The volume of sodium nitrite required to convert the amine groups into diazonium salts is basis for the quantification. Unreacted nitrous acid can be detected by using starch iodide paper or starch paste as an external indicator. Nitrous acid reacts with indicator (HI) and liberates iodine this in turn gives blue colour with starch. Blank titration is performed to determine the nitrous acid consumed by the during diazotization reaction.

Metronidazole $\xrightarrow{Zn/HCl}$ Reduced product of metronidazole $\xrightarrow[\text{0-5 °C, } -H_2O]{HONO \text{ (Nitrous acid)}}$ Diazonium salt ($-N_2^+Cl^-$)

$NaNO_2$ (Sodium nitrite) + HCl $\xrightarrow[\text{-NaCl}]{\text{0 to 5 °C}}$ HONO (Nitrous acid)

KI (Potassium iodide) + HCl ⟶ HI (Hydrogen iodide) + KCl

HI (Hydrogen iodide) + HONO (Nitrous acid) ⟶ I_2 (Iodine) + 2NO + $2H_2O$

I_2 + Starch ⟶ Blue colour (end point)

Procedure

Chemicals Required: Metronidazole tablets, Distilled water, Hydrochloric acid (2 M), Sodium nitrite (0.1 M), Zinc powder, Potassium bromide, Starch-iodide paper (or paste).

Experimental steps

1. Weigh and powder 20 metronidazole tablets.
2. Accurately weigh the powder equivalent to 0.1 g of metronidazole.
3. Transfer the tablet powder into a clean conical flask.
4. Suspend the metronidazole tablet powder with hydrochloric acid (30 mL, 2 M).
5. Add 0.5 g of zinc powder to the suspension and keep it aside with occasional shaking until the reaction completes
   (*filter if any insoluble impurities present and wash the residue with water*).

6. Keep the mixture in an ice bath to reduce temperature below 5 °C (0 to 5 °C).
7. Add potassium bromide (0.5 g) to the flask.
8. Titrate the ice cold mixture with 0.1 M sodium nitrite, shaking continuously using starch iodide paper as an external indicator (**a**).
   (*maintain the ice cold condition throughout the titration*)
9. Appearance of blue colour instantaneously with starch iodide paper, when the drop of titrated solution is placed indicates the end point.
10. Perform a blank determination (**b**).
    Each mL of 0.1 M sodium nitrite is equivalent to 0.01712 g of metronidazole.

$$\text{Amount of metronidazole present in the sample} = \frac{\text{Equivalent weight factor} \times \text{Volume of sodium nitrite (Titre value, } \mathbf{a\text{-}b}\text{)} \times \text{Molarity of sodium nitrite (actual)}}{\text{Weight taken} \times \text{Molarity of sodium nitrite (standard)}}$$

KEY POINTS

- Diazotization titration is useful in the quantitative analysis of sulphonamides, local anaesthetic drugs (benzocaine, procaine), antileprotic drugs (dapsone, solapsone).
- The primary aromatic amines analyzed quantitatively by measuring the volume of sodium nitrite solution required to convert them into diazonium salts.
- Sodium nitrite generates nitrous acid (HONO) *in situ* and the unreacted nitrous acid can be detected by using starch iodide paper.
- The volume of nitrous acid consumed by the drug is basis for the quantification.

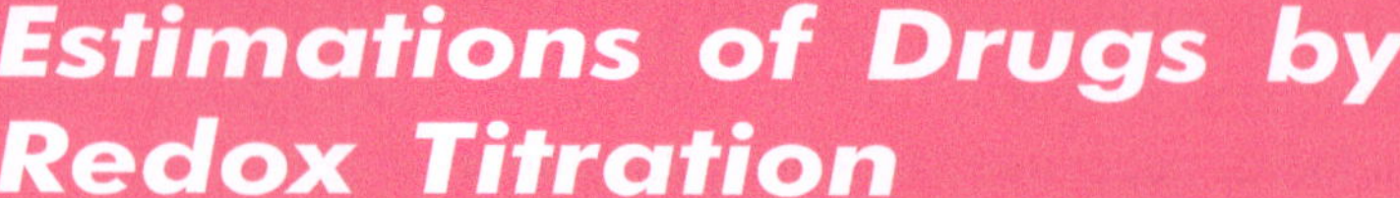

48

Estimations of Drugs by Redox Titration

Redox titration involves simultaneous oxidation and reduction processes. It transfers electron from one species (reducing agent) to another species (oxidizing agent). In redox titrations, a reducing analyte can be titrated against oxidizing agent (e.g., potassium permanganate) or an oxidizing analyte can be titrated against reducing titrant (e.g., sodium thiosulphate). The electron donating species gets oxidized during the course of reducing other species. The species, which accepts electron (oxidizing agent) undergoes reduction.

Important redox titrations

- Permanganometric titrations
- Iodine titrations
- Cerimetric titrations

Permanganometric Titrations

Theory

Potassium permanganate is an oxidizing agent, which accepts electrons and reduces into manganese (Mn^+).

Principle

The oxidation-reduction reaction between potassium permanganate and reducing agent generates nascent oxygen in acidic environment (concentrated sulphuric acid is preferable). In this redox titration, the purple coloured potassium permanganate (reduction) becomes colorless, at the end point.

$$\underset{\text{Potassium permanganate}}{2\,KMnO_4} + \underset{\text{agent}}{\text{Reducing}} + 3\,H_2SO_4 \longrightarrow \underset{\text{Potassium sulphate}}{K_2SO_4} + \underset{\text{Manganese sulphate}}{2\,MnSO_4} + 3\,H_2O + n\,O_2$$

Iodine Titrations

Theory

Iodine (I_2), a mild oxidizing agent and oxidizes other species, which accepts electrons and gets reduced into iodide (I^-). The acidic, neutral and dilute acetic acid medium provides better results.

$$\underset{\text{Iodine}}{I_2} + 2e^- \rightleftharpoons \underset{\text{Iodide}}{2I^-}$$

Principle

Iodine titrations can be explained through the following two major principles.

- ***Iodimetry***: It uses standard iodine solution as an oxidizing agent (titrant, direct). The substances with strong reducing property can be easily estimated through iodimetric titrations. Iodine (I_2), a mild oxidizing agent gets reduced into iodide (I^-) by accepting electrons. Reducing agents like sodium thiosulpahte, ascorbic acid, etc can be estimated by iodimetric titrations. Iodine oxidizes sodium thiosulphate into sodium tetrathionate ion.

$$\underset{\text{Iodine}}{I_2} + \underset{\text{Sodium thiosulphate}}{2Na_2S_2O_3} \longrightarrow \underset{\text{Sodium iodide}}{2NaI} + \underset{\text{Sodium tetrathionate}}{Na_2S_4O_6}$$

- ***Iodometry***: The term iodometry refers to the titrations of liberated iodine (indirect) (opposite to iodimetry, where iodine is used directly). This titration useful in the determination of oxidizing analytes with the help of iodine. The substances with weak reducing property can be easily estimated through iodometric titrations. The titrant in this titration is sodium thiosulphate (reducing agent). The reduction of oxidizing analytes releases the iodine and is basis for the quantification. Iodine oxidizes sodium thiosulphate into sodium tetrathionate ion.

$$\underset{\text{Potassium Iodide}}{KI} + \underset{\text{agent}}{\text{Oxidizing}} \rightleftharpoons \underset{\text{Iodine}}{I_2}$$

$$\underset{\text{Iodine}}{I_2} + \underset{\text{Sodium thiosulphate}}{2Na_2S_2O_3} \longrightarrow \underset{\text{Sodium iodide}}{2NaI} + \underset{\text{Sodium tetrathionate}}{Na_2S_4O_6}$$

Copper sulphate ($CuSO_4.5H_2O$), potassium dichromate ($K_2Cr_2O_7$), cerium sulphate ($Ce(SO_4)_2$), potassium iodate (KIO_3) and potassium bromate ($KBrO_3$) are the important oxidizing agents for liberating the iodine from potassium iodide.

Cerimetric titration

Theory

Ceric ammonium sulphate is highly stable and have high oxidation potential (strong oxidizing agent), hence it is advantageous over potassium permanganate ($KMnO_4$). Cerimetric titration is useful in the estimation of ferrous gluconate, ascorbic acid, chlorpromazine and paracetamol.

Principle

The known excess of ceric ammonium sulphate oxidizes reducing agents and undergoes reduction. For example, ascorbic acid (reducing agent) gets oxidized (loss of electrons) into dehydroascorbic acid (oxidized from). In the reaction, the ceric ion (Ce^{4+}, oxidized state) of ceric ammonium sulphate gains electrons (reduction) and converts into cerous state (Ce^{3+}, reduced state). The unreacted ceric ion (Ce^{4+}) oxidizes ferroin indicator (1,10-phenanthroline-ferrous complex) and gets reduced into cerous ion (Ce^{3+}). The oxidized form of ferroin sulphate develops pale blue colour from initial orange-yellow colour at the end point.

$$\underset{\text{Ceric}}{Ce^{4+}} + e^- \rightleftharpoons \underset{\text{Cerous (reduced)}}{Ce^{3+}}$$

Permanganometry

48.1 Estimation of Hydrogen Peroxide

Hydrogen peroxide is an antimicrobial agent.

Principle

Hydrogen peroxide is a reducing agent and can be quantified by titrating against potassium permanganate (oxidizing agent). The potassium permanganate oxidizes hydrogen peroxide and generates nascent oxygen along with potassium sulphate and manganese sulphate (reduced form of permanganate). The excess of potassium permanganate develops purple colour, at the endpoint.

Procedure

Chemicals Required: Hydrogen peroxide, Sulphuric acid (1 M), Potassium permanganate.

$$\underset{\text{Hydrogen peroxide}}{5\,H_2O_2} + \underset{\text{Potassium permanganate}}{2KMnO_4} + 3H_2SO_4 \longrightarrow \underset{\text{Potassium sulphate}}{K_2SO_4} + \underset{\text{Manganese sulphate}}{MnSO_4} + 8H_2O + 5O_2\uparrow$$

Experimental steps

1. Transfer 20 mL of 1 M sulphuric acid into a conical flask.
2. Add 1 mL of hydrogen peroxide into the conical flask.
3. Titrate the mixture against standard potassium permanganate (self-indicator).
4. The appearance of pale pink colour indicates the end point.

   Each mL of 0.02 M potassium permanganate is equivalent to 0.001701 g of hydrogen peroxide.

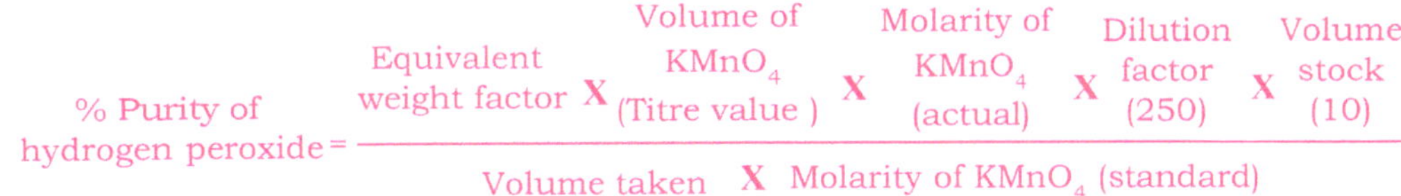

$$\%\text{ Purity of hydrogen peroxide} = \frac{\text{Equivalent weight factor} \times \text{Volume of } KMnO_4 \text{ (Titre value)} \times \text{Molarity of } KMnO_4 \text{ (actual)} \times \text{Dilution factor (250)} \times \text{Volume stock (10)}}{\text{Volume taken} \times \text{Molarity of } KMnO_4 \text{ (standard)}}$$

48.2 Estimation of Ascorbic Acid

Ascorbic acid (vitamin C) is an antioxidant, which plays essential role in the protection of body from infections and diseases.

Principle

The amount of ascorbic acid present in the analyte can be determined by iodimetric titration (redox titration). Ascorbic acid reduces iodine into iodide and gets oxidized to dehydroascorbic acid. Reduction of iodine to iodide will continue as long as ascorbic acid is present. The excess of iodine can be detected by the reaction with starch indicator, which gives blue colour with iodine at end point.

Ascorbic acid (Vitamin C) + I_2 (Iodine) $\rightleftharpoons$ Dehydroascorbic acid + $2I^-$ (Iodide)

This method is applicable for ascorbic acid present in fruits, and pharmaceutical formulations (powder and tablets).

Procedure

Chemicals Required: Ascorbic acid, Sulphuric acid (1 M), Iodine (0.05 M), Starch solution.

Experimental steps

1. Dissolve the accurately weighed ascorbic acid powder (0.1 g) in 100 mL of distilled water (freshly boiled and cooled).

2. Add 25 mL of sulphuric acid (1 M) and immediately titrate the mixture with iodine (0.05 M) using starch solution as an indicator.
3. The appearance of persistent blue colour is the end point.
   Each mL of 0.05 M iodine is equivalent to 0.008806 g of ascorbic acid.

$$\text{Amount of ascorbic acid} = \frac{\text{Equivalent weight factor} \times \text{Volume of Iodine (Titre value)} \times \text{Molarity of Iodine (actual)}}{\text{Weight taken} \times \text{Molarity of Iodine (standard)}}$$

***Note*:** Ascorbic acid is susceptible to oxidation by atmospheric oxygen; hence freshly prepared sample should be used. Alternatively, oxidation can be minimized by adding small amount of oxalic acid.

Cerimetry

48.3 Estimation of Ferrous Sulphate

Ferrous sulphate is a hematinic agent.

Principle

Ferrous sulphate can be assayed by cerimetric titration using ceric ammonium nitrate as titrant. The ceric ammonium nitrate oxidizes ferrous sulphate and reduces into cerous form, hence the titration is known as redox titration. The ceric ion (Ce^{4+}, oxidized state) gains electrons (reduction) and converts into cerous state (Ce^{3+}, reduced state). The unreacted ceric ion (Ce^{4+}) oxidizes ferroin indicator (1,10-phenanthroline-ferrous complex) and gets reduced into cerous ion (Ce^{3+}). The oxidized form of ferroin sulphate develops pale blue colour from initial orange-yellow colour at the end point.

Procedure

$$\underset{\text{Ferrous sulphate}}{2\,FeSO_4} + \underset{\text{Ceric ammonium nitrate}}{Ce(NH_4)_2(NO_3)_6} + H_2SO_4 \longrightarrow \underset{\text{Ferric sulphate}}{Fe_2(SO_4)_3} + \underset{\text{Cerium nitrate}}{Ce(NO_3)_3} + \underset{\text{Ammonium sulphate}}{(NH_4)_2SO_4} + 3HNO_3$$

$$\underset{\text{Cerous (reduced)}}{Ce^{3+}} + \text{Ferroin} \longrightarrow \underset{\text{Red colour}}{\underset{\text{complex}}{Fe^{2+}\text{-Ferroin}}} \longrightarrow \underset{\text{Blue colour}}{\underset{\text{complex}}{Fe^{3+}\text{-Ferroin}}} + \underset{\text{Ceric (oxidized)}}{Ce^{4+}}$$

***Chemicals Required*:** Sodium bicarbonate, Dilute sulphuric acid, Ferrous sulphate, Ceric ammonium nitrate, Ferroin sulphate.

Experimental steps

1. Dissolve 2.5 g of sodium bicarbonate in a mixture of 150 mL of water and 10 mL of dilute sulphuric acid.
2. Add 0.5 g of ferrous sulphate, after the completion of the effervescence.
3. Shake gently to dissolve the contents.
4. Titrate the mixture against 0.1 M ceric ammonium nitrate using 0.1 mL of ferroin sulphate as an indicator.
5. The disappearance of red colour is the end point.

   Each mL of 0.1 M ceric ammonium nitrate is equivalent to 0.02780 g of ferrous sulphate.

$$\text{Amount of ferrous sulphate} = \frac{\text{Equivalent weight factor} \times \text{Volume of } Ce(NH_4)_2(NO_3)_6 \text{ (Titre value)} \times \text{Molarity of } Ce(NH_4)_2(NO_3)_6 \text{ (actual)}}{\text{Weight taken} \times \text{Molarity of } Ce(NH_4)_2(NO_3)_6 \text{ (standard)}}$$

48.4 Estimation of Ascorbic Acid

Ascorbic acid (vitamin C) is an antioxidant, which plays essential role in the protection of body from infections and diseases.

Principle

Ascorbic acid can be assayed by cerimetric titration using ceric ammonium sulphate as titrant. The ceric ammonium sulphate oxidizes ascorbic acid and undergoes reduction. While oxidizing the ascorbic acid into dehydroascorbic acid, ceric ammonium sulphate reduces into cerous form, hence the titration is known as redox titration. The ceric ion (Ce^{4+}, oxidized state) gains electrons (reduction) and converts into cerous state (Ce^{3+}, reduced state). The unreacted ceric ion (Ce^{4+}) oxidizes ferroin indicator (1,10-phenanthroline-ferrous complex) and gets reduced into cerous ion (Ce^{3+}). The oxidized form of ferroin sulphate (1,10-phenanthroline-ferrous complex) develops pale blue colour from initial orange-yellow colour at the end point.

Ascorbic acid (Vitamin C) + Ce^{4+} Ceric (oxidized) ⟶ Dehydroascorbic acid + Ce^{3+} Cerous (reduced)

Ce^{3+} Cerous (reduced) + Ferroin ⟶ Fe^{2+}-Ferroin complex (Red colour) ⟶ Fe^{3+}-Ferroin complex (Blue colour) + Ce^{4+} Ceric (oxidized)

This method is applicable for ascorbic acid present in fruits and pharmaceutical formulations (powder and tablets).

Procedure

Chemicals Required: Ascorbic acid tablets, Sulphuric acid (1M), Ceric ammonium sulphate (0.1M), Ferroin sulphate.

Experimental steps

1. Weigh and powder 20 ascorbic acid tablets.
2. Dissolve accurately weighed ascorbic acid powder (0.15 g) in the mixture of distilled water (30 mL) and sulphuric acid (1M, 20 mL).
3. Titrate the mixture with ceric ammonium sulphate (0.1M) using ferroin sulphate (0.1 mL) as indicator.
4. The colour change of orange-yellow into persistent pale blue colour indicates the end point of titration.
5. Perform the blank titration for necessary correction.

   Each mL of ceric ammonium sulphate (0.1 M) is equivalent to 0.008806 g of ascorbic acid.

$$\text{Amount of ascorbic acid} = \frac{\text{Equivalent weight factor} \times \text{Volume of } Ce(NH_4)_2(NO_3)_6 \text{ (Titre value)} \times \text{Molarity of } Ce(NH_4)_2(NO_3)_6 \text{ (actual)}}{\text{Weight taken} \times \text{Molarity of } Ce(NH_4)_2(NO_3)_6 \text{ (standard)}}$$

48.5 Estimation of Paracetamol

Paracetamol is an analgesic and antipyretic drug.

Principle

Paracetamol can be assayed by cerimetric titration using ceric ammonium sulphate as titrant (cerimetric titration). The quantification procedure requires hydrolysis of paracetamol into *para*-aminophenol using sulphuric acid. The ceric ammonium sulphate oxidizes *para*-aminophenol into *para*-iminoquinone and undergoes reduction. While oxidizing the paracetamol, ceric ammonium sulphate reduces into cerous form, hence the titration is known as redox titration. The ceric ion (Ce^{4+}, oxidized state) gains electrons (reduction) and converts into cerous state (Ce^{3+}, reduced state). The unreacted ceric ion (Ce^{4+}) oxidizes ferroin indicator (1,10-phenanthroline-ferrous complex) and gets reduced into cerous ion (Ce^{3+}). The oxidized form of ferroin sulphate (1,10-phenanthroline-ferrous complex) develops pale blue colour from initial orange-yellow colour at the end point.

Paracetamol + H_2SO_4 ⟶ *para*-Aminophenol + CH_3COOH

para-Aminophenol + Ce^{4+} Ceric (oxidized) ⟶ *para*-Iminoquinone + Ce^{3+} Cerous (reduced)

Ce^{3+} Cerous (reduced) + Ferroin ⟶ Fe^{2+}-Ferroin complex Red colour ⟶ Fe^{3+}-Ferroin complex Blue colour + Ce^{4+} Ceric (oxidized)

Procedure

Chemicals Required: Paracetamol, Distilled water, Sulphuric acid (1 M), Hydrochloric acid (2 M), Ceric ammonium sulphate (0.1 M), Ferroin sulphate.

Experimental steps

1. Dissolve accurately weighed paracetamol powder (0.5 g) in the mixture of water (10 mL) and sulphuric acid (1 M, 50 mL).
2. Boil the mixture under reflux for 1 h, cool and dilute to 100 mL with distilled water.
3. To the 20 mL of above solution add water (40 mL), ice (40 g) and hydrochloric acid (2 M, 15 mL).
4. Titrate the mixture immediately with ceric ammonium sulphate (0.1 M) using ferroin sulphate (0.1 mL) as indicator.
5. The colour change of orange-yellow into persistent pale blue-colour indicates the end point of titration.
6. Perform the blank titration for necessary correction.

   Each mL of ceric ammonium sulphate (0.1 M) is equivalent to 0.00756 g of paracetamol.

$$\text{Amount of paracetamol} = \frac{\text{Equivalent weight factor} \times \text{Volume of } Ce(NH_4)_2(SO_4)_6 \text{ (Titre value)} \times \text{Molarity of } Ce(NH_4)_2(SO_4)_6 \text{ (actual)}}{\text{Weight taken} \times \text{Molarity of } Ce(NH_4)_2(SO_4)_6 \text{ (standard)}}$$

KEY POINTS

- Redox titration involves the transfer of electron from one species (reducing agent) to another species (oxidizing agent).
- Permanganometric, iodine (iodi and iodo) and cerimetric titrations are pharmaceutically important redox reactions.
- The titration of standard iodine (titrant, direct) is referred to as iodimetry and liberated iodine (indirect) is referred to as iodometry.
- Ferrous sulphate, hydrogen peroxide, ascorbic acid and paracetamol can be assayed by redox titrations.

Natural Products Chemistry

Any biological material is strictly a natural product. But, in practice the secondary metabolites of organism in particular plants are known as natural products. These secondary metabolites are essential for the survival of the organism. Dietary supplements and food products of plants are also known natural products.

These natural products have high structural diversity. The diversified structures are responsible for the unique pharmacological functions. Several natural products, such as cocaine, morphine, quinine and artemisinin serve as a lead for the development of drugs. Besides drugs, several natural products are useful as food additives and preservatives.

Natural products can be classified in several ways. The classification based on the chemical constituents is very useful. The most important chemical categories of natural products are given below.

1. Alkaloids (e.g., caffeine, piperine)
2. Proteins (e.g., caseine, albumin)
3. Carbohydrates (e.g., lactose, starch)
4. Flavonoids (e.g., hesperidin)
5. Glycosides (e.g., naringenin)
6. Terpenoids (e.g., trimyristin)
7. Volatile oils (e.g., cinnamon oil, eugenol)

49

Isolation of Plant Alkaloids

Alkaloids are physiologically active nitrogenous secondary metabolites of plant kingdom as well as animal kingdom. In alkaloids, at least one nitrogen atom forms part of a cyclic system (except phenylethylamine). Alkaloids (cyclic organic compounds) contain nitrogen (one/two) in a negative state of oxidation. Alkaloids can be grouped based on the chemical nature and the most important alkaloids are listed given below.

Chemical nature	Alkaloids
Phenylethylamine	Ephedrine
Tropane	Atropine, cocaine
Imidazole	Pilocarpine, pilosine
Indole	Ergotamine, reserpine, strychnine and vincristine
Quinoline	Quinine, cinchonine
Isoquinoline	Papaverine, emetine, berberine and tubocurarine
Phenanthrene	Morphine, codeine and thebaine
Pyridine and piperidine	Piperine, arecoline and pelletierine
Xanthine	Caffeine, theophylline and theobromine

49.1 Isolation of Caffeine from Tea Leaves

Theory

Caffeine is a basic nitrogenous compound found in plants and belongs to purine alkaloids category. It produces stimulant effect in central nervous system, respiratory system and cardiac system. It causes nervousness, insomnia and headache. Tea leaves, coffee seeds and cocoa seeds contain caffeine as one of the major ingredients.

Principle

Tea leaf (*Thea sinensis*) contains methyl derivatives of xanthenes namely, caffeine, theophylline and theobromine. The isolation of caffeine from the tea leaves involves the extraction of water-soluble caffeine present into hot water. The solubility of caffeine in water is 22 mg/mL at 25 °C, 1080 mg/mL at 80 °C and 670 mg/mL at 100 °C. Addition of sodium carbonate to the mixture forms sodium salt of phenolic compounds (tannins). The sodium salt of tannins are more water soluble and remain in the water. Tea leaves consists of cellulose, caffeine, tannins and small amount of chlorophyll. Caffeine is more soluble in dichloromethane (140 mg/mL) than water (22 mg/mL) at 25 °C. Hence, the caffeine present in aqueous layer can be isolated by extraction with dichloromethane.

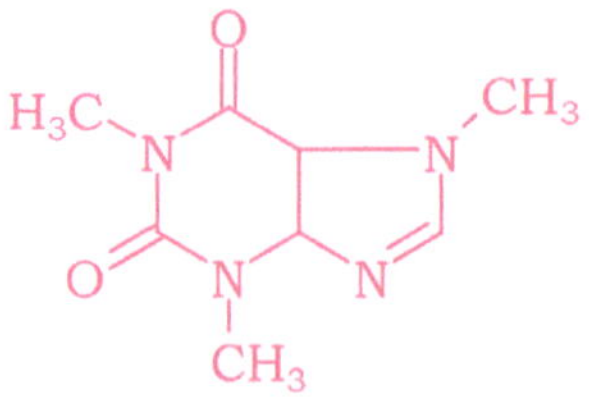

Caffeine

Procedure

Chemicals Required: Tea powder/dust, Sodium carbonate (or calcium carbonate), Dichloromethane, Distilled water, Anhydrous Sodium sulphate, Silver nitrate.

Experimental steps

1. Place the tea bags containing tea powder/dust (5 g) into a beaker, add 30 mL of distilled water and 2 g of sodium carbonate (or calcium carbonate).
2. Gently boil the mixture for 20 min by placing in a water bath (move the tea bag up and down, occasionally).
3. Press tea bags to collect maximum amount of extract.
4. Decant the hot liquid into a flask, add 20 mL of distilled water to the beaker, boil and decant again into the flask.
5. Cool the aqueous tea extract collected in the flask to room temperature and transfer into the separatory funnel.
6. Add 5 mL of dichloromethane to the separatory funnel and swirl the contents.
7. Allow the contents to settle down and to form two distinct layers. (stir with glass rod to break the emulsion, if any forms).
8. Collect the lower organic layer and extract the remaining aqueous layer with dichloromethane (5 mL, second time).
9. Combine the organic layers and add 0.5 g of anhydrous sodium sulphate and swirl the mixture.
10. Decant the liquid into the beaker containing boiling chips and place it in a hot plate.
11. Add petroleum ether (5 mL), when the volume of dichloromethane layer reduces into 3 mL.
12. Allow the beaker to cool to room temperature, when cloudiness appears in the beaker.
13. Isolate the crystals of caffeine by vacuum filtration.

Characterization

(a) The melting point of the pure caffeine is 238 °C.

(b) ***Silver nitrate test*:** Place the sample in a test tube. Add 1 mL of hot water and 3 drops of silver nitrate. Formation of purple colour indicates the presence of caffeine.

49.2 Isolation of Piperine from Pepper

Theory

Piperine can be isolated from black pepper (*Piper nigrum* and *Piper longum*). Piperine is a pungent alkaloid and possess anticancer, antimalarial, antioxidant, neuroprotective and anti-inflammatory effects.

Principle

The isolation of piperine from the black pepper (*Piper nigrum* and *Piper longum*) involves the extraction with dichloromethane (DCM). Piperine is more soluble in dichloromethane and facilitates the isolation.

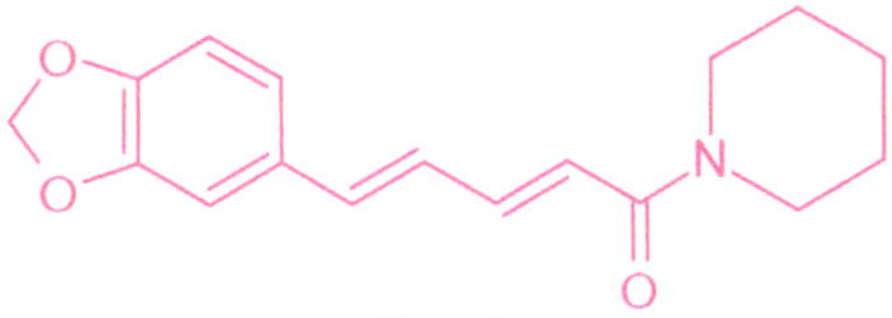

Piperine

Procedure

Chemicals Required : Black pepper, Dichloromethane (DCM), Diethyl ether, Ethanol, Ethanolic potassium hydroxide, Mayer's reagent and Wagner's reagent.

Experimental steps

1. Place the powdered black pepper (10 g) into a flask and add dichloromethane (20 mL) to dissolve the contents.
2. Attach reflux condenser and reflux the mixture for 30 min.
3. Cool the flask, filter and wash the residue with dichloromethane (10 mL).
4. Transfer the filtrate to a round bottom flask and distil to remove the dichloromethane.
5. Place the flask (containing brown oil) in an ice bath and add diethyl ether (2 mL).
6. Stir the mixture to precipitate the solid.
7. Add diethyl ether (2 mL, second volume) and stir the mixture occasionally by keeping in an ice-bath.
8. Dissolve the solid with ethanol (2 mL).

9. Add the ethanolic extract into beaker containing ethanolic potassium hydroxide (10%, 2 mL) to precipitate the acidic resins.
10. Filter to remove the solid and allow it cool to produce yellow precipitate of piperine.
11. Filter and wash the yellow crystals with cold water.

Characterization

(a) The melting point of the pure piperine is 128 to 130°C.

(b) ***Meyer's test:*** Meyer's regent is prepared by dissolving mixture of mercuric chloride and potassium iodide in water. Transfer the sample solution in to a test tube and add Meyer's reagent (1:1). Formation of cream precipitate indicates that the sample in test is an alkaloid.

(c) ***Wagner's test:*** Solution of iodine in potassium iodide is known as Wagner's regent. Transfer the sample solution in to a test tube and add Wagner's reagent (1:1). Formation of reddish-brown precipitate indicates that the sample in test is an alkaloid.

KEY POINTS

- Alkaloids are physiologically active nitrogenous secondary metabolites of plant kingdom as well as animal kingdom.
- Tea leaf (Thea sinensis) contains methyl derivatives of xanthenes namely, caffeine, theophylline and theobromine.
- Caffeine reacts with silver nitrate and develops purple colour.
- Piperine can be isolated from black pepper (Piper nigrum and Piper longum).
- Meyer's test and Wagner's test can be used to detect the presence of piperine.

50

Isolation of Milk Proteins

Milk contains vitamins, minerals, proteins, sugars and lipids. Three major proteins present in the milk are casein, lactalbumin and lactoglobulin. Thiamine, riboflavin, pantothenate, vitamin A, vitamin D and vitamin K are the vitamins present in milk. It contains calcium, potassium, sodium, phosphorous and trace metals. The precipitation of casein from water during destruction is called as protein denaturation.

50.1 Isolation of Casein from Milk

Theory

Casein is a phosphoprotein attached to serine and threonine. Casein exists as calcium salt and composed of α, β and κ caseins. The α and κ caseins are soluble in water. The addition of κ caseins to the mixture of α and β caseins result in micelle.

Principle

Calcium caseinate has isoelectric point at pH 4.6, therefore it is insoluble in solution of pH less than 4.6. The α and β casein can be precipitated by acidification (mineral or organic acids). Denaturation of protein structure by heat or acid (acetic acid, nitric acid) is called as coagulation of protein. Casein bears negative charge at milk pH 6.6, but when acid is added the negative charge gets neutralized and precipitates.

$$\underset{\text{caseinate}}{\text{Calcium}} + CH_3COOH \longrightarrow \text{Casein} + (CH_3COOH)_2Ca$$

Procedure

Chemicals Required: Milk, Acetic acid (10%), Nitric acid, Sulphuric acid, Ammonia, Ammonium molybdate and Distilled water.

Experimental steps

1. Place milk sample (4 g) into a beaker and add 50 mL of distilled water.
2. Warm the aqueous milk sample to 40 °C by placing in a hot plate.

3. Add 5 drops of acetic acid (10%) to the warm milk (after it reaches 40 °C).
4. Stir the solution, on stirring casein precipitates out.
5. Allow the mixture stand for 10 min.
6. Isolate the precipitated casein and wash with distilled water.
7. Remove the milk solution present in the precipitate, and dry the casein by pressing between filter paper.

   Note: Excess of acid hydrolyses lactose to glucose and galactose.

Characterization

- The melting point of the pure casein is 280°C.
- ***Litmus test*:** It turns blue litmus into red (alkaline).
- ***Neumann's test*:** Add 2 drops of nitric acid and 10 drops of sulphuric acid to the sample and heat the contents. Cool and add 2 mL of distilled water, 2 mL of ammonia, 2 mL of ammonium molybdate solution and warm. The development of canary yellow colour precipitate indicates the presence of casein.

50.2 Isolation of Albumin from Milk

Theory

Milk contains water, vitamins, minerals, proteins, sugars and lipids. Three major proteins present in the milk are casein, lactalbumin and lactoglobulin. Albumins are globular proteins soluble in water and dilute salt solutions. The second most abundant protein present in milk is lactalbumin and the other one is lactoglobulins.

Principle

The albumin present in milk can be isolated by acidification (mineral or organic acids) and further neutralization with calcium carbonate. Denaturation of protein structure by heat or acid (acetic acid, nitric acid) is called as coagulation of protein. Albumin and globulin are coagulating proteins. The acidification step helps removing the casein and the next alkalinization isolates the albumin.

Procedure

Chemicals Required: Milk, Acetic acid (10%), Calcium carbonate, Distilled water, Ammonium sulphate and Nitric acid.

Experimental steps

1. Place milk sample (4 g) into a beaker and add 50 mL of distilled water.
2. Warm the aqueous milk sample to 40 °C by placing in a hot plate.
3. Add 5 drops of acetic acid (10%) to the warm milk (after it reaches 40 °C).
4. Stir the solution, on stirring casein precipitates out.
5. Allow the mixture stand for 10 min and isolate the precipitated casein by filtration.

6. Add calcium carbonate to neutralize the milk solution (filtrate).
7. Heat the milk mixture to 75 °C for 5 min by placing on a sand bath.
8. Separate the precipitate of albumin by filtration in hot condition.

Characterization

- **Litmus test:** It shows neutral for litmus test.
- **Full saturation test:** Saturate the sample solution with solid ammonium sulphate. The formation of gelatinous precipitate indicates the presence of albumin.
- **Heller's test:** Appearance of white ring upon addition of nitric acid to the sample solution along the sides of the test tube indicates presence of albumin.

KEY POINTS

- Milk contains casein, lactalbumin and lactoglobulin.
- Thiamine, riboflavin, pantothenate, vitamin A, vitamin D and vitamin K are the vitamins present in milk.
- Denaturation of protein structure by heat or acid (acetic acid, nitric acid) is called as coagulation of protein.
- Ammonium molybdate solution develops canary yellow colour precipitate when reacts with casein, and this test is known as Neumann's test.

51

Isolation of Carbohydrates

Carbohydrates are naturally occurring organic compounds. Chemically they are polyhydroxy aldehydes or polyhydroxy ketones or the compounds that produce these compounds on hydrolysis. Carbohydrates present in foods serve as a primary source of energy. Carbohydrates can be broadly classified into

1. Simple carbohydrates (sugars)
2. Complex carbohydrates (starch and dietary fiber)

Simple Carbohydrates: Simple carbohydrates (sugars) are present in fruits, milk and other foods. The two main types of simple sugars are

1. ***Monosaccharides*:** They contain only one unit of sugar (glucose, fructose).
2. ***Disaccharides*:** Two monosaccharides through condensation produce disaccharides. The important disaccharide sugars present in human nutrition are sucrose (table sugar), lactose (sugar in milk) and maltose (a product of starch breakdown).

Complex Carbohydrates: Complex carbohydrates contain more than two monosaccharide molecules called as oligosaccharides and polysaccharides.

***Polysaccharides*:** Fruits and vegetables are particularly rich in polysaccharides. They are long chain carbohydrates, composed of more than 10 sugar molecules. The polysaccharides include starch, glycogen, inulin and dietary fibers (cellulose, pectin and mucilage).

51.1 Isolation of Pectin from Apples

Theory

Pectin (in *Greek*, congealed and curled) is a hetero polysaccharide found in the middle lamella of cell wall of terrestrial plants. During ripening, pectinase and pectin esterase breaks the pectin and converts the fruit soft. Pectin acts as a soluble fiber and reduces blood cholesterol level. It increases the viscosity of the intestinal tract, there by decreases the absorption of cholesterol from bile and food. Pectin gets converted to short chain fatty acids in large intestine and colon, which have prebiotic effect.

Apple (*Malus domestica*) contains large amount of pectin. Commercial pectins are derived from citrus peel (20-35%) and apple pomace (10-15%). Citrus pectins are light cream/light tan in colour where as apple pectins are darker. Pectins also can be obtained from sugar beet waste, mango waste and sunflower heads.

Principle

Pectin can be extracted with acidified water (pH upto 2) at temperature not more than 70 °C. The sugars found in pectin are D-galactose, L-arabinose and D-xylose. Pectin consists mainly of D-galacturonic acid (GalA) units joined by α-(1-4) glycosidic linkage. In some cases, galacturonic acid is replaced with (1-2)-linked L-rhamnose and this type of pectin is called as rhamnogalacturonan-I. Pectin, monovalent salt of pectinic acid and pectic acid are soluble in water, whereas di and tri valent salts are weakly soluble. Pectin can be isolated by heating the raw materials with water adjusted to pH 3.5-4.0 with tartaric acid. Mineral acids (sulphuric acid, hydrochloric acid and phosphoric acid), oxalic acid, ammonium sulphate, ammonium oxalate, tartaric acid, polyphosphates, Zeolites and Zeocarb can be used for the extraction procedure.

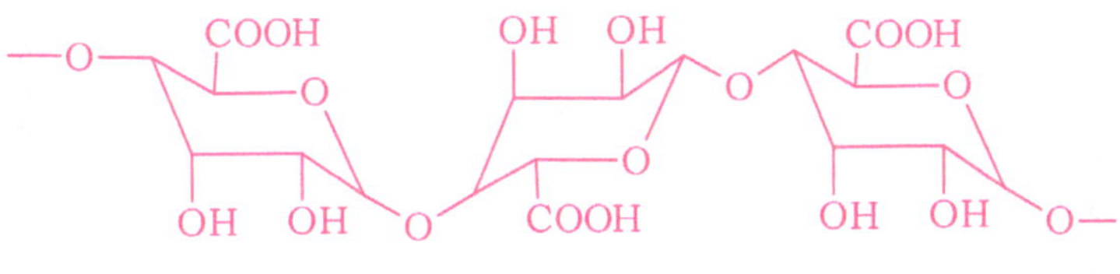

Pectin

Procedure

Chemicals Required: Apple, Tartaric acid, Acetone, Potassium hydroxide.

Experimental steps

1. Place the thin slices of apple (10 g) into a beaker and add 40 mL of distilled water.
2. Adjust the pH 3.5 to 4.0 with tartaric acid (citric acid or ammonium sulphate also can be used).
3. Heat the acidic mixture at 90 to 95 °C for 2 h.
4. Filter the hot mixture and add the filtrate into three volumes of acetone (ethanol or isopropanol also can be used).
5. Filter the precipitate through nylon cloth and wash with organic solvent.
6. Dry the precipitate by keeping in a desiccator, maintaining at 37° C.

Note:

- Longer heating may degrade the pectin.
- Pectin extraction after two hours of extraction gives relatively good yield.

Characterization

Gel formation: Place the sample solution (5 mL, 1%) in a test tube. Add potassium hydroxide (1 mL, 2%). The mixture develops transparent gel after 15 min.

51.2 Isolation of Lactose from Milk

Theory

Milk contains lactalbumin and lactoglobulin. Lactose is the main carbohydrate present in milk.

Principle

The casein and albumin present in the milk can be isolated by acidification and neutralization with calcium carbonate. The remaining liquid contains lactose, which can be isolated by ethanol treatment and heat.

Procedure

Chemicals Required: Milk, Acetic acid (10%), Calcium carbonate, Ethanol (95%), Distilled water, Benedict's reagent.

Experimental steps

1. Place milk sample (4 g) into a beaker and add 50 mL of distilled water.
2. Warm the aqueous milk sample to 40 °C by placing in a hot plate.
3. Add 5 drops of acetic acid (10%) to the warm milk (after it reaches 40 °C).
4. Stir the solution, on stirring casein precipitates out.
5. Allow the mixture stand for 10 min and isolate the precipitated casein.
6. Add calcium carbonate to neutralize the milk solution.
7. Heat the milk mixture to 75 °C for 5 min by placing on a sand bath.
8. Separate the precipitate of albumin by filtration in hot condition.
9. Cool the filtrate to room temperature and centrifuge for 5 min.
10. Decant the liquid into beaker and add 95% ethanol to the beaker (solid get precipitates).
11. Heat the mixture on a sand bath to about 60 °C to dissolve the solid.
12. Centrifuge the solution for 2 min and remove the supernatant, and collect the solid lactose.

Characterization

- ***Reducing sugar test:*** Add 5 mL of Benedict's reagent to the sample solution in a test tube. Place the test tube in a water bath for 10 min. The appearance of red precipitate indicates the presence of reducing sugar.

51.3 Isolation of Starch from Potatoes

Starch is an important polysaccharide. It occurs as granules and insoluble in water.

Principle

Starch can be isolated from raw potatoes. The homogenate obtained by grinding of potatoes and water consists of starch.

Procedure

Chemicals Required: Potatoes, Distilled water, Iodine.

1. Peel the raw potato (5 g) and cut into small slices.
2. Grind the slices with water using mixer (mortar and pestle can also be used).
3. Collect the homogenate into a beaker and add water.
4. Filter the homogenate through muslin cloth to remove particles.
5. Allow the filtrate to settle and decant the supernatant liquid.
6. Wash the residue with water 3 times and decant the supernatant.
7. The solid remains in the flask is polysaccharide starch.

Characterization

Iodine test: Add 2 drops of dilute iodine solution to the sample solution. The development of blue colour indicates the starch.

KEY POINTS

- Carbohydrates are polyhydroxy aldehydes or polyhydroxy ketones or the compounds that produce these compounds on hydrolysis.
- Carbohydrates present in foods serve as a primary source of energy.
- Pectin is a structural hetero polysaccharide found in the middle lamella of cell wall of terrestrial plants.
- Lactose is the main carbohydrate present in milk.

52

Isolation of Essential Oils

Essential oils are generally concentrated in seeds, flowers and also in other parts of plants. These are volatile in nature and can be separated from odoriferous plants by grinding, maceration, solvent extraction, distillation and concentration processes. Combination of all these techniques results in effective and efficient isolation. The most common way of extracting volatile oils are:

- *Steam distillation*: It involves the passage of hot steam into the plants, which extracts the volatile oils from the plant parts.
- *Cold pressing*: It involves the mechanical squeezing of plant material to collect essential oils.

52.1 Isolation of Cinnamon Oil from Cinnamon

Cinnamon is dried barks of *Cinnamomum zeylanicum* (Family: Lauraceae).

Principle

Cinnamon oil can be isolated from cinnamon bark by extracting with ethyl acetate. The cinnamon oil gets into the ethyl acetate layer, upon reflux. Drying the organic layer over anhydrous magnesium sulphate removes the aqueous components, if any present. Cinnamon oil contains 40 to 50% of cinnamaldehyde.

Procedure

Chemicals required: Cinnamon bark, Ethyl acetate, Anhydrous magnesium sulphate (or Calcium chloride), Osmic acid .

Experimental steps

1. Weigh 5 g of dry cinnamon bark and grind them into a coarse powder with the aid of mixer.
2. Transfer the grinded mass into a round bottom flask.
3. Add 35 mL of ethyl acetate to the flask and reflux the mixture for 20 min.
4. Cool the mixture to room temperature and decant the solution to flask.
5. Rinse the residue with ethyl acetate and combine the organic layers.
6. Add anhydrous magnesium sulphate (or calcium chloride) and swirl the flask for about 30 sec.

7. Filter the mixture into the round bottom flask and remove the ethyl acetate by distillation.
8. The cinnamon oil remains in the flask.

Characterization

- Cinnamon oil with 1% solution of osmic acid gives brown colour.

52.2 Isolation of Clove Oil from Clove

Cloves are dried flower buds of *Eugenia caryophyllata*. Clove oil has analgesic, antibacterial, antifungal, insecticidal and antioxidant properties. Clove oil is also useful in the treatment of asthma and allergic disorders. Clove oil used as flavouring agent and perfume.

Principle

Eugenol is the major component (85-90%) in the clove along with eugenol acetate (9-10%). Clove oil can be isolated by organic extraction, hydrodistillation and distillation in Clevenger.

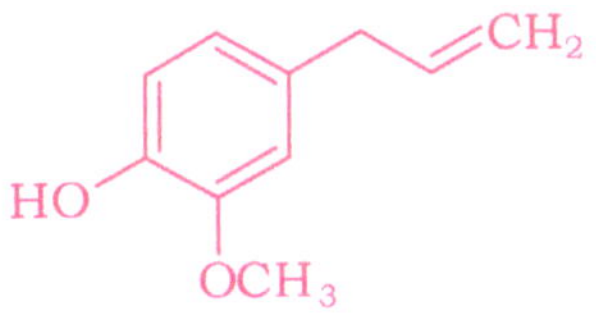

CH_2 HO OCH_3

Eugenol

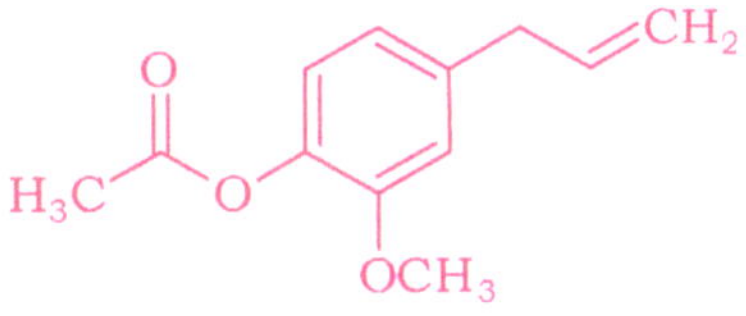

CH_2 O H_3C O OCH_3

Eugenol acetate

Procedure

Experimental steps

Method 1: Isolation of clove oil by organic extraction

Chemicals Required: Clove, Anhydrous magnesium sulphate (or calcium chloride), Ethyl acetate.

1. Weigh 5 g of dry clove and grind them into a coarse powder with the aid of mixer (mortar and pestle also can be used).
2. Transfer the grinded mass into a round bottom flask loaded with boiling chips.
3. Add 35 mL of ethyl acetate to the flask and reflux the mixture for 20 min.
4. Cool the mixture to room temperature and decant the solution to flask.
5. Rinse the residue with ethyl acetate and combine the organic layers.
6. Add anhydrous magnesium sulphate (or calcium chloride) and swirl the flask for about 30 sec.
7. Filter the mixture into round bottom flask and remove the ethyl acetate by distillation.
8. The oil remains in the flask is clove oil.

Method 2: Isolation of clove oil by hydrodistillation

Chemicals required: Cloves, Dichloromethane, Sodium chloride, Anhydrous sodium sulphate, Distilled water.

1. Weigh 5 g of dry cloves and grind them into a coarse powder with the aid of mixer (mortar and pestle also can be used).
2. Transfer the grinded mass into round bottom flask, loaded with boiling chips and add 50 mL of distilled water to the flask.
3. Distil the mixture ($3/4^{th}$) and allow the distillate to cool to room temperature.
4. Transfer the distillate into separating funnel and add 10 mL of saturated sodium chloride solution.
5. Rinse the condenser and flask with 10 mL of dichloromethane and pour into a separatory funnel.
6. Swirl the contents of separating funnel gently, and allow the two layers to separate.
7. Collect the dichloromethane layer into flask and extract the aqueous layer further with two portions of dichloromethane.
8. Combine the organic layer, dry with anhydrous sodium sulphate, decant the dichloromethane layer and evaporate the dichloromethane by placing in water bath.
9. Clove oil remains in the evaporation dish after complete evaporation.

Method 3: Isolation of clove oil by distillation in Clevenger

Requirement: Cloves, Sodium chloride

1. Place 5 g of clove previously grinded into coarse powder in the round bottom flask.
2. Add boiling chips to the flask and attach Clevenger and distil the contents of the flask for 12 h (until no oil drop comes out).
3. Wash the distillate with saturated sodium chloride and separate the hydro layer.
4. The oil remains in the separatory funnel.

Characterization

- **Boiling point:** 254 °C

KEY POINTS

- Essential oils are generally concentrated in seeds and flowers which can be separated from by grinding, maceration, solvent extraction, distillation and concentration.
- Drying the organic layer over anhydrous magnesium sulphate removes the aqueous components.
- Clove oil is useful in the treatment of asthma and allergic disorders.

53

Isolation of Glycosides

Glycosides are composed of both sugar moiety (glycone, genin) and non-sugar moiety (aglycone, agenin). Sugar moieties establishes link with non-sugar moieties through glycosidic bond. The sugar can be mono (e.g., glucose, L-rhamnose, L-fructose, l-arabinose and D-xylose), di (e.g., galactose, mannose and gentiobiose) and tri (e.g., strophanthotriose) saccharide.

53.1 Isolation of Naringin from Grapes

Theory

Naringin a flavone glycoside abundant in grapes and trace in orange which gives the grape juice bitter taste. In the commercial production of grapefruit juice the enzyme naringinase removes the bitterness of naringin. Naringin inhibits cytochrome P450 enzymes (CYP3A4 and CYP1A2) and results in drug-drug interactions.

Naringin also shown neuroprotective in diabetes induced neuropathy, protective effects on cognition and antioxidant effects.

Principle

Naringin can be isolated from grape fruits and orange. Soxhlet extraction and Kesterson (Hendrickson) methods isolates naringin through aqueous and ethanol extraction. Alkali mixture of naringin in diethylene glycol produces yellow colour and the melting point is 71 °C.

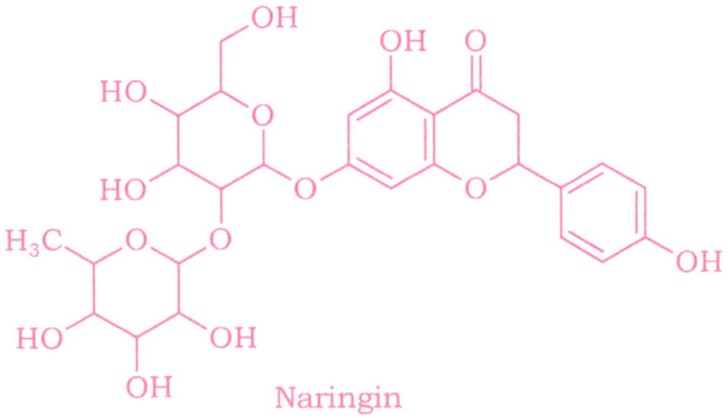

OH
OH O
HO
O
HO O O
H_3C O O
OH
HO OH
OH

Naringin

Method 1

Procedure

Chemicals Required: Grapes, Ethanol, Calcium oxide, Diethylene glycol.

Experimental steps

1. Remove the grapefruit rind with cork borer and blend 40 g with 100 mL of ethanol.
2. Filter the mixture and dry the residue to remove alcohol.
3. Divide the dry residue into two equal portions and use in different extraction procedures.

Soxhlet extraction:

- Transfer one portion of the residue to an extraction thimble and add 50 mL of ethanol.
- Extract the mixture for 3 h and filter the contents of flask.
- Make up the volume of filtrate to 250 mL with ethanol and dilute to 1 to 100 for analysis.

Kesterson (Hendrickson) extraction:

- Allow the combined mixture of portion of filtrate and residue to stand for 16 h with occasional stirring.
- Extract the residue with water containing calcium oxide for 2 h and then with water heated to 95 °C immediately and allowed to stand for 2 h.
- Combine the three filtrates make up the volume to 500 mL, and diluted 1 to 50 for analysis.

Analysis

- The analysis depends upon the production of yellow colour on the addition of alkali to the mixture in presence of diethylene glycol.
- Measure the absorbance of the yellow colour.

Method 2

Procedure

Chemicals Required: Grapes, Ethanol, Isopropanol, Distilled water, Celite.

1. Heat one part of chopped grape peel and four parts of water to 90 °C, and allow it stand at this temperature for 5 min.
2. Filter the water extract and add two parts of water to the solid.
3. Repeat the extraction at 80 °C and filter immediately.
4. Boil the combined extracts with 1% celite, filter and concentrate *in vacuo* to approximately $1/9^{th}$ of original volume.
5. Crystallize the concentrated extract in a refrigerator and filter.
6. Dissolve the naringin in 100 mL of boiling isopropanol and filter while hot.

7. Heat the filtrate to initiate crystallization, cool, filter and wash with cold isopropanol (hot water).
8. The melting point of pure naringin is 171 °C.

KEY POINTS

- Glycosides are composed of both sugar moiety (glycone, genin) and non-sugar moiety (aglycone, agenin).
- Naringin, a flavone glycoside abundant in grapes and trace in oranges.
- Naringin inhibit cytochrome P450 enzymes (CYP3A4 and CYP1A2) and results in drug-drug interactions.

54

Isolation of Flavanoids

Flavanoids are low-molecular weight polyphenolic compounds containing benzo-γ-pyrone nucleus. They are widely distributed in plant kingdom (leaves, flowers and fruits). Flavanoids include the subgroups of anthocyanins, favones, flavonols, flavanolols, flavanols (catechin), isoflavanoids, neoflavanoids and chalcones.

54.1 Isolation of Hesperidin from Oranges

Theory

Hesperidin (rhamnoglucoside of hesperitin) was identified from oranges of Hesperides family, hence given the name Hesperidin. Later its presence in citrus fruits was also identified. Hesperidin decreases the fragility of blood capillaries. Neohesperidin, an isomer of hesperidin also found in these fruits. Hesperidin is non-bitter compound, whereas neohesperidin is a bitter compound.

Principle

Hesperidin can be isolated by two methods.

1. **Petroleum ether extraction:** In this method hesperidin is isolated by extracting dried citrus peel with petroleum ether followed by methanol. Petroleum ether removes the essential oils present in the peel and the methanol extracts the glycoside-hesperidin.
2. **Alkaline extraction:** In this method, alkaline extraction of chopped orange peel followed by acidification gives crystals of hesperidin.

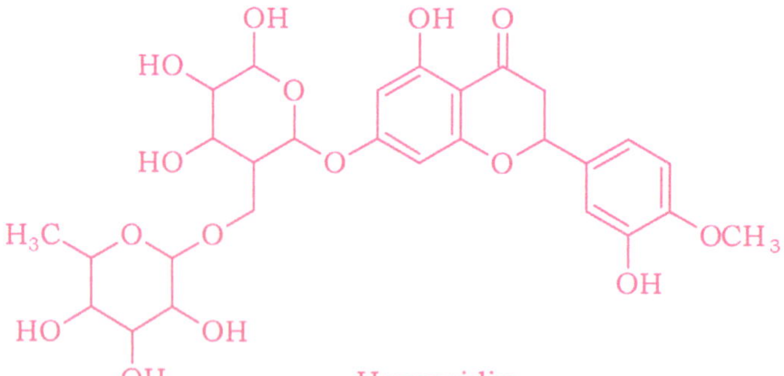

Hesperidin

Procedure

Chemicals Required:Oranges, Calcium hydroxide (10%), Hydrochloric acid, Formamide solution (20 to 25% v/v).

Experimental steps

1. Place dried and chopped orange peel (20 g) and calcium hydroxide (10%, 75 mL) in an Erlenmeyer flask and allow it to remain in room temperature for overnight.
2. Filter the mixture through celite placed on the Buchner funnel.
3. Acidify the yellow-orange filtrate obtained with hydrochloric acid to bring the pH 4 to 5.
4. Filter the solid, wash with water and dry.
5. Purify the hesperidin by recrystallization with aqueous formamide solution (20 to 25% v/v).

   (Concentrate the solution under reduced pressure, in case if there are no crystals formed after acidification).

Characterization

- The melting range of the pure hesperidin is 252 to 254 °C.

KEY POINTS

- Flavanoids, a polyphenolic compounds containing benzo-γ-pyrone nucleus are widely distributed in leaves, flowers and fruits.
- Flavanoids include anthocyanins, favones, flavonols, flavanolols, flavanols (catechin), isoflavanoids, neoflavanoids and chalcones.
- Hesperidin (rhamnoglucoside of hesperitin) decreases the fragility of blood capillaries.

55

Isolation of Terpenoids

Terpenoids (isoprenoids) are a large and diverse class of naturally-occurring organic chemicals, derived from five-carbon isoprene units. The term terpene is applied to a mixture of isomeric hydrocarbons of molecular formula $C_{10}H_{16}$ occurring in turpentine and many other essential oils.

55.1 Isolation of Trimyristin and Myristin from Nutmeg

Theory

Nutmeg is the fruit of *Myristica fragrans* houtt (Family: Myristicaceae) and has carminative and stimulative properties. At maturity, the fruit of the tree splits into two, exposing a single seed sheathed in a crimson aril. The aril, a fibrous covering, constitutes the spice known as mace, and the seed is a whole nutmeg. Nutmeg oil is obtained by steam distillation of kernels of the fruit and consists of approximately 90% of terpene hydrocarbons. Major components are sabinene and α, β-pinene. Nutmeg oil is used primarily for food flavoring. Its characteristic odour is due to safrole derivatives like myristicin and elemicin. Hot extraction of nutmeg with diethyl ether will produce trimyristin (glyceryl trimyristate) along with a small quantity of myristicin. Nutmeg oil generally consists of over 80% trimyristin. Myristicin is toxic and has narcotic activity which may also cause convulsions.

Principle

Trimyristin is an ester with the chemical formula $C_{45}H_{86}O_6$. It is a saturated fat which is the triglyceride of myristic acid. Trimyristin is found naturally in many vegetable fats and oils. Trimyristin is a white to yellowish-gray solid that is insoluble in water, but soluble in ethanol, benzene, chloroform, dichloromethane and ether. Trimyristin makes up between 20-25% of the overall mass of dried, ground nutmeg. Separation is generally carried out by steam distillation and purification uses extraction from ether followed by distillation or rotary evaporator to remove the volatile solvent. The extraction of trimyristin can also be done with diethyl ether at room temperature, due to its high solubility in the ether. Pure trimyristin can easily be isolated by recrystallization from ethanol.

$$
\begin{array}{l}
H_2C—O—CO\text{-}C_{13}H_{17} \\
\quad | \\
HC—O—CO\text{-}C_{13}H_{17} \\
\quad | \\
H_2C—O—CO\text{-}C_{13}H_{17}
\end{array}
$$

Trimyristin

Procedure

Chemicals Required: Ground nutmeg, Diethyl ether, Ethanol (95%).

Experimental steps

1. Weigh 20 g of ground nutmeg, and place in a 250 mL round bottom flask.
2. Add 50 mL of diethyl ether to the above flask and reflux the mixture on water bath at 45 °C in a fume hood for 30 min.
3. Cool the flask to room temperature, and decant the supernatant liquid containing the impure trimyristin into a clean 100 mL beaker.
4. Wash the solid residue with 20 mL of diethyl ether, and add that liquid to the beaker.
5. Evaporate the liquid ether to recover the yellow solid residue which melts at 56 °C (If the product melts during evaporation of the solvent, solidify in an ice bath before adding ethanol).
6. Dissolve the residue in small portion of 95% ethanol at room temperature. If necessary, decant to separate solution from insoluble solids.
7. Cool in ice bath to recrystallize, and vacuum filter. Rinse crystals with cold ethanol.
8. The melting range of the pure trimyristin is in the range of 56 to 58 °C.

55.2 Isolation of Carotenoids from Tomatoes and Carrots

Theory

Carotenoids are natural phytochemicals of the tetraterpenoid (8 isoprene units). Carotenoids naturally occur in the chloroplasts of plants and other photosynthetic organisms. Carotenoids provides antioxidant function, stimulate the immune system, and are required for the production of provitamin A. β-Caroteneand lycopene are the most studied carotenoids since they are the most abundant in human diet.

- β-Carotene is yellow-orange in color and can be isolated from the roots of carrots. Dietary levels of β-carotene have been known to reduce the risk of many types of cancer.
- Lycopene is a red-orange color. Lycopene is two times more effective antioxidant than β-carotene; and it is associated with the reduced risk of prostate, lung and stomach cancers.

Procedure

Chemicals Required: Tomatoes (or Carrots), Ethanol, Dichloromethane, Sodium chloride, Sodium sulfate, Hexane.

Experimental steps

1. Place the 10 g tomato paste (or carrot paste) into a beaker containing 30 mL of 95% ethanol.
2. Stir the solution for about 6 min, isolate the solid by vacuum filtration and place into a 25 mL round-bottom flask loaded with 10 mL of dichloromethane.
3. Reflux the solution for about 5 min and collect the solid by vacuum filtration (repeat the operation for 2 times).
4. Combine the organic layers, wash with brine solution and dry with sodium sulfate.
5. Evaporate the organic layer, add 1 mL of hexane (or benzene) and place it in a ice-bath for the crystallization.

KEY POINTS

- The terpenoids are derived from five-carbon isoprene units.
- Nutmeg, a fruit of *Myristica fragrans* houtt has carminative and stimulative properties.
- Trimyristin is the triglyceride of myristic acid.
- Carotenoids provides antioxidant function, stimulate the immune system, and are precursor for provitamin A.
- β-Carotene and lycopene are two important terpenoids, known for reducing risk of prostate, lung and stomach cancers.

56

Qualitative Analysis of Carbohydrates

Carbohydrates are most important and abundant class of natural organic compounds. Naturally occurring polyhydroxy aldehydes or ketones are known as carbohydrates. Chemically carbohydrates are hydrates of carbons (named accordingly), and the molecular composition is C:H:O (1:2:1), for example glucose ($C_6H_{12}O_6$). Food carbohydrates serve as a primary source of energy and are essential for the biosynthesis of glycoproteins and glycolipids.

Classification

In general, carbohydrates can be classified into four major categories, and are:

1. Monosaccharides
2. Disaccharides
3. Oligosaccharides
4. Polysaccharides

The *Latin* word 'Saccharum' and the *Greek* word '*Sakkharon*' refers to the sugars, which in turn means sweet substances. The term 'Saccharides' is derived from these two words.

1. **Monosaccharides:** The simplest form of carbohydrates (sugars) present in the food materials, such as fruits and milk are known as monosaccharides. They cannot be hydrolyzed into smaller units, further. The most common monosaccharides found in the human diet are named as aldoses (e.g., glucose and galactose) and ketoses (e.g., fructose) based on the functional groups present in it. Based on the number of carbons present in the monosaccharides, they are grouped pentoses (e.g., ribose) and hexoses (e.g., glucose). Monosaccharides reduce the oxidizing agents, and undergo reduction; hence they are all known as reducing sugars.

Ribose	Glucose
CHO	CHO
H—C—OH	H—C—OH
H—C—OH	HO—C—H
H—C—OH	H—C—OH
CH_2OH	H—C—OH
	CH_2OH

Ribose Glucose

2. **Disaccharides:** The condensation of two mono saccharides through glycosidic bond forms a disaccharide. The condensation of two monomeric units of glucose (monosaccaride) forms a disaccharide called as maltose. The important disaccharide sugars present in human nutrition are sucrose (table sugar), lactose (sugar in milk) and maltose (a hydrolysis product of starch, polysaccharide). Disaccharides undergo hydrolysis and release monosaccharides. The disaccharides containing free anomeric carbon atoms are known as reducing sugars. The compounds, such as sucrose, where two monosaccharides are joined through anomeric carbon atoms are known as non-reducing sugars.

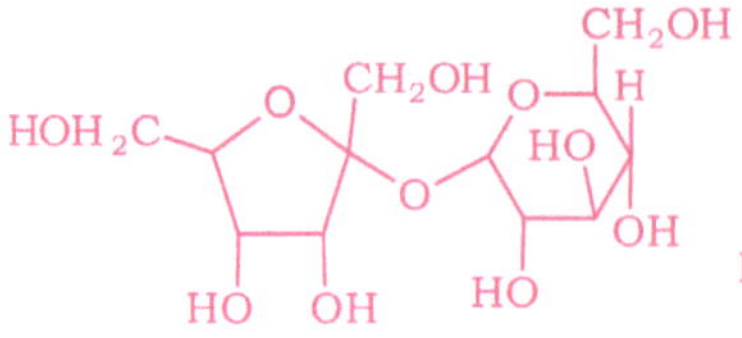

Sucrose 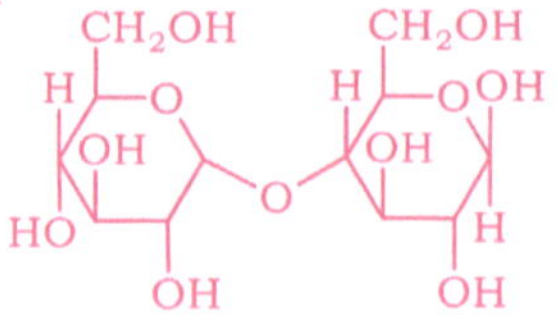 Maltose 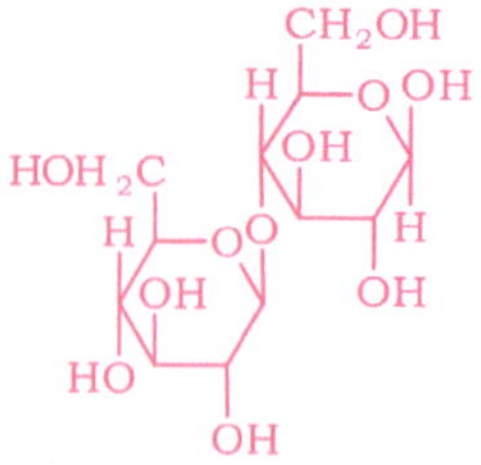 Lactose

3. **Oligosaccharides**: The condensation of three to ten monosaccharides through glycosidic bond forms oligosaccharide. Raffinose is composed of glucose, fructose and galactose, which is a trisaccharide present in the beans and cereals.

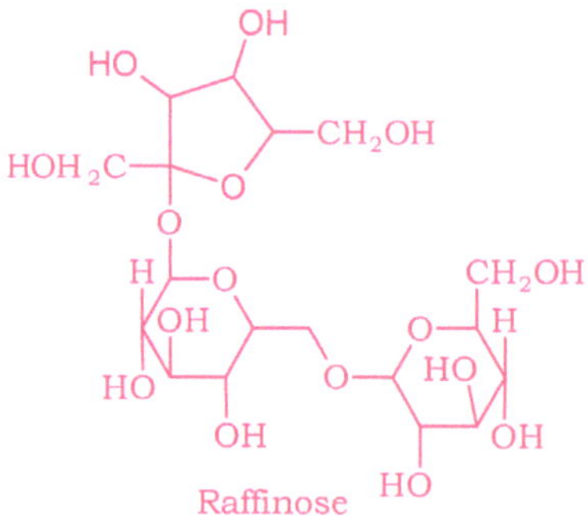

Raffinose

4. **Polysaccharides**: A long chain carbohydrates, composed of more than 10 sugar molecules are known as polysaccharides. Fruits and vegetables are rich in polysaccharides. The two common polysaccharides are storage polysaccharides and dietary fibers.
   - ***Storage polysaccharides:*** It includes starch, glycogen, inulin and glucosamine glycans.
   - ***Dietary fibers (non-starch polysaccharides):*** It includes cellulose, hemicellulose, pectin, gums, chitin and mucilage, which provides structure to plant cell wall. The fibrous carbohydrates promote the elimination of

digestive waste from the gut and lower the absorption of both glucose and bile salt in humans.

Complex carbohydrates are chains of more than two sugar molecules. They may be oligosaccharides or polysaccharides depending upon the chain length.

Starch

Identification tests for carbohydrates

1. General Test: Molisch Test
2. Test for monosaccharides
3. Test for disaccharides
4. Test for oligosaccharides
5. Test for reducing sugars
6. Test for polysaccharides

56.1 General Test for Carbohydrates

S. No.	Experiment	Observation	Inference
1.	**Molisch Test:** Place 1 mL of the carbohydrate solution in a clean test tube. Add 2 drops of Molisch reagent (10% alcoholic α-Naphthol) and mix well. Incline the test tube and slowly add 0.5 mL of concentrated sulfuric acid in drops along the sides of the test tube.	Violet (or purple) colour ring develops at the junction of two liquids. ***Note***: Concentrated solutions may give a red colour instead of violet due to the charing action of the sulphuric acid.	Indicates the presence of Carbohydrates.
	Mechanism: Concentrated sulphuric acid dehydrates pentoses and hexoses to form furfural and 5-hydroxymethyl furfural, respectively. The furfural derivatives condense with alcoholic α-naphthol (Molisch reagent) and form violet colored products. Di, oligo and polysaccharides undergo acid hydrolysis (forms monosaccharides) and dehydration to form furfural. Glucose $\xrightarrow{\text{Con } H_2SO_4}$ 5-Hydroxymethyl furfural + H_2O		

Table *Contd...*

S. No.	Experiment	Observation	Inference
2.	5-Hydroxymethyl furfural + 2 α-Naphthol → Purple coloured dye		
	Solubility Test: Dissolve the carbohydrate sample in distilled water.	Soluble	May be Mono and Disaccharides.
		Insoluble	May be Polysaccharides.

56.2 Tests for Reducing Sugars

Monosaccharides and disaccharides with free anomeric carbons (aldehyde or ketone groups) have reducing properties. These saccharides reduce the weak oxidizing agents like copper (Cu^{2+}) ion in alkaline medium. This reaction produces characteristic colour changes and is unique for different carbohydrates.

S. No.	Experiment	Observation	Inference
1.	**Fehling's test:** Place 2 mL of the carbohydrate solution in a test tube. Add 2 mL of each of Fehling's solution A and B. Mix well and place the test tube into the water-bath for 5 min.	Appearance of yellow or brick red (brown) precipitate. Note: Fehling's A and Fehling's B should be used separately to avoid the formation of black precipitate of cupric oxide.	Indicates the presence of Reducing sugars. Fructose gets converted to aldose and produces the positive result.
	Fehling's solution A: Copper sulphate (7 g, $CuSO_4.5H_2O$) in of distilled water (100 mL) containing 2 drops of dilute sulphuric acid. ***Fehling's solution B:*** Potassium tartrate (35 g) and sodium hydroxide (12 g) in distilled water (100 mL).		
	Mechanism: The alkali converts glucose to enediol, which in turn reduces copper sulphate to cupric hydroxide. Cupric hydroxide is unstable and decomposes to cuprous oxide on boiling. The precipitated cuprous oxide will have different shades of colour depending upon the glucose concentration. The potassium tartrate (Rochelle salt) dissolves the precipitate of cupric hydroxide and avoids the interference.		
	$\underset{\text{Copper sulphate}}{CuSO_4} + 2\,NaOH \xrightarrow{-2\,Na_2SO_4} \underset{\text{Cupric hydroxide}}{Cu(OH)_2} \xrightarrow[-H_2O]{\Delta} \underset{\text{Cupric oxide}}{CuO}$ $\underset{\text{(aldehyde or ketone)}}{\text{Reducing sugar}} + \underset{\text{Cupric oxide}}{CuO} \xrightarrow[NaOH]{\Delta} \underset{\text{Cuprous oxide (red precipitate)}}{Cu_2O\downarrow} + \text{Oxidized sugar}$		

Table ***Contd...***

S. No.	Experiment	Observation	Inference
2.	**Benedict's test:** Place 8 drops of the carbohydrate solution in a test tube. Add 5 mL of Benedict's reagent to the test tube. Place the test tube in the water-bath for 10 min.	Appearance of precipitate. • Green (Low sugar) • Yellow • Orange • Red • Brick red (high sugar)	Indicates the presence of Reducing sugars. Fructose gets converted to aldose and produces the positive result.
	Benedict's test is based on the reduction of alkaline copper sulphate. *Note*: Benedict's test is more specific than Fehling's test because strong alkali in Fehling's solution may destroy small amounts of reducing sugar.		
	Mechanism: Benedict's reagent contains copper sulphate, sodium carbonate and sodium citrate. Copper sulphate: Generate cuprous oxide under sodium carbonate medium. Sodium citrate: Prevents the precipitation of cupric hydroxide by forming cupric sodium citrate complex.		
	$\underset{\text{Copper sulphate}}{CuSO_4} + 2\,NaOH \xrightarrow[-2\,Na_2SO_4]{} \underset{\text{Cupric hydroxide}}{Cu(OH)_2} \xrightarrow[-H_2O]{\Delta} \underset{\text{Cupric oxide}}{CuO}$ $\underset{\text{(aldehyde or ketone)}}{\text{Reducing sugar}} + \underset{\text{Cupric oxide}}{CuO} \xrightarrow[NaOH]{\Delta} \underset{\text{Cuprous oxide (red precipitate)}}{Cu_2O\downarrow} + \text{Oxidized sugar}$		
	Note: Sucrose does not react under normal conditions. Hence, inverse test is required.		
3.	**Tollen's test (Silver mirror test):** Place 2 mL of Tollen's reagent and 2 mL sugar solution in a test tube. Boil for 5 min and cool.	Silver mirror will appear on the sides of test tube.	Indicates the presence of Reducing sugars.
	Note: Acidify the mixture with dilute acid before disposal to prevent the formation of highly explosive silver azide.		
	Tollen's reagent: Ammoniacal silver nitrate, $(Ag(NH_3)_2NO_3)$		
	Mechanism: Silver ions (Ag^+) of Tollen's reagent reacts with aqueous ammonia and forms silver diamine complex $(Ag(NH_3)_2)^+$. The reducing sugars reduce the silver diamine complex into metallic silver.		
	$\underset{\text{(aldehyde or ketone)}}{\text{Reducing sugar}} + \underset{\text{Tollens reagent}}{Ag(NH_3)_2NO_3} \xrightarrow{\Delta} \underset{\text{Silver mirror}}{2Ag\downarrow} + \text{Oxidized sugar}$		
4.	**Tommer's test:** Place 2 mL of Tommer's reagent in to a test tube. Add 3 mL of sugar solution, boil for 2 min and cool.	Formation of yellow or red precipitate.	Indicates the presence of Reducing sugars.
	Tommer's reagent: Copper sulphate (5%) and sodium hydroxide solution.		
	Mechanism: The alkali reduces copper sulphate into cupric hydroxide. The unstable cupric hydroxide decomposes to cupric oxide on boiling. The later upon reduced to cuprous oxide by reducing sugar. The precipitated cuprous oxide will have different shades of colour depending upon the glucose concentration.		
	$\underset{\text{Copper sulphate}}{CuSO_4} + 2\,NaOH \xrightarrow[-2\,Na_2SO_4]{} \underset{\text{Cupric hydroxide}}{Cu(OH)_2} \xrightarrow[-H_2O]{\Delta} \underset{\text{Cupric oxide}}{CuO}$ $\underset{\text{(aldehyde or ketone)}}{\text{Reducing sugar}} + \underset{\text{Cupric oxide}}{CuO} \xrightarrow[NaOH]{\Delta} \underset{\text{Cuprous oxide (red precipitate)}}{Cu_2O\downarrow} + \text{Oxidized sugar}$		

56.3 Test to Distinguish Monosaccharides from Disaccharides

S. No.	Experiment	Observation	Inference
1.	**Barfoed's test:** Place 2 mL of carbohydrate solution in a test tube. Add 5 mL of Barfoed's reagent. Place the test tube on the water-bath.	Formation of light red precipitate • Precipitate within 2-3 min.	Indicates the presence of Monosaccharides.
		• Precipitate within 4-10 min. Disaccharides respond much slower.	Indicates the presence of Disaccharides.
	***Barfoed's reagent*:** Copper (II) acetate in acetic acid.		
	***Mechanism*:** Copper ions of reagent oxidizes Monosaccharides and forms brick red cuprous oxide (Cu_2O) within 3 min. Reduction of cupric ions will affect only in mild acidic condition (*difference from Benedict's test*). Disaccharides may give positive result on prolonged boiling.		
	$(CH_3COO)_2Cu + 2H_2O \longrightarrow Cu(OH)_2 \xrightarrow[-H_2O]{\Delta} CuO$ Copper acetate; Cupric hydroxide; Cupric oxide Reducing sugar (aldehyde or ketone) + $CuO \xrightarrow[NaOH]{\Delta} Cu_2O\downarrow$ + Oxidized sugar Cupric oxide; Cuprous oxide (red precipitate)		

56.4 Test to Distinguish Ketoses and Aldoses

S. No.	Experiment	Observation	Inference
1.	**Seliwanoff's test:** Place 1 mL of the sample solution in a test tube. Add Seliwanoff's reagent (3 mL) and mix well. Place the test tube into the water-bath for 30 sec and cool.	Formation of deep red precipitate.	Indicates the presence of Ketose. (Fructose and sucrose give positive result).
	Seliwanoff' reagent: Resorcinol and hydrochloric acid.		
	Mechanism: The concentrated hydrochloric acid dehydrates ketoses into 5-hydroxymethyl furfural. 5-Hydroxymethyl furfural reacts with resorcinol and forms red complex within 2 min. Ketoses will form deep red colour, while aldoses will show light pink colour (requires longer time than ketoses). Acid hydrolysis of oligo and polysaccharides gives deep cherry red colour.		
	Glucose (CHO; H–OH; HO–H; H–OH; H–OH; CH_2OH) $\xrightarrow{\text{Con HCl}}$ 5-Hydroxymethyl furfural (HOH_2C–furan–CHO) + H_2O 5-Hydroxymethyl furfural + 2 Resorcinol $\xrightarrow{HCl}$ Red coloured dye		

Table *Contd...*

2.	**Rapid furfural test:** Place 1 mL of the carbohydrate solution in a clean test tube. Add 2 drops of Molisch reagent (1% alcoholic α-naphthol) and mix well. Add 5 mL of concentrated hydrochloric acid to the test tube. Boil the solution for few min.	Development of deep purple colour.	Indicates the presence of Ketoses (fructose and sucrose).

56.5 Tests to Distinguish Pentoses and Hexoses

S. No.	Experiment	Observation	Inference
1.	**Bial's test:** Place 2 mL of a sample solution in a test tube. Add 2 mL of Bial's reagent and heat the solution by placing in a hot water-bath.	• Formation of bluish-green colour within 5 min (no precipitate).	• Indicates the presence of Pentoses.
		• Formation of green, red and brown colour.	• Indicates the presence of Hexoses.
	Bial's reagent: Solution of orcinol, hydrochloric acid and ferric chloride.		
	Hexose (CHO; H–C–OH; HO–C–H; H–C–OH; CH_2OH) —Con H_2SO_4→ Furfural + H_2O		
	Bial's reagent dehydrates pentoses to furfural, which reacts with the orcinol and the Ferric ion to produce a bluish-green color, without the formation of a precipitate.		
2.	**Taubers's benzidine test:** Place 4 drops of sugar solution and benzidene reagent (1 mL) into a test tube. Boil the mixture vigorously on open flame and cool on ice bath. ***Benzidine reagent:*** Benzidine in acetic acid.	Development of red to violet colour.	Indicates the presence of Pentoses.

56.6 Confirmatory Tests for Reducing Sugars

Reducing sugars (glucose, fructose, lactose and maltose) when treated with phenylhydrazine hydrochloride in the presence of acetate buffer (pH 5.0) produces characteristic yellow colored crystals of osazones.

S. No.	Experiment	Observation	Inference
1	**Osazone test:** Place solid sample (0.2 g), phenylhydrazine hydrochloride (0.4 g), sodium acetate (0.6 g), and distilled water (4 mL) in a test tube. Place the tube in a beaker containing boiling water for 20 min. Remove the test tube and set it aside to cool. Pour a small amount of the liquid on a watch glass and spread out the crystals. Absorb the mother liquid with a piece of filter paper. Examine the crystals under a low-power microscope.	• Broom shape crystals within 5 min. • Broom shape crystals within 2 min. • Spherical shape crystals within 15 min. • Ball of prickles shape crystals within 15 min.	• Indicates the formation of Glucosazone. • Indicates the formation of Fructosazone. • Indicates the formation of Maltosazone. • Indicates the formation of Lactosazone.
	***Note*:** The addition of saturated sodium bisulfite solution (0.5 mL) before heating avoids the formation of tarry products due to oxidation of the phenylhydrazine hydrochloride.		
	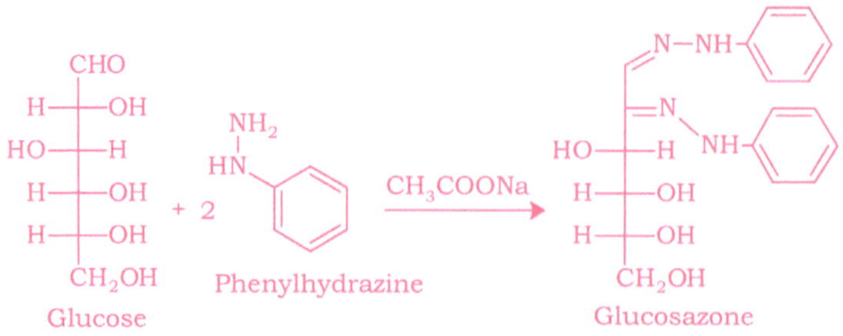 Glucose + 2 Phenylhydrazine $\xrightarrow{CH_3COONa}$ Glucosazone		

56.7 Test for Non-reducing Sugar (Sucrose)

Sucrose is a non-reducing disaccharide and gives negative results for Fehling's, Benedict's, Tommer's and Barfoed's tests.

S. No.	Experiment	Observation	Inference
1.	**Inversion test:** Add 2 drops of hydrochloric acid and one drop of thymol blue to 5 mL of sucrose solution. The development of pink colour indicates the acidity. Divide it into two equal parts. • Boil one portion for about 1 min and then cool it under the tap. Neutralize both portions with 2% sodium carbonate solution. Neutralization develops blue colour.		
	Sucrose on acid hydrolysis splits into monosaccharides (glucose and fructose). These monosaccharides (reducing sugars) can be detected by reducing sugar tests.		
		• The boiled portion gives positive results for Benedict's and Seliwanoff's test. • The unboiled portion does not reduce Benedict's reagent.	
	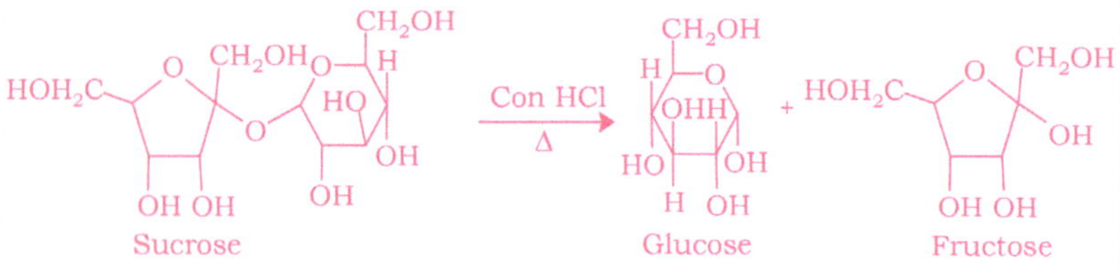 Sucrose $\xrightarrow[\Delta]{\text{Con HCl}}$ Glucose + Fructose		

56.8 Test for Starch and Non-Starch Polysaccharides

S. No.	Experiment	Observation	Inference
1.	**Iodine test:** Add 2 drops of dilute iodine solution to 3 mL of dilute sample solution. *Note*: Polysaccharides, such as starch forms coloured adsorption complexes.	Formation of • Deep blue colour	Indicates the presence of • Starch
		• Deep red colour	• Dextrin
		• Deep reddish brown colour	• Glycogen
	Iodine solution: Iodine dissolved in an aqueous solution of potassium iodide.		
	The amylose fraction of starch gives blue colour. The amylopectin portion of starch forms orange or yellow colour.		
2.	**Precipitation reaction:** Take 5 mL of saturated solution of ammonium sulphate in a test tube. Add 5 mL of sample solution. Mix well by inverting the test tube and allow it to stand for 5 min. Filter the flocculent precipitate of sugar (polysaccharide) formed and perform iodine test with the residue as well as with the filtrate.	(see table below)	

Sugar	Residue	Filter	Inference
Starch	Blue	No blue	Complete precipitation
Glycogen	Brown	No brown	Incomplete precipitation
Dextrin	Red	Red	Incomplete precipitation

Results of Benedict's, Seliwanoff's and Iodine Tests

Carbohydrates	Benedict's Test	Seliwanoff's Test	Iodine Test
Glucose	Red	Peach	Orange-Red
Fructose	Red	Deep Red	Orange-Red
Sucrose	Blue	Deep Red	Orange-Red
Lactose	Red	Red	Orange-Red
Starch	Blue	Pinkish	Blue
Water	Blue	Almost clear	Orange-Red

Tests of foods

Sample	Benedict's Test	Seliwanoff's Test	Iodine Test
Honey	Red	Deep Red	Orange-Red
Brown Sugar	Red	Deep Red	Orange-Red
Teddy Grahams	Red	Deep Red	Black

56.9 Scheme for Identification of Unknown Sugar

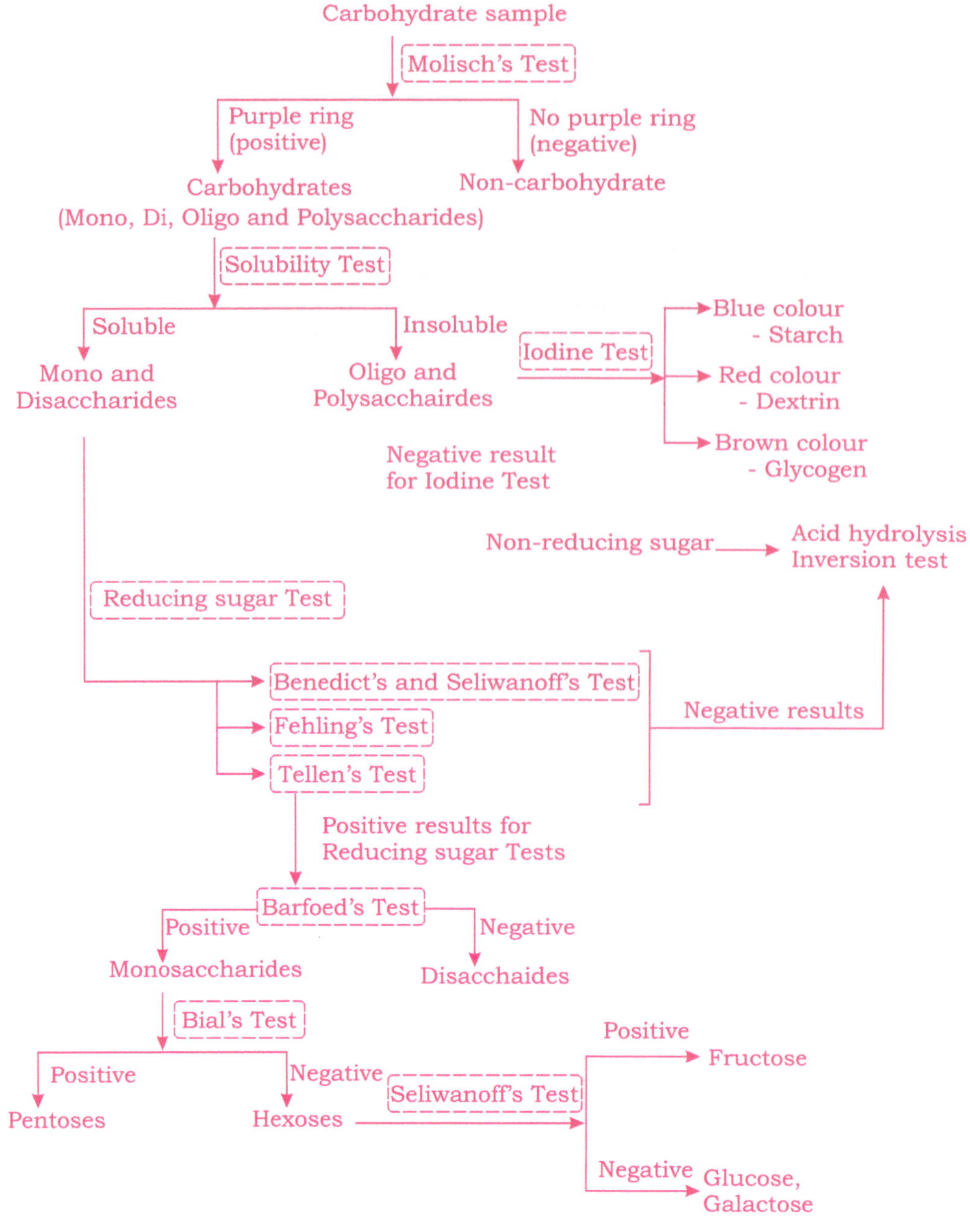

57

Qualitative Analysis of Amino Acids and Proteins

α-Amino acids are the building blocks of proteins. They are essential for the vital functions, such as protein synthesis. Amino acids contain amino (-NH_2) and carboxyl group (-COOH), on the α-carbon. Hence, they are known as α-amino acids, which alone can constitute the protein molecules. α-Amino acids are zwitterionic in nature, as they contain both acidic (carboxylic) and basic (amino) groups.

Amino group ⟶ $H_2N-CH(R)-COOH$ ⟵ Carboxylic group

↑ α-Carbon

Classification

Based on solubility

1. Polar amino acids

1a) *Acidic amino acids*

$HOOC-CH_2-CH(NH_2)-COOH$

Aspartic acid

$HOOC-CH_2-CH_2-CH(NH_2)-COOH$

Glutamic acid

1b) *Basic amino acids*

$H_2N-CH_2-CH_2-CH_2-CH_2-CH(NH_2)-COOH$

Lysine

$HN{=}C(NH_2)-NH-CH_2-CH_2-CH_2-CH(NH_2)-COOH$

Arginine

(Imidazol-4-yl)$-CH_2-CH(NH_2)-COOH$

Histidine

1c) *Neutral amino acids*

Alcohol amino acids

Serine

Threonine

Thiol amino acids

Cysteine

Amide amino acids

Asparagine

Glutamine

2. Non-polar amino acids

2a) *Aliphatic amino acids*

Glycine

Alanine

Valine

Leucine

Isoleucine

Methionine

2b) *Aromatic amino acids*

Phenylalanine

Tyrosine

Tryptophan

2c) Proteinogenic amino acid

Proline

Based on nutritional value

α-Amino acids can be broadly classified into following categories.

1. **Essential amino acids:** Certain amino acids (e.g., threonine) cannot be synthesised in the human physiological system and they should be supplied through the diet. These amino acids are known as essential amino acids. They are also known as indispensable amino acids.
2. **Non-essential amino acids:** The amino acids which can be synthesised in our body (e.g., glycine) are known as non-essential amino acids. They are also known as dispensable amino acids.
3. **Conditionally essential amino acids:** The amino acids which can be synthesised by the human, but number of factors limits the biological synthesis are known as conditional essential amino acids.

Essential	Non-essential	Conditionally (semi) essential
Arginine	Alanine	Arginine
Histidine	Asparagine	Cysteine
Isoleucine	Aspartic acid	Glutamine
Leucine	Glutamic acid	Glycine
Lysine	Glutamine	Proline
Methionine	Glycine	Tyrosine
Phenylalanine	Lysine	
Threonine	Proline	
Tryptophan	Serine	
Valine	Tyrosine	

Proteins

Proteins are nitrogenous macromolecules composed of carbon, hydrogen, oxygen, nitrogen and phosphorous. The word protein is derived from *Greek* word '*Proteios*', and refers to primary. Proteins are linear polymers of α-amino acids, where α-amino acids are polymerized through peptide linkages (covalent bond, amide bond). Protein polymers composed with more than 50 amino acids are called as polypeptides and more than 50 amino acids are known as proteins.

Functions

1. **Buffer:** Proteins are amphoteric in nature, hence they act as a buffer in maintaining the desired pH of body fluids and tissues.

2. **Catalyst:** Proteins mediate variety of biochemical reactions, for example salivary amylase is the protein responsible for digestion.
3. **Protection:** Proteins constitute biological structures such as cell membrane, collagen (provides mechanical strength to skin and bone) and keratin (provides strength to hair, skin, fingernails).
4. **Immunity:** Proteins such as immunoglobulins offer immunity to the host from various pathogens.
5. **Blood clotting:** Proteins regulate the blood clotting by controlling the fibrinolytic function.
6. **Storage function:** Ovalbumin and casein are the storage form of proteins.
7. **Regulatory proteins:** Growth hormone and thyroid hormones are essential for the maintenance of several biochemical functions.
8. **Nerve impulse transmission:** Rhodopsin, a protein molecule transmits impulses across the synapses and assists in the vision.

57.1 General Tests for Proteins

Physicochemical Tests

S No	Experiment	Observation	Inference
1	Appearance	• Turbid solution	• Albumin, Globulin, Casein
		• Clear solution	• Gelatin, Peptone
		• Milky opalescent	• Albumin, Casein
2	Colour	• Faint yellow • Faint brown	• Peptone • Gelatin
3	Smell	• Egg smell • Milk like smell • Meat like smell	• Albumin • Casein • Peptone, Gelatin
4	Litmus test	• Neutral • Acidic • Alkaline	• Albumin, Gelatin • Peptone • Casein and Metaproteins

57.2 Colour Reactions of Proteins

General tests for proteins

S No	Experiment	Observation	Inference
1	**Biuret test:** Place 2 mL of protein solution in a test tube. Add 1 mL of 40% sodium hydroxide and 1 drop of 1% copper sulphate solution.	Development of violet colour	Indicates the presence of peptide (protein).
		Development of rosy pink colour	Indicates the presence of peptide (peptone).
	Mechanism: Biuret test detects the peptide bonds (-CO-NH-) of protein and their hydrolytic products (peptides and metaproteins). The alkaline environment reduce the copper (II) ion of the reagent into cuprous. The cuprous forms a complex with nitrogen of the peptide and produces violet colour. The colour depends upon the number of peptide groups (pink to purple to violet).		

Table *Contd...*

S No	Experiment	Observation	Inference
	$CuSO_4$ (Copper sulphate) + 2 NaOH $\xrightarrow{-2\,Na_2SO_4}$ Cu_2O (Cuprous oxide) —NH·CH(R)–C(=O)—NH·CH(R)–COOH (Peptide/Protein) $\xrightarrow[NaOH]{Cu^{2+}}$ Biuret complex (violet colour)		
2	**Ninhydrin test (*Triketohydrindene hydrate test*):** Place 2 mL of protein solution in a test tube. Add 2 drops of 0.2% ninhydrin solution. Boil the mixture for 2 min and then cool.	Development of purple colour	Indicates the presence of Peptides.
		Development of yellow colour	Indicates the presence of Proline and Hydroxy proline.
	Mechanism: This test is characteristic for amino acids containing free amino group and carboxylic group. The ninhydrin (triketohydrindene hydrate) forms a complex with the amino or carboxylic group. This complex upon reduction gives diketoamino derivative, which further complex with another molecule of ninhydrin and gives purple colour. Proline and hydroxy proline gives yellow colour due to the presence of secondary amino group.		
	Ninhydrin + H_2N–CH(R)–C(=O)–NH– → =N–CH(R)– → –NH_2 Ninhydrin + –NH_2 → –N= (Purple colour complex)		

57.3 Colour Reactions of Amino Acids

Test for Aromatic Amino Acids

S No	Experiment	Observation	Inference
1	**Pauly's test:** Mix 1 mL of sulphanilic acid (1% solution in 10% hydrochloric acid) with 2 mL of test solution and cool in ice. Add 1 mL of 5% sodium nitrite solution to cool solution and add 2 mL of 1% sodium carbonate solution after 5 min.	• Development of red colour	• Indicates the presence of Histidine and tyrosine.
		• Development of orange-red colour	• Indicates the presence of Tryptophan.

Table ***Contd...***

S No	Experiment	Observation	Inference
2	**Xanthoprotic test:** Place 2 mL of protein solution in a test tube. Add 1 mL of concentrated nitric acid. Boil the white precipitate in water-bath (colour changes to yellow). Cool the tube and add 2 mL sodium hydroxide (40%) drop wise to make it alkaline.	Development of orange colour.	Indicates the presence of Aromatic amino acids.
	Mechanism: Aromatic group gets converted to yellow coloured aromatic nitro derivative on treatment with nitric acid (nitration). Alkaline pH (sodium hydroxide) changes yellow colour to orange colour, due to ionization.		
	Phenyl alanine (H_2C–CH–COOH, H_2N) —Con HNO_3→ Nitro derivative of Phenyl alanine (Yellow in colour) (NO_2)		
3	**Millon's test (*for Tyrosine*):** Place a few drops of the reagent in the test tube. Add 1 mL of the acidified protein solution. Boil the mixture by placing in water-bath for 10 min at 100 °C. Cool, add few drops of 1% sodium nitrite solution and warm gently.	Development of red colour	Indicates the presence of Phenolic group (Tyrosine).
	Millon's reagent: 10% mercuric sulphate in 10% sulphuric acid, 1% sodium nitrite solution. Solution of mercuric and mercurous nitrates in nitric acid contains little nitrous acid.		
	Mechanism: The neutral protein solution reacts with acidified mercuric nitrate to form a yellow precipitate of mercury-protein complex. This complex forms a nitrite complex with nitrite solution on warming and develops red colour.		
	Tyrosine (OH, H_2C–CH–COOH, H_2N) —$HgNO_3$ (Hg + HNO_3)→ Tyrosine-Nitrite complex (Red in colour)		
4	**Hopkins-Cole Adam-MicKiewicz reaction-Aldehyde test (*for Tryptophan*):** Place 1 mL protein solution in a test tube. Add 1 drop of 10% mercuric sulphate solution (in 10% sulphuric acid) and 1 drop of 40% formaline. Mix well, incline the test tube and add 1 mL sulphuric acid from the sides of the test tube.	Development of purple ring at the juction of two liquids.	Indicates the presence of Tryptophan.
	Mechanism: The amino acid tryptophan condenses with formaldehyde in presence of concentrated sulphuric acid and forms violet coloured compound.		

Table ***Contd...***

S No	Experiment	Observation	Inference
3	**Glyoxalic Acid Reation - Hopkin's cole test (*for Tryptophan*):** Place 2 mL of the protein solution in a test tube. Add 2 mL of glyoxalic acid reagent. Pour this mixture to another test tube containing 4 mL of sulphuric acid from the sides of the tube. Rotate the test tube gently.	Development of purple ring at the juction of two liquids.	Indicates the presence of Tryptophan.
	Glyoxalic acid reagent: Exposing glacial acetic acid to sunlight for a few minutes offers glyoxalic acid.		
4	**Echrlich's test (*for Tryptophan*):** Place 1 mL of the protein solution in a test tube. Add 1 mL of Echrlich's reagent.	Development of red colour.	Indicates the presence of Tryptophan.
	Echrlich's reagent: *para*-Dimethylamino benzaldehyde (10%) in hydrochloric acid (10%).		

Test for basic Amino Acids

S No	Experiment	Observation	Inference
1	**Sakaguchi test (*for Arginine*):** Place 3 mL of the protein solution in a test tube. Add 1 mL of 10% sodium hydroxide, 5 drops of 1% alcoholic α-naphthol and mix. Then add 5 drops of bromine water (or 5 drops of freshly prepared sodium hypobromide solution).	Development of bright orange red colour.	Indicates the presence of Arginine.
	Mechanism: Guanidine group of arginine reacts with α-naphthol in presence of bromine (or sodium hypobromide) solution and produces red orange condensation product.		

Test for sulphur containing Amino Acids

S No	Experiment	Observation	Inference
1	**Sulphur test:** Boil 1 mL of the protein solution with 1 mL of 40% sodium hydroxide for 1 min and add a drop of lead acetate solution.	Formation of black (or brown precipitate (insoluble in dilute hydrochloric acid).	Indicates the presence of sulphur containing amino acids.
	Mechanism: Sulphur (present in amino acids) reacts with sodium hydroxide and forms sodium sulphide. Sodium sulphide upon reaction with lead acetate produces black (or brown precipitate, lead suphide), which is insoluble in dilute hydrochloric acid.		

57.4 Test for Proteins

Heat coagulation tests

S No	Experiment	Observation	Inference
1	Take protein solution about 2/3rd of the test tube and heat the upper portion of the solution.	Appearance of opalescent (becomes deep with few drops of 2% acetic acid).	Indicates the presence of heat Coagulating Proteins (Albumin and Globulin).
	Mechanism: Denaturation of protein structure by heat or acids (acetic acid, nitric acid) is called as coagulation of protein. Albumin and globulin are coagulating proteins.		
2	Take 2 mL of nitric acid in a test tube and add the protein solution by the side of the test tube.	Appearance of white ring at the junction of the two liquids.	Indicates the presence of Coagulating Proteins

57.5 Test for Phosphorous Present in Proteins (Casein)

S No	Experiment	Observation	Inference
1	**Neumann's test:** Place the sample in dry test tube add 2 drops of nitric acid and 10 drops of sulphuric acid. Heat the contents strongly over a flame in a fume cupboard with constant stirring to avoid spurting. Allow the contents to cool, add 2 mL of distilled water and 2 mL of ammonia. Mix, add 2 mL of ammonium molybdate solution and warm.	Development of lemon yellow/ Shining yellow/Canary yellow colour precipitate of ammonium phosphomolybdate.	Indicates the presence of Phosphorous present in protein (e.g., Casein).

57.6 Test for Carbohydrates Present in Protein (Glycoprotein)

S No	Experiment	Observation	Inference
1	**Molish test**: Place 1 mL of the carbohydrate solution in a clean test tube. Add 2 drops of Molisch reagent (10% alcoholic α-Naphthol) and mix well. Incline the test tube and add 0.5 mL of concentrated sulfuric acid in drops along the sides of the test tube.	Violet (or purple) colour ring develops at the junction of two liquids. ***Note***: Concentrated solutions may give a red colour instead of violet due to the charing action of the sulphuric acid.	Indicates the presence of Carbohydrates in the Protein sample.
	Glucose (CHO; H–OH; HO–H; H–OH; H–OH; CH_2OH) $\xrightarrow{\text{Con } H_2SO_4}$ 5-Hydroxymethyl furfural (HOH_2C–furan–CHO) + H_2O 5-Hydroxymethyl + 2 α-Naphthol ⟶ Purple coloured dye		

57.7 Precipitation Reactions for Proteins

Proteins are precipitated from their solutions by variety of reagents and these precipitates are useful in isolation, identification and derivatization of proteins. Heavy metals (mercuric chloride, silver nitrate and copper sulphate), alkaloidal reagents (picric acid, phosphotungstic acid and tannic acid), acids (nitric acid and metaphosphoric acid) and concentrated solutions of ammonium sulphate and sodium chloride precipitates the proteins by 'salting out' methods. Dehydrating agents such as alcohols and acetone also can precipitate by converting them into suspensoids (which flocculate by few drops of salt solution). Alcohols bring protein solution into isoelectric point at which it is precipitated.

S No	Experiment	Observation	Inference
1	**Heller's test:** Place 3 mL of the nitric acidin a test tube. Add 3 mL of protein solution along the sides of test tube.	Appearance of white precipitate at the junction of the two liquids (excess of acid dissolves the precipitate).	Indicates the precipitation of Proteins.
	Mechanism: Mineral acids precipitates the protein by changing the pH and/inducing the protein denaturation (coagulation).		
2	**Precipitation by heavy metals:** Alkalify the protein solution by adding 1% sodium carbonate solution. To the 2 mL of alkaline protein solution add few drops of 5% heavy metal solution.	• Copper sulphate gives bluish white precipitate • Zinc sulphate gives white precipitate • Lead acetate gives white precipitate • Mercuric nitrate gives brown precipitate • Ferric chloride produces opalescence (disappears with excess of ferric chloride)	Indicates the presence of Proteins
3	**Sulphosalicylic acid test:** Place 2 mL of the dilute protein solution in a test tube. Add a drop of 20% solution of sulphosalicylic acid in sulphuric acid.	Formation of white precipitate (or turbidity).	Indicates the precipitation of Protein.
4	**Esbach's test:** Place 1 mL of the dilute protein solution in a test tube. Add 1 mL Esbach's reagent (mixture of picric acid and citric acid, 10%).	Formation of yellow precipitate.	Indicates the precipitation of Protein.
5	**Trichloroacetic acid test:** Place 2 mL of the dilute protein solution in a test tube. Add 2 mL of 10% trichloroacetic acid.	Formation of white precipitate.	Indicates the precipitation of Protein.
6	**Tannic acid test:** Place 2 mL of the dilute protein solution in a test tube. Add 5 drops of 2% tannic acid.	Formation of white precipitate.	Indicates the precipitation of Protein.
7	**Precipitation by alcohol:** Place 1 mL of protein solution in a test tube. Add 3 ml of ethanol.	Formation of white opalescence.	Indicates the presence of Protein
	Saturation tests		
8	**Full saturation test:** Place 5 mL protein solution in a test tube. Add solid ammonium sulphate, until it becomes saturated.	Formation of gelatinous precipitate.	Indicates the presence of Albumin.
9	**Half saturation test:** Place 3 mL saturated solution of ammonium sulphate in a test tube. Add 3 mL of saturated protein solution and shake vigrously.	Formation of gelatinous precipitate.	Indicates the presence of Albumin

Scheme

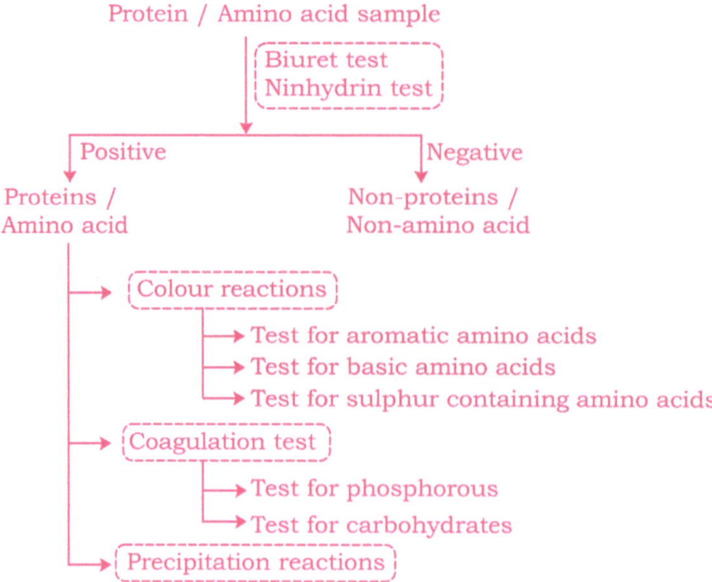
Protein / Amino acid sample
Biuret test
Ninhydrin test
Positive
Negative
Proteins / Amino acid
Non-proteins / Non-amino acid
Colour reactions
Test for aromatic amino acids
Test for basic amino acids
Test for sulphur containing amino acids
Coagulation test
Test for phosphorous
Test for carbohydrates
Precipitation reactions

58

Qualitative Analysis of Alkaloids

Alkaloids are physiologically active nitrogenous secondary metabolites of plant as well as animal kingdom. Alkaloids are derived from amino acids, such as lysine, tyrosine and tryptophan. They contain at least one nitrogen atom as a part of a cyclic or acyclic system in a negative state of oxidation.

- **True alkaloids:** Metabolites of amino acids containing nitrogen in a heterocyclic ring.
- **Proto alkaloids:** Metabolites of amino acids, but do not have nitrogen in a heterocyclic ring.
- **Pseudo alkaloids:** Metabolites of non-amino acid sources, but have nitrogen in a heterocyclic ring.

Morphine (analgesic), cocaine (local anesthetic) and quinine (anti-malarial) are the most important alkaloids, and serves as leads for the drug discovery.

Functions of alkaloids

The following are the functions of alkaloids:

- Nitrogen reservoirs for protein synthesis and in case of nitrogen deficiency.
- Plant stimulants or regulators involve in growth, metabolism and reproduction.
- Source of energy in case of deficiency in carbon dioxide assimilation.
- Protective against insects and herbivores due to their bitterness and toxicity.
  - Detoxication by methylation, condensation and cyclization of the compounds.

Classification

Based on the source

1) **Plant alkaloids:** Nicotine, Ephedrine
2) **Animal alkaloids:** Bufotenine (*Bufo alvarius*), Muscopyridine (*Moschus moschiferus*)

Based on the nucleus

1) Phenylethylamine alkaloids

Ephedrine
Pseudo ephedrine
(*Ephedra sinica, Ephedra vulgaris*)

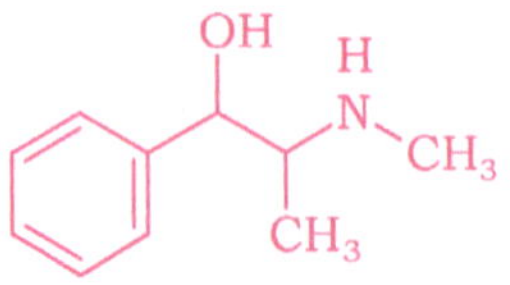

OH, H, N, CH_3, CH_3

Hordenine
(*Ariocarpusfissuratum, Hordeum vulgare*)

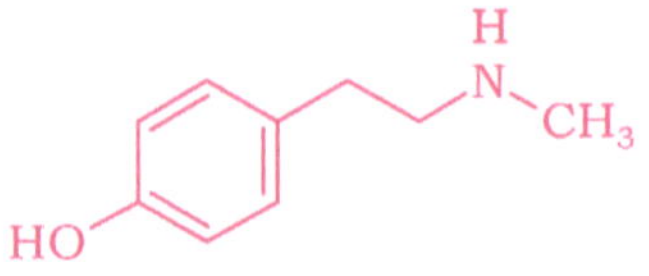

H, N, CH_3, HO

Mescaline
(*Lophophora williamsii, Echianopsispachanoi Echianopsis peruviana*)

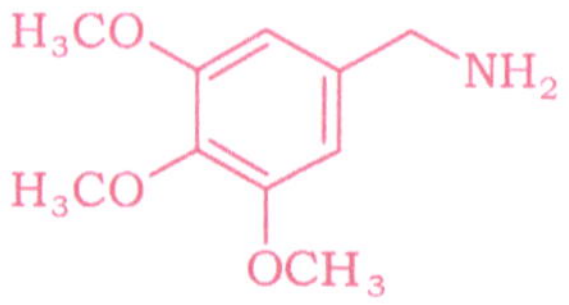

H_3CO, NH_2, H_3CO, OCH_3

Narceine
(*Papaver somniferum*)

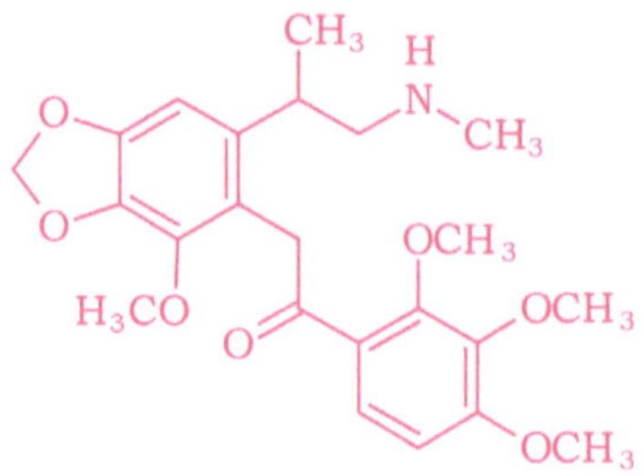

CH_3, H, N, CH_3, O, O, OCH_3, H_3CO, OCH_3, O, OCH_3

2) Tropane Alkaloids

Atropine
Hyoscyamine (*levo* atropine)
(*Atropa belladonna*)

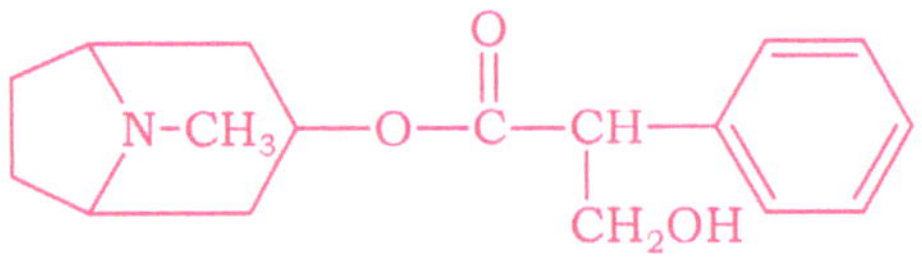

N-CH_3—O—C(=O)—CH(—CH_2OH)—

Hyoscine
(*Atropa belladonna, Hyoscyamus niger Datura stramonium*)

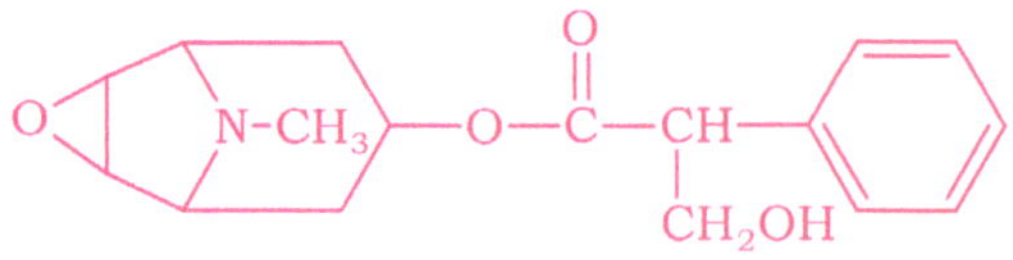

O, N-CH_3—O—C(=O)—CH(—CH_2OH)—

Cocaine
(*Erythroxylon coca*)

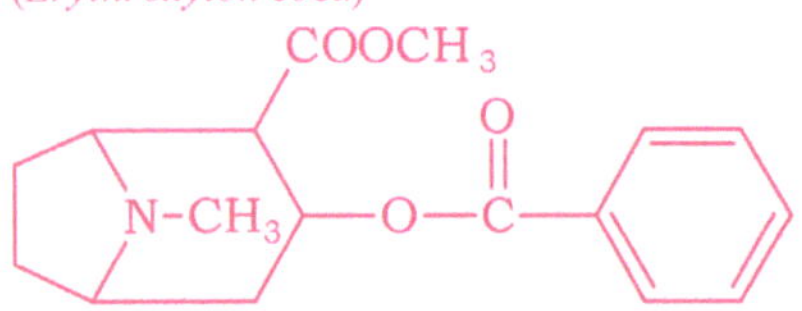

$COOCH_3$, N-CH_3—O—C(=O)—

Ecgonine
(*Erythroxylon coca*)

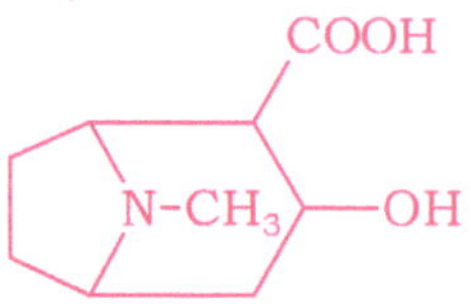

COOH, N-CH_3—OH

3) Imidazole (glyoxaline) alkaloids

Pilocarpine
Pilocarpidine
(*Pilocarpus jaborandi*)

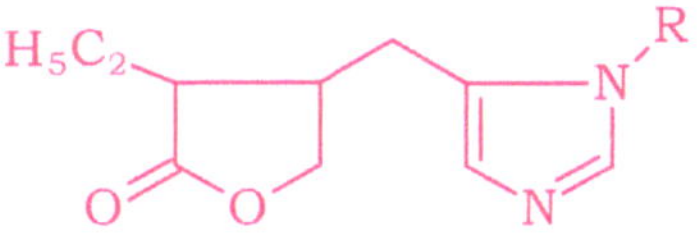

Pilocarpine, R = CH_3
Pilocarpidine, R = H

Pilosine
(*Pilocarpusmicrophyllus*)

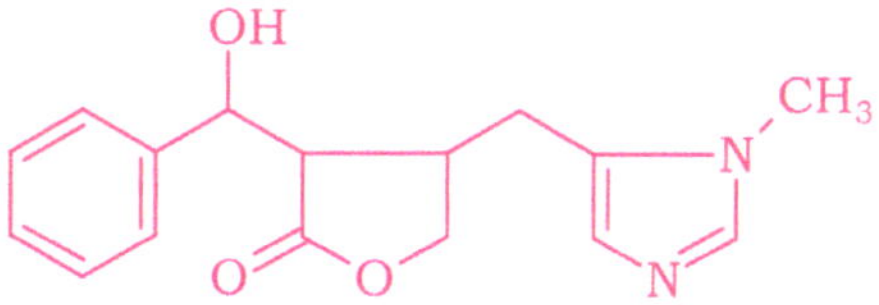

4) Indole alkaloids

Ergotamine
(*Claviceps purpurea*)

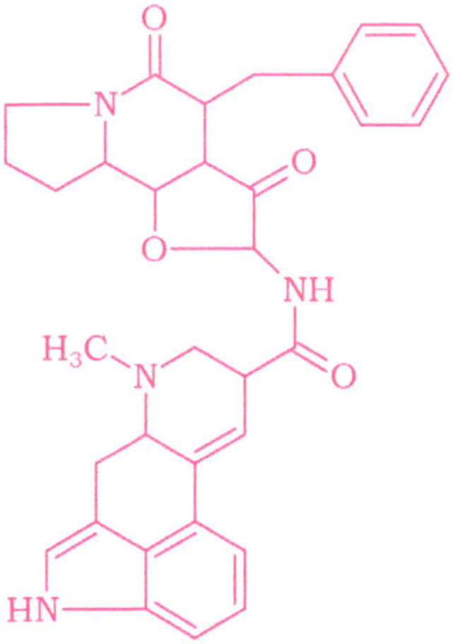

Reserpine
(*Catharanthus roseus, Rauwolfia serpentina*)

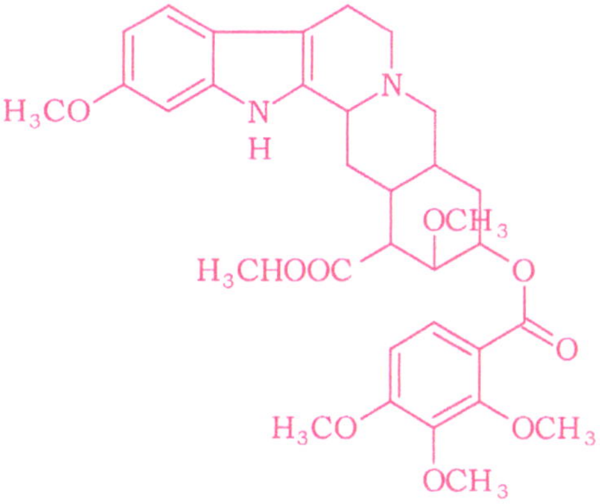

Strychnine and Brucine
(*Strychnusnuxvomica*)

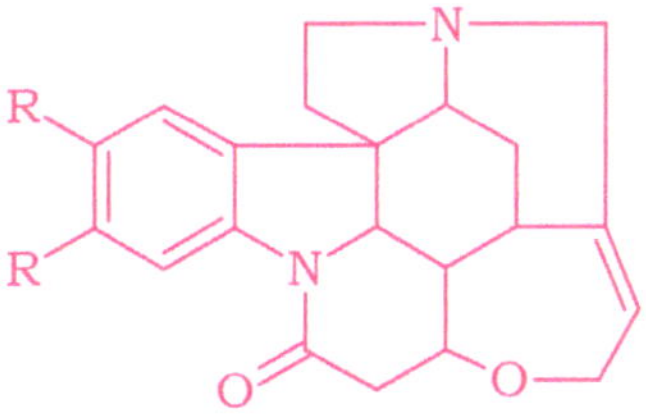

Strychnine, R = H
Brucine, R = OCH_3

Vincristine
(*Vinca rosea*)

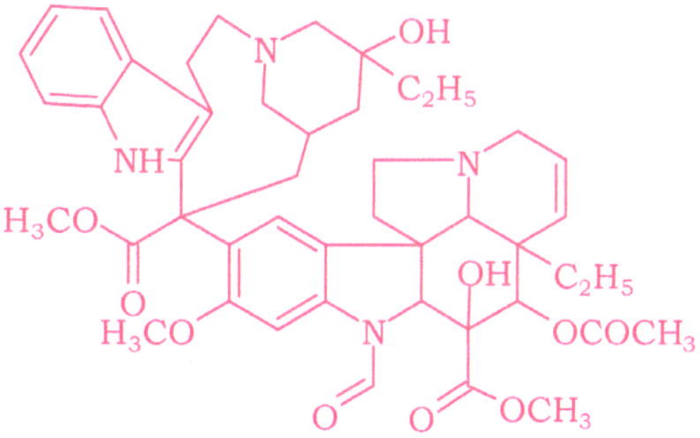

Physostigmine
(*Physostigmavenenosum*)

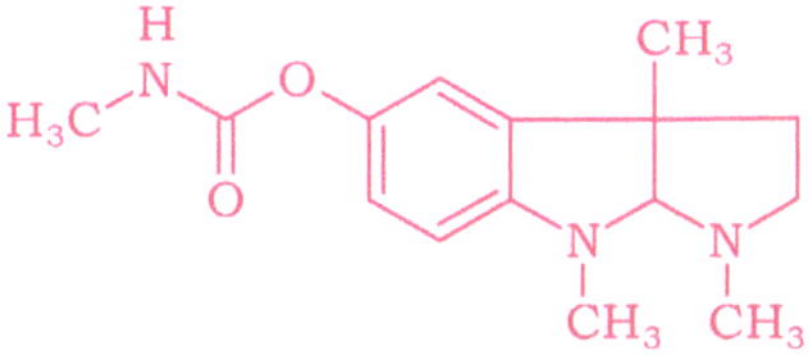

5) Quinoline alkaloids

(-)-Quinine
(+)-Quinidine
(*Cinchona officinalis*)

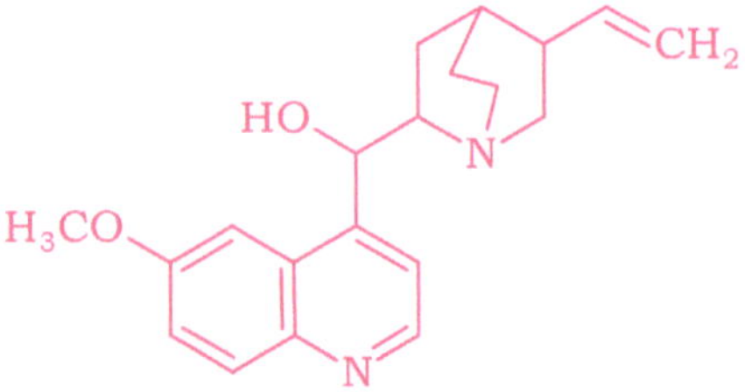

(+)-Cinchonine
(-)-Cinchonidine
(*Cinchona officinalis*)

HO, H_3CO, N, N, CH_2

H_3C, N, N, CH_2

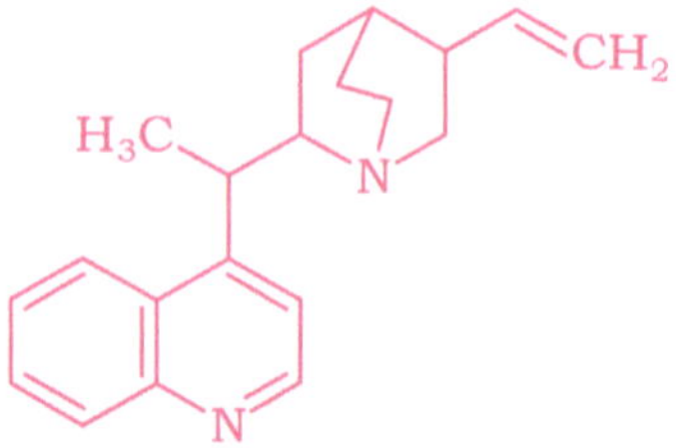

6) Tetrahydroisoquinoline alkaloids

Papaverine
(*Papaver somniferum*)

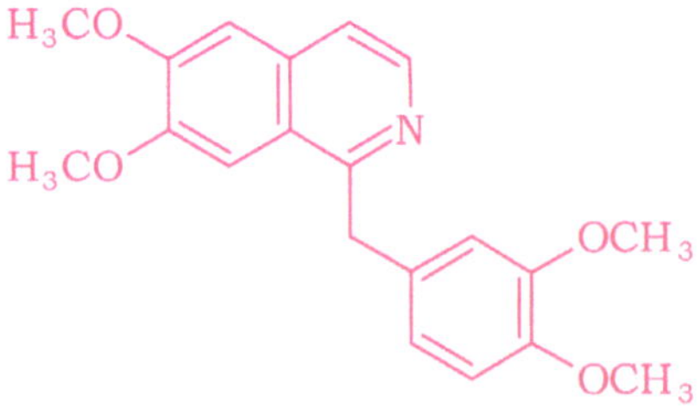

H_3CO, H_3CO, N, OCH_3, OCH_3

Emetine
(*Cephaelis ipecacuanha*)

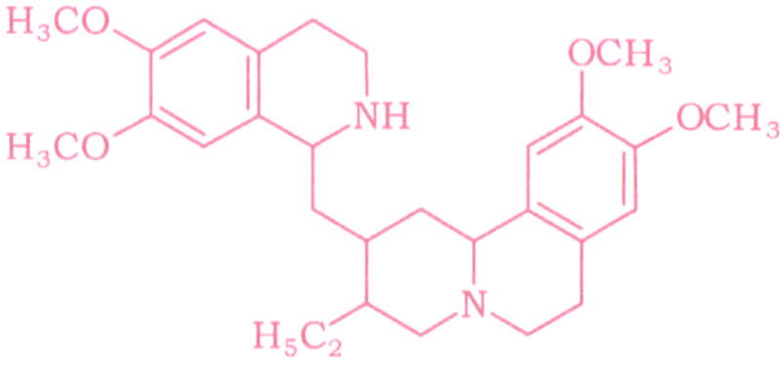

H_3CO, H_3CO, NH, OCH_3, OCH_3, N, H_5C_2

Berberine
(*Berberis vulgaris*)

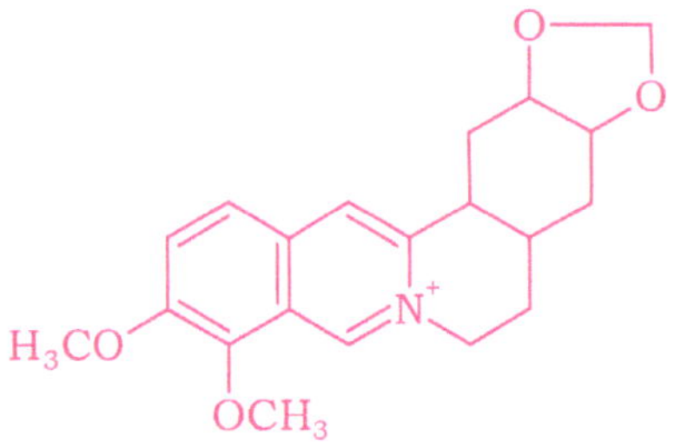

O, O, N^+, H_3CO, OCH_3

Tubocurarine (*Chondrodendrontomentosum*)

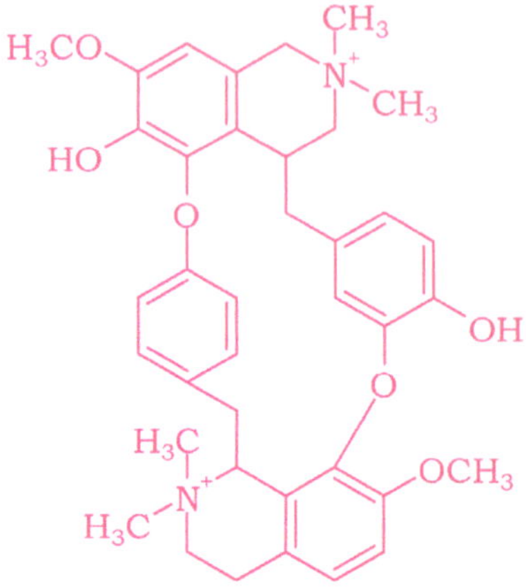

H_3CO, HO, CH_3, N^+, CH_3, O, OH, O, H_3C, N^+, H_3C, OCH_3

7) Phenanthrene alkaloids: Morphine, Codeine, Heroin

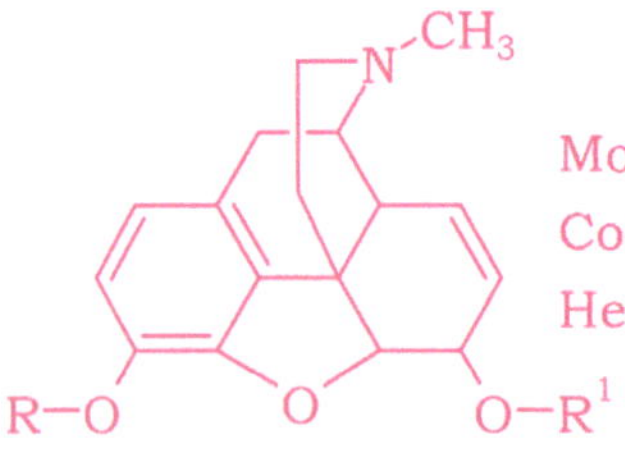

N, CH_3, R–O, O, O–R^1

Morphine, R = R^1 = H
Codeine, R = CH_3, R^1 = H
Heroin, R = R^1 = $COCH_3$

8) Pyridine and piperidine alkaloids: Nicotine, Piperine,

Nicotine

Piperine

9) Purine (Xanthine) alkaloids

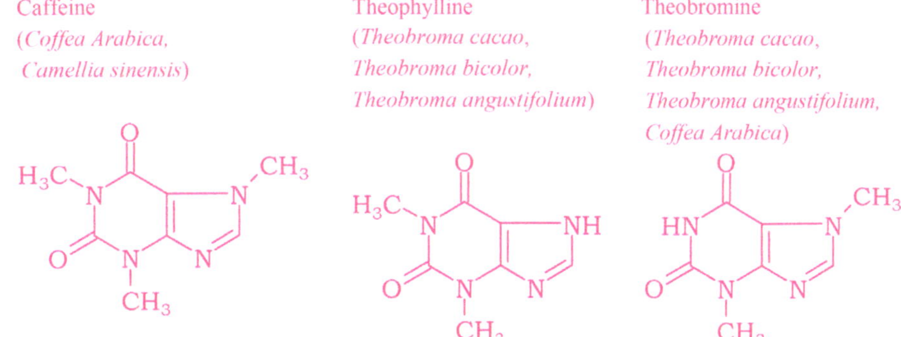

10) Tropolone alkaloids: Colchicine (*Colchicum autumnale*)

11) Pyrrolizidine alkaloids

Retronecine
(*Senecio vulgaris, Heliotropiumeuropaeum*)

Senecionine
(*Senecio aureus, Tussilago farfara*)

Based on the amino acid (from which it is derived)

Alkaloids are also classified according to the amino acid from which they are derived as

1. ***Histidine alkaloids:*** Pilocarpine, pilosine(imidazole alkaloids)
2. ***Tryptophan alkaloids:*** Ajmalin, Ajmalicin, Yohimbine, Reserpine, Vincristine, Srychnine.
3. ***Phenylalanine alkaloids***: Ephedrine, Papaverine, Emetine, Berberine, Tubocurarine, Morphine, Codeine, Thebaine
4. ***Tyrosine alkaloids:*** Morphine, Codeine, Thebaine, Berberine, Papaverine, Emetine, Tubocurarine
5. ***Lysine alkaloids:*** Piperidine, Lobeline, Pelletierine
6. ***Proline alkaloids:*** Nicotine
7. ***Ornithine alkaloids:*** Senecionin, Cocaine, Scopolamine, Nicotine

58.1 General Tests for Alkaloids

Physical Properties

S. No.	Experiment	Observation	Inference
1.	*Physical state*	• Crystalline solids • Amorphous solids • Liquids – Volatile – Non-volatile	• Cocaine • Emetine • Nicotine • Pilocarpine
2	*Color*	• Yellow	• Colchicine, Berberine
		• Orange	• Canadine
		• Copper-red	• Sanguinarine
3	*Solubility:* • Water	• Soluble	• Caffeine, Ephedrine, Codeine, Colchicine, Pilocarpine, Coniine, Quinine
	• Chloroform	• Soluble	• Lobeline, Apoatropine
	• Ether	• Sparingly soluble	• Morphine
	• Benzene	• Insoluble	• Theobromine, Theophylline
	Note: Alkaloidal salts are soluble in water and insoluble in organic solvents. But, alkaloidal bases are soluble in organic solvents and insoluble in water.		

Characteristic chemical tests

General: Place the sample in test tube and add dilute hydrochloric acid. Shake well to dissolve (or disperse) and filter the solution. The filtrate is useful in the following general tests.

S. No.	Experiment	Observation	Inference
1.	**Mayer's test:** Place 2 mL of the filtrate in a test tube. Add 2 drops of Mayer's reagent.	Development of creamy white (or yellow) precipitate.	Indicates the presence of Alkaloids.
	Mayer's reagent: Potassio-mercuric iodide solution.		
	Note: Ephedrine, caffeine and theobromine give negative result.		
2	**Dragendorff's test:** Place 2 mL of the filtrate in a test tube. Add 2 drops of Dragendroff's reagent.	Development of orange or orange red precipitate.	Indicates the presence of Alkaloids.
	Dragendorff's reagent: Potassium bismuth iodide solution		
3	**Wagner's test:** Place 2 mL of the filtrate in a test tube. Add 2 drops of Wagner's reagent.	Development of reddish-brown precipitate.	Indicates the presence of Alkaloids.
	Wagner's reagent: Solution of iodine in potassium iodide		
4	**Hager's test:** Place 2 mL of the filtrate in a test tube. Add 2 mL of Hager's reagent.	Development of yellow precipitate.	Indicates the presence of Alkaloids.
	Hager's reagent: Solution of picric acid (1 g) in water (100 mL)		
5	**Tannic acid test:** Place 2 mL of the filtrate in a test tube. Add 2 drops of tannic acid reagent.	Development of yellowish white precipitate.	Indicates the presence of Alkaloids.
	Tannic acid reagent: Solution of tannic acid (10 g) in alcohol (10 mL), diluted to 100 mL with water.		
6	**Mercuric chloride test:** Place 2 mL of the filtrate in a test tube. Add 2 drops of Mercuric chloride reagent.	Development of white precipitate.	Indicates the presence of Alkaloids.

Colour change test

A simple colour change of the following reagents indicates the alkaloids.

- ***Mandelin's reagent (sulphovanadic acid):***Ammonium vanadate (1 g) in concentrated sulphuric acid (100 mL).
- ***Froehde's reagent:*** Molybdic acid (5 g, or sodium molybdate) in hot concentrated sulphuric acid (5 mL).
- ***Marquis reagent:*** Concentrated sulphuric acid (3 mL) containing 3 drops of formaldehyde (40%).
- ***Erdmann's reagent:*** A mixture of 10 drops of concentrated nitric acid and sulphuric acid.
- ***Mecke's reagent (selenious-sulphuric acid):*** Selenious acid (1 g) in concentrated sulphuric acid (200 mL).
- ***Modified Dragendroff's reagent (Kraut's reagent):*** Bismuth subnitrate (1.6 g) in glacial acetic acid (60 mL, 20%), potassium iodide solution (5 mL, 40%) and water.
- ***Rosenthaler's reagent (selenious-sulphuric acid):*** Potassium arsenate (1 g) in concentrated sulphuric acid (200 mL).

58.2 Identification of Phenylethylamine Alkaloids

S. No.	Experiment	Observation	Inference
	Test for Ephedrine		
1	**Chen's test:** Place 2 mL of sample solution in to a test tube. Add few drops of dilute hydrochloric acid, 1 mL of copper sulphate (5%), 1 mL sodium hydroxide (20%) and 1 mL petroleum ether.	Reddish colour develops and shake well the contents. Formation of purple colour in organic layer and blue colour in aqueous layer.	Indicates the presence of Ephedrine.
2	Dissolve sample in chloroform in a stoppered flask. Shake the contents vigorously and allow it stand at room temperature for 12 h. Evaporate the chloroform layer.	Crystals (ephedrine hydrochloride) separates out.	Indicates the presence of Ephedrine.
3	Triturate the sample with crystals of potassium ferricyanide. Add few drops of water and heat on a water-bath.	Odour of Bitter almonds (benzaldehyde odour).	Indicates the presence of Ephedrine.

58.3 Identification of Tropane Alkaloids

S. No.	Experiment	Observation	Inference
1	**Vitali-Morin's Test:** Evaporate 1 mL of sample solution to dryness and cool. Add 2 drops of fuming nitric acid and evaporate to dryness. Cool and add acetone and ethanolic potassium hydroxide (10%).	Development of violet colour.	Indicates the presence of Tropane alkaloids (Atropine, Cocaine).
2	***p*-Dimethylamino benzaldehyde (DMAB) test:** Place 1 mL of sample solution in to a test tube. Add 3 drops of *p*-dimethylamino-benzaldehyde in H_2SO_4/HCl and heat the mixture by placing in hot plate with continuous stirring.	Development of cherry red colour.	Indicates the presence of Tropane alkaloids (Atropine, Cocaine).
	Test for Atropine		
3	**Gerrard reaction:** Place sample in a test tube. Add 2% w/v ethanolic mercuric chloride solution.	Produces instant red colour.	Indicates the presence of Atropine.
	Test for Cocaine		
4	**Permanganate test:** To the sample solution prepared in the saturated alum add few drops of potassium permnganate.	Formation of violet crystalline precipitate (cocaine permanganate).	Indicates the presence of Cocaine.
	Test for Hyoscyamine		
5	**Schaer's test:** Place the sample in a test tube. Add drop of hydrogen peroxide (30%) and 1 mL of concentrated sulphuric acid.	Formation of distinct green colour.	Indicates the presence of Hyoscyamine.
6	**Gerrard reaction:** Place the sample in a test tube. Add 2% w/v ethanolic mercuric chloride solution.	Produces red colour after warming.	Indicates the presence of Hyoscyamine.

Table *Contd...*

S. No.	Experiment	Observation	Inference
	Test for Hyoscine		
7	**Silver nitrate test:** To the sample solution add few drops of silver nitrate solution.	Formation of yellowish white precipitate (*Insoluble* in nitric acid and *soluble* in dilute ammonia).	Indicates the presence of Hyoscine.
8	**Gerrard reaction:** To the sample solution present in a test tube. Add 2% w/v ethanolic mercuric chloride solution.	Produces white colour.	Indicates the presence of Hyoscine.

58.4 Identification of Imidazole Alkaloids

S. No.	Experiment	Observation	Inference
1	**Helch's test:** Place the aqueous solution in a test tube. Add 3 drops of hydrogen peroxide and 3 drops of potassium dichromate.	Development of violet colour.	Indicates the presence Imidazole alkaloids.
2	**Ekkerts test:** Place the aqueous sample solution in a test tube. Add sodium nitroprusside, 3 drops of dilute sodium hydroxide to the tube. After 5 min, add dilute hydrochloric acid.	Development of wine red colour. (addition of sodium thiosulphate changes into green).	Indicates the presence Imidazole alkaloids.

58.5 Identification of Indole Alkaloids

S. No.	Experiment	Observation	Inference
Test for Ergot alkaloids			
1	**Ehrlich test:** Place 2 mL of sample solution in a test tube. Add few drops of Ehrlich reagent.	Formation of deep blue colour.	Indicates the presence of Ergot alkaloids. (Polypeptide alkaloids also give positive test).
	Ehrlich regent: Mixture of *p*-dimethylamino benzaldehyde (DMAB) in 15% sulphuricacid, containing trace of ferric chloride.		
2	**Van-Urk's test:** Place 2 mL of sample solution in a test tube. Add few drops of Van-Urk's reagent.D	Formation of red colour.	Indicates the presence of Pyrrolizidine alkaloids.
	Van-Urk's *regent:* Mixture of 4–dimethylaminobenzaldehyde (DMAB), perchloric acid (60%) in glacial acetic acid.		
3	**Keller's test:** Place the sample solution in acetic acid with traces of ferric chlorideìn a test tube. Add sulphuric acidalong the wall of the test tube.	Formation of intense blue colour between two phases.	Indicates the presence of Ergot alkaloids. (Polypeptide alkaloids also give positive test).
Test for Vinca alkaloids			
4	**Vanillin-hydrochloric acid test:** Place the powdered sample in a test tube. Add vanillin in hydrochloric acid.	Development of pink or orange-yellowcolour.	Indicates the presence Vincristine.

Table *Contd...*

S. No.	Experiment	Observation	Inference
Test for Vinca alkaloids			
5	**Van-Urk's test:** Place 2 mL of sample solution in a test tube. Add few drops of Van-Urk's reagent.	Development of reddish brown colour.	Indicates the presence of Vinca alkaloids.
Test for Physostigma alkaloids			
6	**Eserine blue test:** Place 2 mL of sample solution in a test tube. Add strong ammonia solution.	Development of yellowish red colour (upon evaporation forms bluish residue (*eserine blue*)).	Indicates the presence of Physostigmine.
7	**Alkali hydrolysis test:** Place 2 mL of sample in a test tube. Divide into two parts.		Indicates the formation of Eserine hydroxides.
	To one part add ammonium hydroxide solution.	Produces red colour	
	To another part add potassium hydroxide solution.	Produces yellow colour	
8	**Fuming nitric acid test:** Place 1 mL sample in a test tube. Add 5 drops of potassium ferricyanide and 2 drops of ferric chloride (1%).	Develops blue colour.	Indicates the formation of Chloroeserine.
9	**Potassium ferric cyanide test:** Place small quantity of sample solution in a porcelain dish. Add 5 drops of fuming nitric acid.	Develops yellow colour (upon evaporation produces green residue).	Indicates the presence of Physostigmine.
Test for Nux-vomica alkaloids			
10	**Nitric acid test:** Place few crystals of sample in a china dish. Add drops of nitric acid.	Development of faint yellow colour.	Indicates the presence of Strychnine.
		Development of intense red colour (turns to violet on addition of Stannous chloride).	Indicates the presence of Brucine.
Tests for Strychnine			
11	**Sulfuric acid-dichromate test:** Place few crystals of sample in a test tube. Add 3 drops of concentrated sulphuric acid and few crystals of potassium dichromate.	Development of deep blue colour. (gradually changes to violet to purple to red to orange to yellow)	Indicates the presence of Strychnine.
12	**Mandelin's reagent test:** Place few crystals of sample in a test tube. Add 1 mL of Mandelin's reagent to the tube.	Development of deep violet colour. (changes to red to cherry red on addition of water)	Indicates the presence of Strychnine.
Tests for Brucine			
13	Transfer 5 mL of the sample solution to separating funnel. Add 2 mL of ammonia and 5 mL of chloroform. Shake well and separate the chloroform layer. Evaporate 1 mL of chloroform layer to dryness, which gives residue after evaporation. The residue is useful for the following tests.		

Table *Contd...*

S. No.	Experiment	Observation	Inference
Tests for Brucine			
13a	**Erdmann's reagent test:** To the part of residue add 2 drops of Erdmann's reagent.	Development of orange red colour.	Indicates the presence of Brucine.
13b	**Nitric acid test:** To another part of residue add 2 drops of nitric acid.	Development of orange red colour	Indicates the presence of Brucine.
13c	**Stannous chloride test:** To the above residue add freshly prepared Stannous chloride solution.	Development of violet colour.	Indicates the presence of Brucine
	Test for Rauwolfia alkaloids		
14	**Vanillin test:** Place the powdered sample in a watch glass. Add vanillin solution in hydrochloric acid.	Development of red or orange-yellow colour.	Indicates the presence Rauwolfia alkaloids.
Test for Quinine			
15	**Fluorescence test:** Place 1 mL of the sample solution in a test tube. Add concentrated sulphuric acid (1 mL) and 5 mL of water.	Appearance of blue fluorescence under ultra violet light.	Indicates the presence of Quinine.
16	**Thalleoquin test:** Place 1 mL of sample solution in a test tube. Add 5 drops of bromine water (or chlorine water) and 1 mL of ammonia. This produces greenish resinous mass, called as Thalleoquin.	Development of emerald green colour.	Indicates the presence of Quinine.
17	**Herapathite test:** Place pinch of sample in a test tube. Add glacial acetic acid (7.5 mL) and ethanol (3 mL) ato the tube and boil the mixture. Add 5 drops of concentrated sulphuric acid, add ethanolic iodine (1%, 3.5 mL).	Formation of crystals on standing. (appears dark in reflected light and green in transmitted light)	Indicates the formation of iodosulphate of Quinine.
18	**Glacial acetic acid test:** Place pinch of powdered sample in a test tube. Add few drops of glacial acetic acid.	Development of purple colour.	Indicates the presence of Quinine.
19	**Silver nitrate test:** Place 1 mL of sample solution in a test tube. Add 5 drops of silver nitrate solution to the tube.	Formation of white precipitate (soluble in nitric acid).	Indicates the presence of Quinine.

58.6 Identification of Quinoline Alkaloids

S. No.	Experiment	Observation	Inference
1	**Erythroquinine test (Rosequin/Ferrocyanide test):** Dissolve pinch of sample in dilute acetic acid in a test tube. Add few drops of bromine water (freshly prepared). Add drop of 10% potassium ferrocyanide and concentrated ammonium hydroxide.	Formation of instant red colour. Shake the above mixture with 2 mL of chloroform. The organic layer becomes red colour.	Indicates the presence of Quinine. (Formation of Erythroquinine/ Rosequin/Ferrocyanide)

58.7 Identification of Isoquinoline Alkaloids

S. No.	Experiment	Observation	Inference
1	Transfer 5 mL of the sample solution to separating funnel. Add 2 mL of ammonia and 5 mL of chloroform. Shake well and separate the chloroform layer. Evaporate 1 mL of chloroform layer to dryness, which gives residue after evaporation. The residue is useful for the following tests.		
2	**Marquis test:** Place part of residue in a test tube. Add 2 drops of Marquis reagent.	Formation of greenish-violet colour.	Indicates the presence of Isoquinoline alkaloid.
3	**Froehd's test:** Place part of residue in a test tube. Add 2 drops of Froehd's reagent.	Formation of green colour.	Indicates the presence of Papaverine.
		Development of dirty green colour.	Indicates the presence of Emetine.
4	**Warren's test:** Place part of residue in porcelain dish. Add few crystals of potassium permanganate and crush them. To the mixture add 3 drops of Marquis reagent (mixture of formaldehyde and concentrated sulfuric acid).	Formation of purple colour. (changes to bluish green to violet blue)	Indicates the presence of Papaverine.
5	**Schaer's test:** Place the sample in a test tube. Add 2 drops of hydrogen peroxide (30%) and 1 mL of sulphuric acid. Heat the mixture for 2 min.	Development of orange colour.	Indicates the presence of Emetine.

58.8 Identification of Pyridine Alkaloids

S. No.	Experiment	Observation	Inference
1	***p*-Dimethylamino benzaldehyde (DMAB) test:** Place 1 ml alkaloid solution in a test tube. Add few drops of *p*-dimethylamino benzaldehyde and heat the mixture by placing in hot plate with continuous stirring.	Development of red colour. (changes to violet)	Indicates the presence of Nicotine.
2	**Vanillin-hydrochloric acid test:** To the powdered sample add vanillin in hydrochloric acid.	Development of red colour.	Indicates the presence Nicotine.

58.9 Identification of Purine Alkaloids

S. No.	Experiment	Observation	Inference
1	**Murexide Test:** Transfer 5 mL of the sample solution to separating funne. Add 2 mL of ammonia and 5 mL of chloroform. Shake well and separate the chloroform layer. Evaporate 1 mL of chloroform layer to dryness, which gives residue after evaporation. To the residue add 0.5 mL of hydrochloric acid and 0.5 mL of potassium chlorate solution. Evaporate the mixture to dryness.	Formation of yellow residue, which becomes crimson on exposure to few drops of ammonia and finally to purple.	Indicates the presence of Purine alkaloids. (caffeine, theophylline)
2	**Schaer's test:** Place the sample in a test tube. Add 1 drop of hydrogen peroxide (30%) and 1 mL of concentrated sulphuric acid.	Formation of orange residue. (changes into violet after the addition of ammonia)	Indicates the presence of Purines.
3	**Silver nitrate test:** Place the sample in a test tube. Add 1 mL of hot water and 3 drops of silver nitrate. It forms Jelly like floccules, then add ammonia.	Formation of purple colour (disappears by the addition of sodium hydroxide).	Indicates the presence of Caffeine.
		Formation of violet red colour solution.	Indicates the presence of Theophylline.
		Colourless solution.	Indicates the presence of Theobromine

Test Name	Ephedrine	Atropine	Cocaine	Reserpine	Brucine	Strychnine	Quinine	Papaverine	Theobromine/ Caffeine
Mayer's reagent	-	Creamy white ppt	Creamy white ppt	Creamy white ppt	Creamy white ppt	Creamy white ppt	Creamy white ppt	Creamy white ppt	No ppt
Wagner's reagent	Brown ppt	Brown ppt	Brown ppt	Brown ppt	Brown ppt	Brown ppt	Brown ppt	Brown ppt	Brown ppt for caffeine only
Tannic acid	- -	- -	-	White ppt	White ppt	White ppt	White ppt	White ppt	White ppt
Mandelin's reagent	-	-	-	Violet turns into orange red on adding water	-	Violet turns into orange red on adding water	-	-	-
Froehde's reagent	- -	- -	-	-	-	-	-	Green	-
Marquis reagent	- -	-	-	-	-	-	-	Greenish to violet	-
Erdmann's reagent	- -	-	-	-	Orange red color	-	-	-	-
Confirmatory test	**Chen's test** Purple color in $CHCl_3$ layer, Blue color in the H_2O layer	**Vitali-Morin's test** Violet colour	**Permanganate test** Violet crystalline precipitate Cocaine with sulfuric acid gives smell of methyl benzoate.	**Vanillin-hydrochloric acid test** Red or orange yellow color	**Stannous chloride** Violet color	**Dichromate test** Intense violet streaks appear	**Thalleoquine test** emerald green color is produced **Blue** fluorescence under UV light	**Warren's test** purple color to blue green to intense violet-blue to brown Papaverine gives lemon yellow colour upon reaction with HCl and potassium ferricyanide.	**Murexide test** a purple residue upon reaction of caffein with potassium chlorate and drops of hydrochloric acid.

KEY POINTS

- Alkaloids are physiologically active nitrogenous secondary metabolites of plant as well as animal kingdom.
- Morphine (analgesic), cocaine (local anesthetic) and quinine (anti-malarial) are the most important alkaloids, and serves as leads for the drug discovery.
- Alkaloids acts as a nitrogen reservoirs for protein synthesis and regulators for growth, metabolism and reproduction of plants.

59

Qualitative Analysis of Steroids

The term steroids refer to group of secondary metabolites of plants, animals and fungi, which includes alkaloids and sex hormones. These metabolites with diversified chemical structures produce several beneficial functions, and serve as a lead in the drug design. Steroids contains cyclopentanoperhydrophenanthrene (CPP) skeleton with four fused rings (designated as A, B, C and D) in 6-6-6-5 pattern. All these steroids are cyclization products of triterpene squalene. The precursor of animal and fungi steroids is lanosterol, whereas plant sterols derived from cycloartenol. Steroids include bile acids and hormones (gonadal and adrenal).

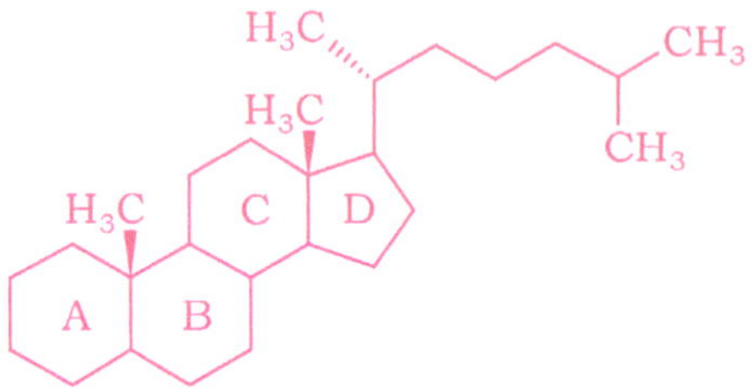

Steroid skeleton

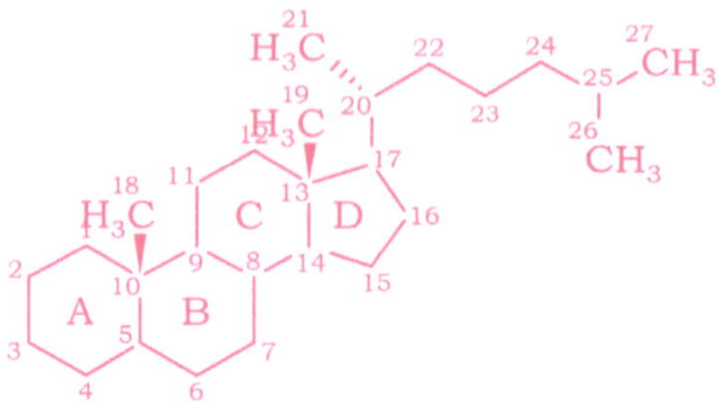

Steroidal skeleton with numbering

Steroids are synthesized from squalene (product of mevalonate pathway). In plants squalene gets converted into cycloartenol and forms phytosterols. In fungi and animals, lanosterol synthesis from squalene and further steroid synthesis results.

Classification

Steroids can be grouped based on the organism from which they are derived.

1. Plant steroids
2. Fungal steroids
3. Animal steroids
4. Insect steroids

Plant steroids

The steroids derived from plant sources, such as withanolides are known as plant steroids. It can be grouped into phytosterols and brassinosteroids.

Phytosterols**:** A steroid alcohols, such as withaferin A,ergosterol and stigmastrol

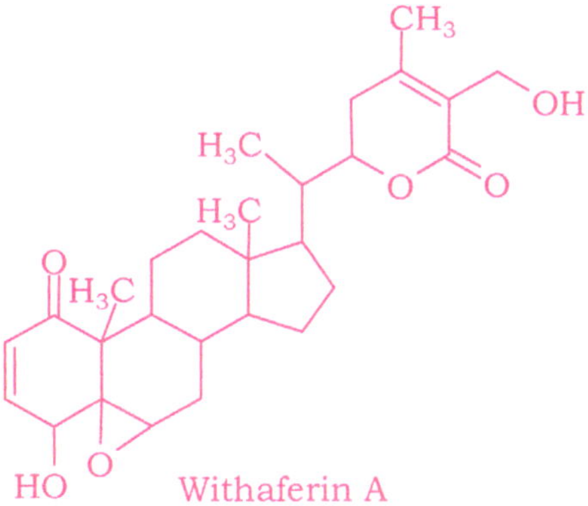

Withaferin A

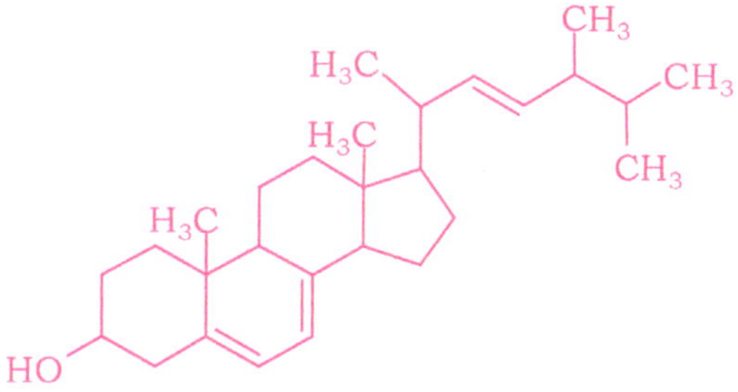

Ergosterol

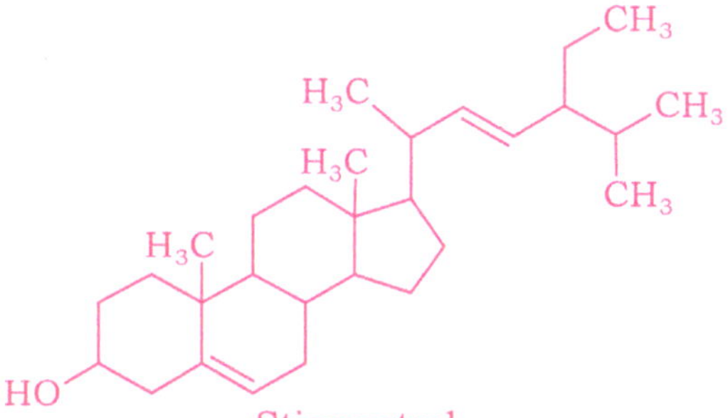

Stigmastrol

Brassinosteroids**:** These are endogenous plant hormones (e.g., brassinolide).

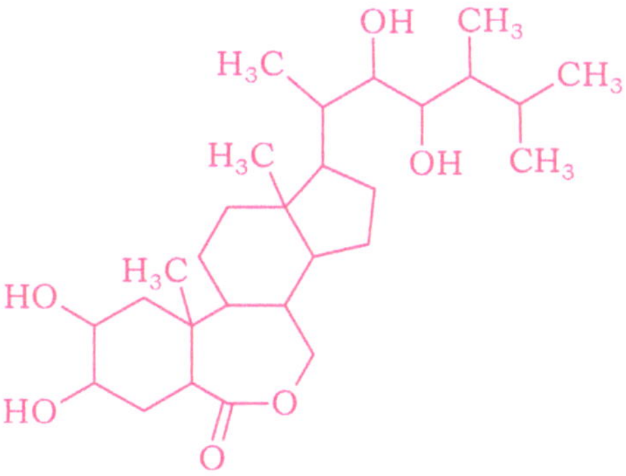

Brassinolide

Fungal steroids

The steroids derived from fungi are known as mycosterol, which includes ergosterol and zymosterol.

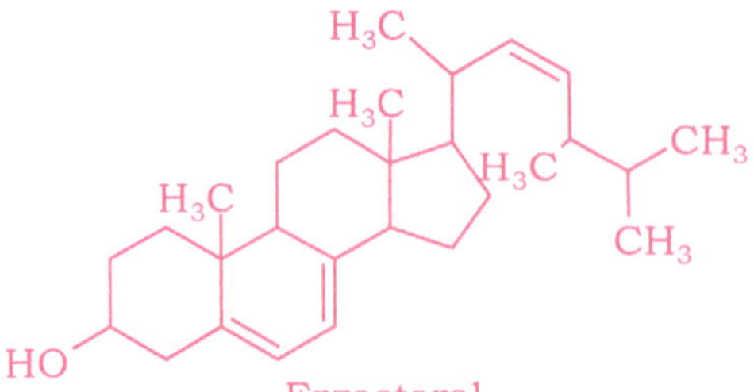

Ergosterol 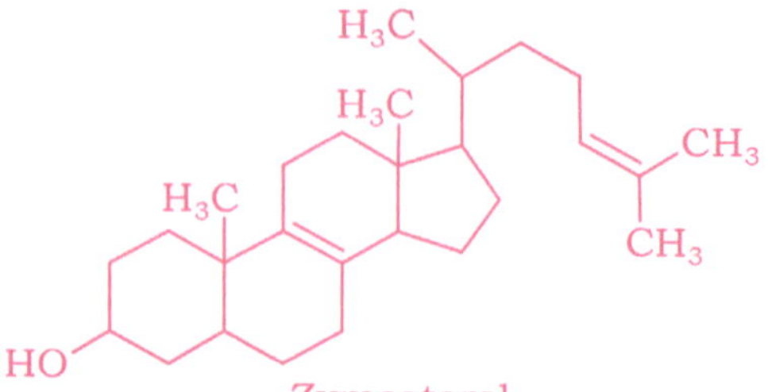 Zymosterol

Animal steroids

This includes steroid hormones, corticosteroids, sterols and bile acids.

Steroid hormones: The gonadal hormones namely estrogen, androgen and progesterones are essential for the sexual characteristics.

Corticosteroids: This includes glucocorticoids (e.g., cortisol) and mineralocorticoids (e.g., aldosterone). They regulate the biochemical functions, such as immunity and metabolism.

Sterols: Cholesterol is the good example. It plays central role in the maintenance of biological membranes, vitamin D synthesis, bile acid synthesis and immunity functions.

Bile acids: These are the steroid acids predominantly found in the bile of mammals and vertebrates. They are conjugated with taurine or glycine to give bile salts. Bile acids are synthesized in the liver.

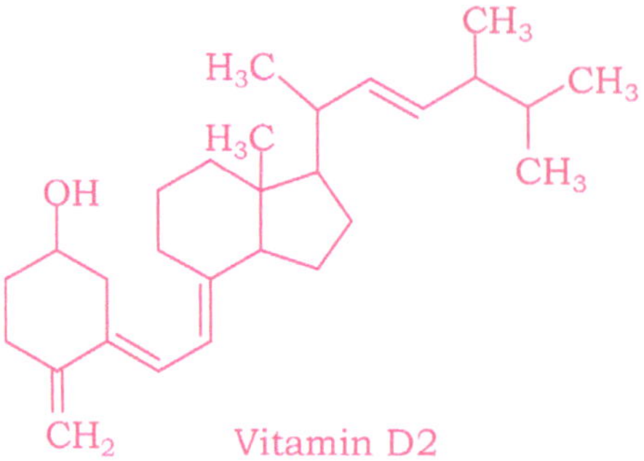

Vitamin D2 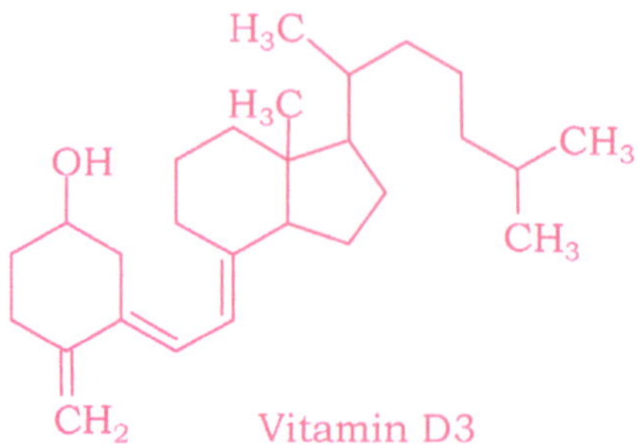 Vitamin D3

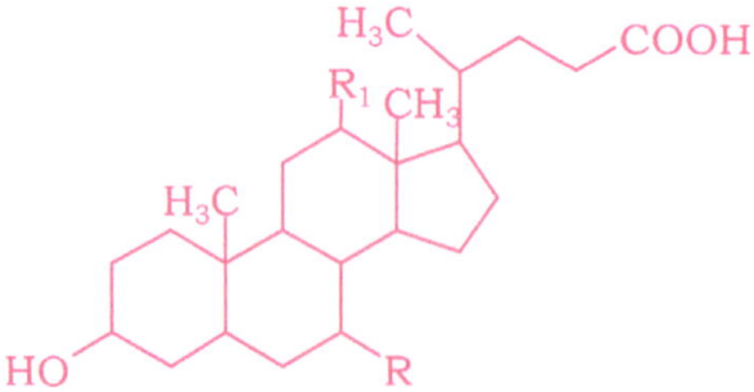

Cholic acid, R and R_1 = OH
Dexoyholic acid, R = H; R_1 = OH
Chenodeoxycholic acid, R = OH, R_1 = H

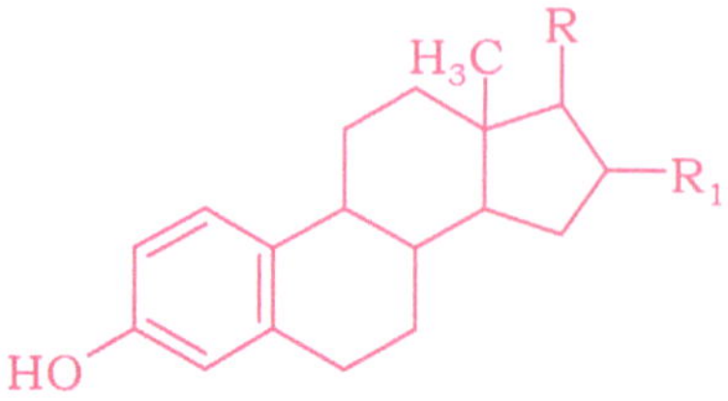

Estrone, R = =O; R_1 = H
Estradiol, R = OH; R_1 = H
Estriol, R = OH, R_1 = OH

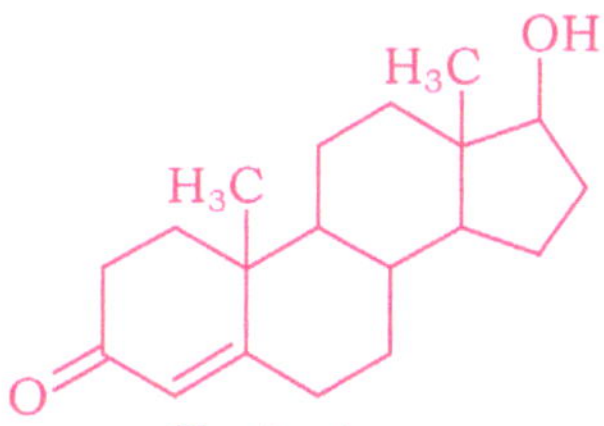

Testosterone

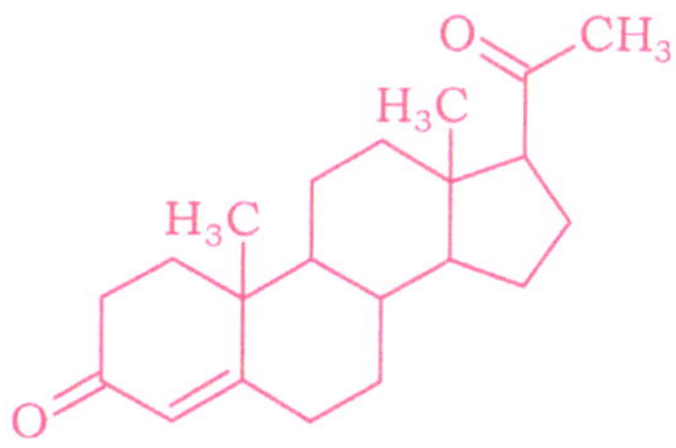

Progesterone

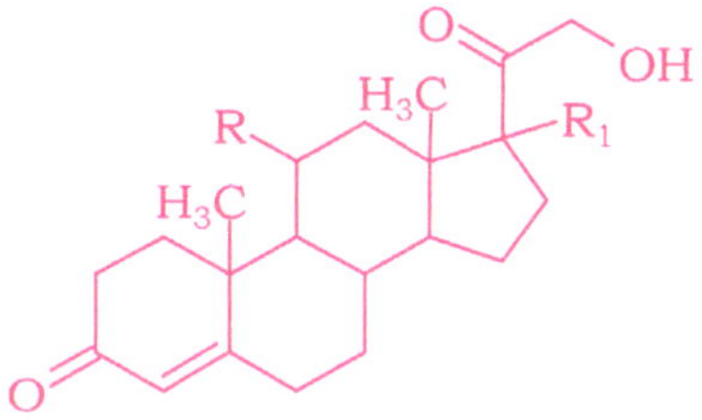

Corticosterone, R = OH; R_1 = H

Cortisone, R = =O; R_1 = OH

Cortisol, R = OH, R_1 = OH

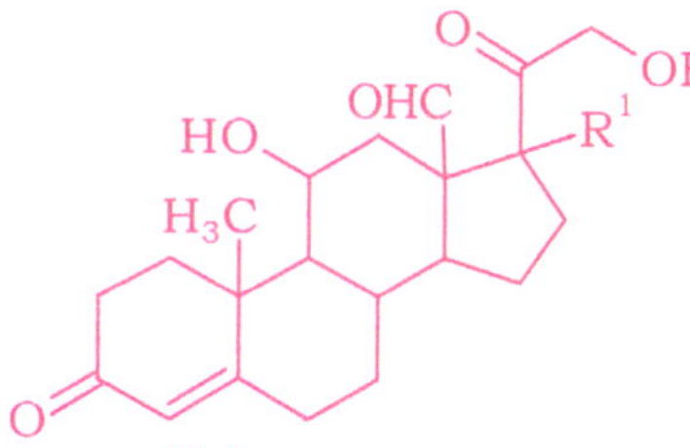

Aldosterone

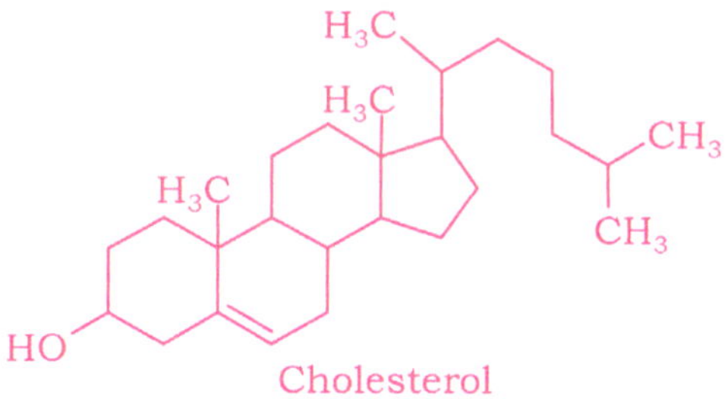

Cholesterol

Insect steroids (Ecdysteroids)

These are polyhydroxy steroids and are essential for the cell proliferation and growth of insects.

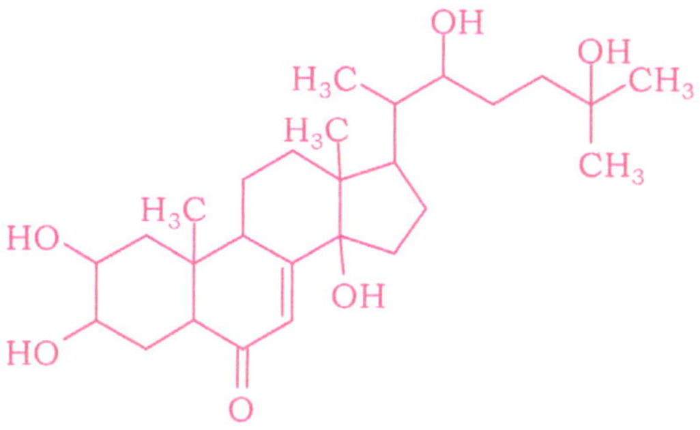

Ecdysteroid

59.1 General Tests for Steroids

Physicochemical tests

Heat test

All the steroids on dehydrogenation with selenium at 360 °C give 'diels hydrocarbon'.

H$_3$C CH$_3$ H$_3$C CH$_3$ H$_3$C C D A B

Steroid

Selenium Dehydrogenation 360 °C

CH$_3$

Diels hydrocarbon

S. No.	Experiment	Observation	Inference
1.	**Salkowski reaction (sulphuric acid test):** Dissolve a little cholesterol in 2 mL of chloroform contained in a dry test tube. Add 2 mL of sulphuric acid and shake gently.	Chloroform layer (upper) appears as bluish red which changes to cherry red and then to purple. Sulphuric acid layer (lower) shows yellowish-green colour with green fluorescence.	Indicates the presence of Steroids.
2	**Liebermann-Burchard reaction (Acetic anhydride-sulfuric acid test):** Place few crystals of sample in a dry test tube. Add 2 mL of chloroform and dissolve the sample. Add 10 drops of acetic anhydride, 3 drops of concentrated sulfuric acid and mix well.	Formation of rose red colour, which quickly changes to blue then to green.	Indicates the presence of Steroids.
3	**Zak's test:** Place few crystals of sample in a dry test tube. Add 2 mL of chloroform and dissolve the sample. Evaporate the chloroform solution to dryness. Add 3 mL of ferric chloride (0.05%) in glacial acetic acid and 1 mL of concentrated sulfuric acid.	Formation of red colour.	Indicates the presence of Steroids.
4	**Formaldehyde- H_2SO_4 test:** Place 2 mL of sample (in chloroform) in a test tube. Add 2 mL of formaldehyde -sulfuric acid solution (1 part of 40% formaldehyde to 50 parts of the sulfuric acid).	Formation of cherry red colour in chloroform layer.	Indicates the presence of Steroids.
	Decant the chloroform layer into test tube containing 3 drops of acetic anhydride	Formation of blue colour.	Indicates the presence of Steroids.

Table *Contd...*

S. No.	Experiment	Observation	Inference
5	**Rosenheim test:** Place 1 mL of sample (in chloroform) in a test tube. Add 1 mL of 90% trichloroacetic acid to the tube.	Appearance of blue or pink colour.	Indicates the presence of Steroids.
6	**Lifschutz test:** Place 1 mL of sample and few mg of perbenzoic acid in glacial acetic acid in a test tube. Heat the mixture and add 0.5 mL of concentrated sulphuric acid.	Appearance of intense blue or green colour.	Indicates the presence of Steroids.

Test for sterols

S. No.	Experiment	Observation	Inference
1	**Fieser test:** Place 1 mL of sample (in benzene) in a test tube. Add few mg of selenium dioxide in benzene to the tube and maintain the temperature at 20 °C.	Appearance of yellow colour.	Indicates the presence of 5α series Sterols. (5β series does not give any colour).
2	**Tortelli-Jaffe test:** Place 1 mL of sample (in acetic acid) in a test tube. Add 1 mL of 2% bromine in chloroform.	Appearance of green colour at the interface.	Indicates the presence of Sterols.
3	**Zlatkis test:** Place 1 mL of sample (in acetic acid) in a test tube. Add 1 mL of solution of ferric chloride (in concentrated sulphuric acid) and glacial acetic acid.	Appearance of purple colour. (This test is used in the determination of plasma cholesterol)	Indicates the presence of Sterols.

Test for vitamin D

S. No.	Experiment	Observation	Inference
1	**Antimony trichloride test:** Place 1 mL of sample in a test tube. Add 1 mL of solution of antimony trichloride in chloroform.	Appearance of intense yellow colour.	Presence of Vitamin D.
2	**Dichlorohydrin test:** Place 1 mL of sample in a test tube. Add 1 mL of solution of dichlorohydrin and acetyl chloride in chloroform.	Appearance of green colour.	Presence of Vitamin D.
3	Place 1 mL of sample in a test tube. Add 1 mL of solution of aluminum chloride in ethanol.	Appearance of violet colour.	Presence of Vitamin D.
4	Place 1 mL of sample (in chloroform) in a test tube. Add 1 mL of acetic anhydride and concentrated sulphuric acid.	Appearance of bright red colour. (red colour changes to violet and green)	Presence of Vitamin D.

Test for bile acids

S. No.	Experiment	Observation	Inference
1	**Mylius reaction:** Place 1 mL of sample in a test tube. Add 2 mL of ethanol and 3 drops of iodine solution. Warm the mixture.	Appearance of blue colourin transmitted light and needles. (appear yellow in reflected light)	Presence of Cholic acid.
2	**Hammersten test:** Place 1 mL sample in a test tube. Add 1 mL of hydrochloric acid (25%) and 1 mL of cholic acid.	Appearance of violet colour. (changes to yellow on heating)	Presence of Cholic acid.
3	**Pettenkofer reaction:** Place 1 mL of sample solution in a test tube. Add 1mL of sucrose (or furfural) and 3 drops of concentrated sulfuric acid. Warm the mixture.	Appearance of red colour.	Presence of Cholic acid.

Test for estrogens

S. No.	Experiment	Observation	Inference
1	**Kober test:** Place 1 mL of sample in a test tube. Heat and add 2 mL of sulfuric acid (60%) containing phenol, hydroquinone/ β-naphthol.	Appearance of yellow colour with green fluorescence. (on dilution with water and reheating produces pink colour)	Presence of Estrogens.

S. No.	Experiment	Observation	Inference
1	**Diazo coupling test:** Place 1 mL of sample in a test tube. Add diazotized p-nitroaniline/ sulphanilic acid.	Development of orange or red colour	Presence of Estrogens.
2	**David test for estriol:** Place 1 mL of sample in a test tube. Add 3 drops of concentrated sulfuric acid and arsenic acids.	Development of blue colour.	Presence of Estrogens.

S. No.	Experiment	Observation	Inference
1	**Bachmann test for estriol:** Place 1 mL of sample in a test tube. Add 1 mL of mixture of sodium p-toluene sulphonate and phosphoric acid.	Development of violet colour.	Presence of Estriol.
2	**Zimmermann reaction:** Place 1 mL of alcoholic solution of sample in a test tube. Add 1 mL of m-dinitrobenzene and 1 mL of potassium hydroxide.	Development of coloured complex. • Brown colour • Purple colour	Presence of Keto steroid. • Testosterone • Androsterone
3	**Pinus reaction:** Place 1 mL of the sample solution in a test tube. Add a solution of antimony trichloride in acetic acid.	Produces blue colour.	Presence of Androsterone.
4	**Pettenkofer reaction:** Place 1 mL of sample solution in a test tube. Add solution furfural in acetic acid. And add 3 drops of concentrated sulfuric acid. Warm the mixture.	Appearance of red colour.	Presence of Dihydroepiandro-sterone.

KEY POINTS

- Steroids contains cyclopentanoperhydrophenanthrene (CPP) skeleton with four fused rings (designated as A, B, C and D) in 6-6-6-5 pattern.
- The precursor of animal and fungi steroids is lanosterol, whereas plant sterols derived from cycloartenol.
- Steroids on dehydrogenation with selenium at 360 °C give 'Diels hydrocarbon'.

60

Qualitative Analysis of Terpenes and Terpenoids

Terpenes and terpenoids are a large and diverse class of naturally-occurring hydrocarbons, derived from five-carbon isoprene unit (2-methyl-1,3-butadiene, C_5H_8). They are major secondary metabolites (essential oils) of plants, fungi, marine organisms and insects. These phytochemicals are lipophilic in nature (insoluble in water). They possess anthelmintic, antibacterial, antineoplastic and insecticidal functions.

CH_3
H_2C CH_2
Terpene

Terpenes: A mixture of isomeric hydrocarbons derived from isoprene units. The term is derived from turpentine (obsolete spelling of terpentine), the first terpene product isolated. Multiples of isoprene units, through head-to-tail linkage forms cyclic hydrocarbons called as terpene. Mono and diterpenes are important components of essential oils.

Classification

Terpenoids are classified on the basis of the number of isoprene units which they contain.

Terpenes	Isoprene unit(s)	Examples
Hemiterpenes	1	Prenol, Isovaleric acid
Monoterpenes	2	Citral, Camphor
Sequiterpenes	3	Farnesol, Zingiberene
Diterpenes	4	Retinol, Retinal, Abietic acid
Sesterpenes	5	Geranylfarnesol
Triterpenes	6	Squalene, Amyrins
Tetraterpenes	8	Carotenoids
Polyterpenes	*n*	Rubber

Terpenoids (Isoprenoids): Terpenoids are group of naturally occurring oxygenated or rearrangement derivatives of terpenes. Terpenoids deviate from the isoprene rule (loss or shift of methyl group) and also forms multicyclic structures (e.g., sterols). Citral, menthol, camphor, salvinorin A and cannbinoids are the important terpenoids. Terpenoids, particularly mono and sesqui-terpenoids contribute to the scent of eucalyptus, the flavors of cinnamon, cloves and ginger. Hence, they are useful in perfume industry. The color of sunflower and tomato are due to the presence of terpenoids. The important terpenoid constituents of essential oils are given in the Table.

Essential oils	Terpenoids	Essential oils	Terpenoids
Turpentine	Pinene	Jasmine	Linalool
Caraway	Carvone, ά-Limonene	Lemon	D-Limonene, Citral
Coriander	Linalool, Pinene	Sandalwood	Santalol
Eucalyptus	Cineole	Camphor	Cineole, Eugenol

60.1 General Tests for Terpenoids

Properties

Terpenoids are mostly colourless, pleasant smelling liquids or solids, insoluble in water and readily volatile in steam. Most terpenoids are optically active compounds. All of the terpenoids have one or more double bonds and they add on halogens, hydrogen halides and Tilden reagent (nitrosyl chloride). Some of the terpenoids having conjugated system of double bonds undergo Diel's - Alder reaction, and due to the presence of olefinic bonds easily undergo oxidization by all the oxidizing agents.

General Tests

S No	Experiment	Observation	Inference
1.	Place 1 mL of the sample solution in a test tube. Add 1 mL of alcoholic Sudan III.	Development of red colour.	Indicates the presence of Terpenoids.
2	Place 1 mL of the sample solution in a test tube. Add 3 drops of tincture alkane.	Development of red colodur.	Indicates the presence of Terpenoids.
3	**Salkowski test:** Place 1 mL of the sample solution in a test tube. Add few drops of chloroform and 3 mL of concentrated sulphuric acid.	Greyish or reddish brown colour appears.	Indicates the presence of Terpenoids.

Tests for camphor

S No	Experiment	Observation	Inference
1.	**Vanillin test:** Place the powdered sample in a test tube. Add drop of vanillin in hydrochloride (1:100 fresh) and 2 drops of concentrated sulphuric acid.	Development of red colour.	Indicates the presence of Terpenoids.
		Development of instant yellow colour	Indicates the presence of Camphor (natural).
		Colour changes into red to violet and blue	

Tests for menthol/ thymol

S No	Experiment	Observation	Inference
1.	Place 10 mg of sample crystals in a test tube. Add 4 drops of concentrated sulphuric acid and drop of vanillin sulphuric acid reagent to the tube.	Development of orange yellow colour.	Indicates the presence of Menthol.
		Colour changes into violet on the addition of water	
2	Place 10 mg of sample crystals in a test tube. Add 1 mL glacial acetic acid, 2 drops of concentrated sulphuric acid and 2 drops of concentrated nitric acid.	No colour change	Indicates the presence of Menthol.
		Appearance of green/bluish colour.	Indicates the presence of Thymol.
3	Place 1 mL of sample in a test tube. Add pinch of phthalic anhydride.	Development of violet red colour (addition of dilute alkali forms blue colour)	Indicates the presence of Thymol.

Tests for eucalyptus oil/cineole

S. No	Experiment	Observation	Inference
1.	Place the sample (drop of oil) in microslide. Add drop of 5% alcoholic hydroquinone.	Appearance of colourless prisms (rhomboids).	Indicates the presence of Eucalyptus oil and Cineole.
2	Place the sample (drop of oil) in microslide. Add drop of 50% resorcinol.	Appearance of leaf like crystals.	Indicates the presence of Eucalyptus oil and Cineole.

Tests for asafoetida

S. No	Experiment	Observation	Inference
1.	Triturate the sample with water.	Formation of milky white emulsion.	Indicates the presence of Umbelliferone.
2	Place drop of sulphuric acid on the freshly fractured surface.	Appearance of reddish brown colour.	Indicates the presence of umbelliferone.
3	Place drop of nitric acid on the freshly fractured surface.	Appearance of green colour. (turns into violet after washing with water)	Indicates the presence of Umbelliferone.
4	**Umbelliferone test:** Boil the sample with 50% hydrochloric acid, filter and alkalify with ammonium hydroxide.	Produces blue fluorescence.	Indicates the presence of Umbelliferone.

Tests for colophony resin

S. No	Experiment	Observation	Inference
1.	Test the alcoholic resin for the acidity with litmus paper.	Turns blue litmus red.	Indicates the acidic property of resin.
2	Place the powdered resin in a test tube. Add 10 mL of acetic anhydride and 2 drop of sulphuric acid. Shake well the mixture.	Appearance of purple colour.	Indicates the presence of Colophony resin.
3	**Tollen's test (Silver mirror test):** Place 2 mL of Tollen's reagent and 2 mL sugar solution in a test tube. Boil for 5 min and cool.	Formation of silver mirror.	Indicates the presence of resin.

Tests for carotenoids

S. No	Experiment	Observation	Inference
1.	Stratify the ether (or chloroform) solution of sample with 85% sulphuric acid.	Appearance of blue colour between the junction of two layer.	Indicates the presence of Carotenoids.
2	**Carr-price test:** To the sample add antimony trichloride in chloroform	Appearance of blue colour.	Indicates the presence of Carotenoids.

Tests for curcumin

S. No	Experiment	Observation	Inference
1.	Place the powdered sample in a watch glass. Add 2 drops of sulphuric acid.	Appearance of crimson red colour.	Indicates the presence of Curcumin.
2	Place the aqueous solution of sample in a test tube. Add pinch of boric acid and 2 drops of alkali solution.	Appearance of reddish brown colour. (changes in to greenish blue on the addition of alcohol)	Indicates the presence of Curcumin.
3	**Fluorescence test:** Place the sample powder in a test tube. Add 2 drops of acetic anhydride and 2 drops of sulphuric acid.	Appearance of violet colour produces red fluorescence	Indicates the presence of Curcumin.

Tests for eugenol

S. No	Experiment	Observation	Inference
1.	**Bromine test:** Place 1 mL of sample solution in a test tube. Add 1 mL of bromine in dichlromethane.	Decolurization of yellow colour of bromine.	Indicates the presence of carbon-carbon double bond (C=C) in Eugenol.
2	**Potassium permanganate test:** Place 1 mL of sample solution in a test tube. Add 1 mL of potassium permanganate.	Decolurization of purple colour of bromine.	Indicates the presence of carbon-carbon double bond (C=C) in Eugenol.
3	**Ferric chloride test:** To the 1 mL of sample solution add 1 mL of 5% alcoholic ferric chloride.	Development of blue colour.	Indicates the presence of phenolic group of Eugenol.

KEY POINTS

- Terpenes and terpenoids are diverse class of natural hydrocarbons, derived from five-carbon isoprene units (2-methyl-1,3-butadiene).
- Multiple isoprene unit, through head-to-tail linkage forms cyclic hydrocarbons called as terpene.
- Mono and diterpenes are important components of essential oils.

61

Qualitative Analysis of Glycosides

Glycosides are metabolic products of plants. They have nutritional value for both humans and animals. Glycosides are composed of sugar and non-sugar moiety. A sugar part is linked to non-sugar portion through glycosidic bond.

- Sugar moiety of glycosides is known as glycone or genin.
- Non-sugar moiety of glycosides is known as aglycone or agenin.

The sugar can be monosaccharide (e.g., glucose, L-rhamnose, L-fructose, L-arabinose and D-xylose), disaccharide (e.g., galactose, mannose and gentiobiose) and trisaccharide (e.g., strophanthotriose). Several plant glycosides, upon enzymatic hydrolysis releases sugar moiety and becomes functionally active.

- ***Flavanoids***: Glycosides with terpene as aglycone part (non-sugar moiety) are named as flavanoids (e.g., hesperidin).
- ***Saponins***: Glycosides possessing soap properties are known as saponins (e.g., glycyrrhizin).

Classification

Based on the glycosidic bond**:** Glycosides can be classified, depending upon type of functional group to which sugar moiety bond (glycosidic bond).

(a) O-Glycosides: A glycosidic bond between hydroxyl group of sugar and non-sugar moieties. e.g., Salicin

(b) N-Glycosides: A glycosidic bond between hydroxyl group of sugar moiety and amino group of non-sugar moiety. e.g., Adenine

(c) S-Glycosides: A glycosidic bond between hydroxyl group of sugar moiety and sulphur group of non-sugar moiety. e.g., Sinigrin

(d) C-Glycosides: A glycosidic bond between hydroxyl group of sugar moiety and carbon group of non-sugar moiety. e.g., Barbaloin

Based on the chemical nucleus**:** Glycosides can be further classified based on basic nucleus (functionality) of aglycone.

Glycosides	Examples
Alcoholic glycosides	Salicin
Aldehyde glycosides	Glucovanillin (vanniloside)
Anthraquinone glycosides	Sennoside, Barbaloin, Cascaroside
Coumarin glycosides	Umbelliferone
Cyanogenic glycosides	Amigdalin, Prunasin
Flavanoid glycosides	Quercetin, Vitexin, Naringin
Phenolic glycosides	Arbutin, Sennoside, Barbaloin, Cascaroside
Saponin glycosides	Diosgenin
Steroidal glycosides (Cardiac glycosides)	Lannatoside A, Digitoxin, Gitoxin, Quabain
Steviol glycosides	Stevioside
Thioglycosides	Allicin

Aldehyde glycosides

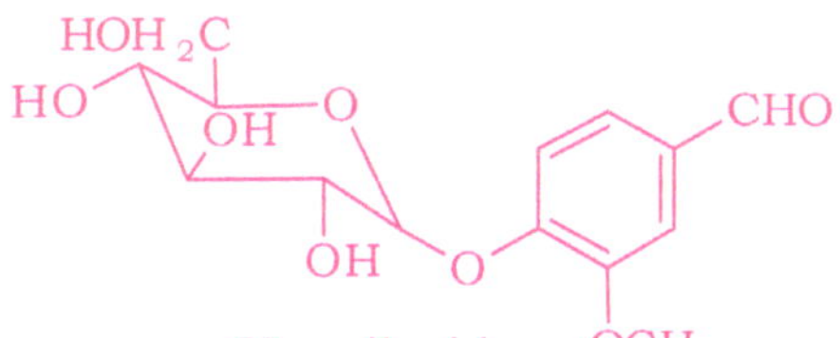

Vanniloside
(Glucovannillin)

Steroidal glycosides (Cardiac glycosides)

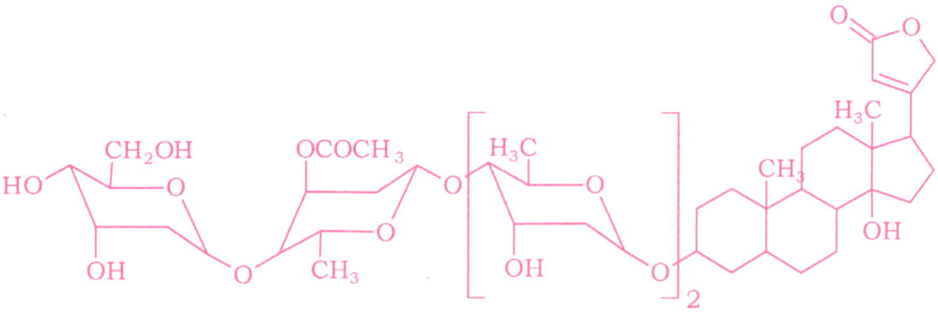

Lanatoside A

Digitoxin (Digitalis pupurea)

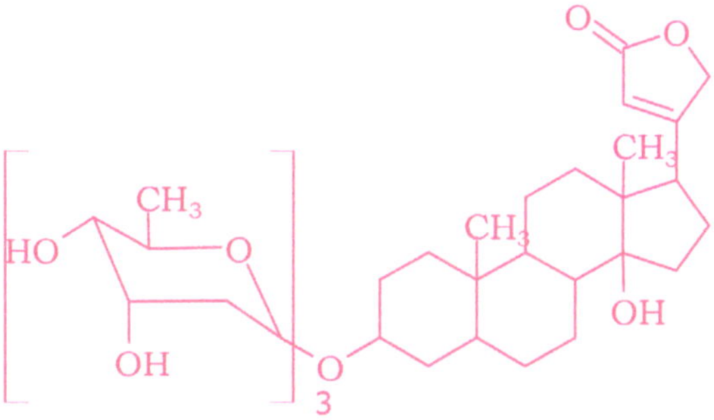

Digitoxin

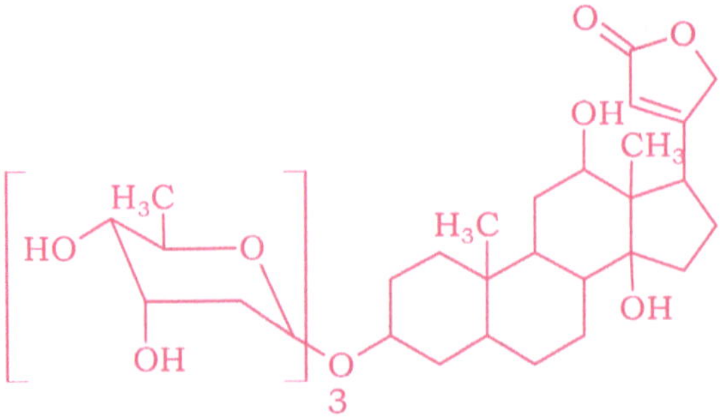

Digoxin

Ouabain *(Strophanthus kombe)*

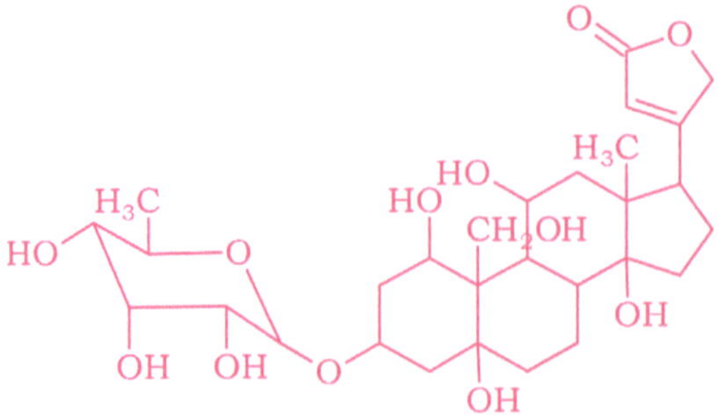

Ouabain

Anthraquinone glycosides

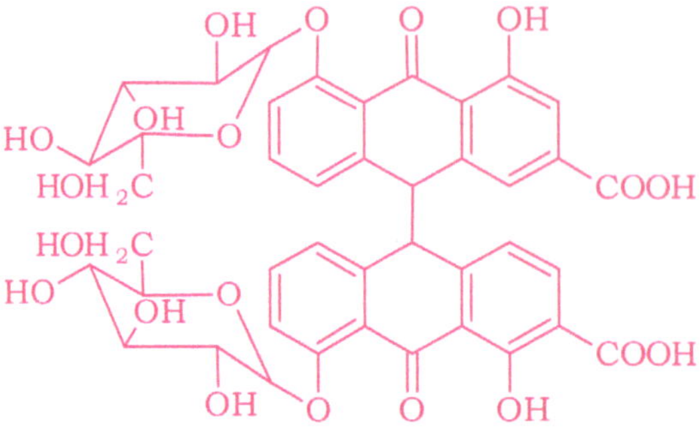

Sennoside

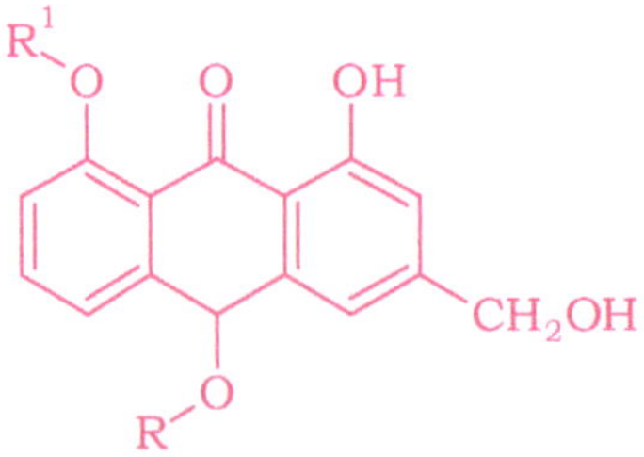

Barbaloin, R = Glucose; R_1 = H

Cascaroside, R = R_1 = Glucose

Phenolic glycosides (includes Sennoside, Barbaloin and Cascaroside)

61.1 General Tests for Glycosides

Physicochemical properties

- Colour: Glycosides are colourless (flavanoid: yellow, anthraquinone: red/orange)
- Texture: Solid, amorpous, non-volatile (except glycyrrhizin, stevioside and populin).
- Solubility: Most compounds are water soluble and insoluble in organic solvents.
- Reducing power: Glycosides are non-reducing sugars and gives positive results with Benedict's test and Fehling's test (after hydrolysis).

S No	Experiment	Observation	Inference
1	**Legal's test:** Place 1 mL of sample solution in a test tube. Add drops of pyridine, sodium nitroprusside (92%, w/v) and sodium hydroxide (20%, w/v).	Development of pink/red colour.	Indicates the presence of Gycosides.
2	**Baljet test:** To the fractured part of sample add alkaline picric acid.	Development of yellow to orange colour.	Indicates the presence of Glycosides.
3	**Raymond test:** To the solution of glycoside in 1 mL of ethanol (50%) add 0.1 mL of Raymond reagent and 3 drops of sodium hydroxide (20%, w/v).	Development of violet colour. (changes into blue)	Indicates the presence of Gycosides.
	Raymond reagent: 1% w/v *m*-Nitrobenzene in ethanol		
4	**Tollen's test:** To the 1 mL solution of the sample in pyridine and 1 mL of Tollen's reagent and heat.	Formation of silver mirror.	Indicates the presence of Sugar portion of Glycosides.

Table *Contd...*

S No	Experiment	Observation	Inference
5	**Antimony trichloride test:** To the 1 mL solution of the sample add 1 mL of antimony trichloride and 1 mL of trichloroacetic acid and heat the mixture.	Development of blue/ violet colour.	Indicates the presence of Gycosides.
6	**Kedde test:** To the 1 mL solution of the sample add equal volume of Kedde reagent.	Development of blue/ violet colour (1-2 h).	Indicates the presence of Gycosides.
	Kedde reagent: Equal volume of 2% w/v 3,5-Dinitro benzoic acid in methanol and 75% w/v of aqueous potassium hydroxide.		

Test for Aldehyde Glycosides

S No	Experiment	Observation	Inference
1	**Vanillin test:** To the sample add 10 mL of water and dissolve by warming. Add 3 drops of ferric chloride solution to the mixture.	Development of blue-purple colour. (changes to brown and white to grey-white precipitate)	Indicates the presence of Vanillin.
2	To the sample add 5 mL of sodium hydrogen sulphate and dissolve by warming. Add 10 mL of dilute sulphuric acid and warm the mixture at 60-70 °C for 5 min.	Formation of crystals.	Indicates the presence of Vannilin.

61.2 Identification of Cardiac Glycosides

S No	Experiment	Observation	Inference
1	**Keller-Killiani test (for deoxy sugar):** To the 2 mL of glycoside solution add glacial acetic acid and trace of ferric chloride in sulphuric acid along the sides of the test tube.	Development of reddish brown to bluish brown colour at the junction of the two liquids (2-5 min).	Indicates the presence of Cardiac glycosides (deoxy sugars).
	Cardiac glycosides are steroid in nature, hence give positive results for the following steroidal identification tests.		
2	**Salkowski reaction (sulphuric acid test):** Dissolve a little sample in 2 mL of chloroform in a dry test tube, add an equal volume of sulphuric acid and shake gently.	Chloroform layer (upper) appears as bluish red which changes to cherry red and then to purple. Sulphuric acid layer (lower) shows yellowish-green colour with green fluorescence.	Indicates the presence of Steroids.
3	**Liebermann-Burchard reaction:** Dissolve a little sample in 2 mL of chloroform in a dry test tube. Add 10 drops of acetic anhydride, 3 drops sulphuric acid and mix well.	Formation of rose red colour, which quickly changes to blue then to green.	Indicates the presence of Steroids.

61.3 Identification of Anthraquinone Glycosides

S No	Experiment	Observation	Inference
1	**Borntrager test:** To the sample add 2 mL of dilute sulphuric acid and heat (hydrolysis). Filter, cool, add benzene/ carbon tetra-chloride and shake the mixture. Separate the organic layer and add equal volume of ammonia solution to it.	Development of pink/cherry-red colour in ammoniacal layer.	Indicates the presence of anthraquinone glycosides
		Development of yellow-orange colour (rapidly changes to red).	Indicates the presence of anthranol (Addition of hydrogen peroxide produces rapid result)
2	**Borax test:** To the 5 mL of filtrate add 0.2 gm of borax and heat to dissolve. Pour few drops of the liquid into test tube containing water (full).	Produces green colour fluorescence.	Indicates the presence of Aloe glycosides.
3	**Bromine test:** To the 2 mL of filtrate add 2 mL of bromine solution (fresh).	Forms yellow colour precipitate.	Indicates the presence of aloe glycoside tetra Bromaloin.
4	**Nitric acid tes:** To 5 mL of filtrate add 2 mL of concentrated nitric acid.	Brown to green	Indicates the cape aloe
		Deep brownish red	Indicates the barbados
		Pale brownish to yellow	Indicates the socotrine
		Yellow to brown	Indicates the zanzibar
5	**Klunge's test:** To the 20 mL of filtrate add drop of saturated copper sulphate solution, 1 g of sodium chloride and 10 mL of ethanol (90%).	Formation of wine red colour	Indicates the presence of barbados
		No colour develops	Indicates zanzibar and socotrine
6	**Nitrous acid test:** To the 1 mL of filtrate add few crystals of sodium nitrite and 1 mL of acetic acid.	Produces rich pink to carmine colour	Indicates the presence of barbados
		Produces lemon pink colour	Indicates the presence of cape aloe
7	**Modified Borntrager test (for C-glycosides):** To the sample add 5 mL of dilute sulphuric acid and 2 mL of aqueous ferric chloride (5%). Boil the mixture for 5 min in water bath. Filter, cool, add benzene (or carbon tetrachloride) and shake the mixture. Separate the organic layer and add equal volume of ammonia solution to it.	Development of yellow to orange colour.	Indicates the presence of anthraquinone glycosides
		Development of pink/red colour in ammoniacal layer.	Indicates the presence of anthraquinone glycosides.

61.4 Identification of Phenolic Glycosides

S No	Experiment	Observation	Inference
1	**Mandelin's test:** To the 1 mL of sample add few drops of Mandelin's reagent.	Produces purple red colour.	Indicates the presence of phenolic glycosides.
	Mandelin's reagent (sulphovanadic acid): 1 gm of ammonium vanadate in 100 mL of concentrated sulphuric acid (Sulphovanadic acid).		
2	**Froehde's test:** To the 1 mL of sample add few drops of Froehde's reagent.	Produces violet colour.	Indicates the presence of phenolic glycosides.
	Froehde's reagent: 5 g of molybdic acid or sodium molybdate in 5 mL of hot concentrated sulphuric acid.		
3	**Erdmann's test:** To the 1 mL of sample add few drops of Erdmann's reagent.	Produces bright red colour	Indicates the presence of phenolic glycosides.
	Erdmann's reagent: A mixture of 10 drops of concentrated nitric acid and sulphuric acid.		

61.5 Identification of Cyanogenic Glycosides

S No	Experiment	Observation	Inference
1	**Ferri ferrocyanide test:** Macerate 1 g of sample with 5 mL of alcoholic potassium hydroxide (5%) for 5 min. Transfer the contents into test tube containing aqueous solution of ferrous sulphate (2.5%) and ferric chloride (91%). Allow the mixture to stand at 60-70 °C for about 10 min. Transfer the contents into test tube containing hydrochloric acid (20%).	Appearance of prussian blue colour.	Indicates the presence of Cyanogenic glycoside.
2	**Grignard test (Sodium picrate test):** Soak the filter paper with picric acid (10%) (drain the excess reagent). Dip this paper into solution of sodium carbonate (10%) and dry. Place the paper in the flask containing moistened sample in warm condition for 1 h.	Filter paper turns into brick red or maroon. (liberated cyanide reacts with sodium picrate and produces brick red or maroon colour)	Indicates the presence of Cyanogenic glycoside.

61.6 Identification of Coumarin Glycosides

S No	Experiment	Observation	Inference
1	**Alkali test:** Place the alcoholic sample solution in a test tube. Add alkali hydroxide.	Development of blue or green fluorescence.	Indicates the presence of Coumarin glycoside.
2	**Guaicum test (Benzidine test):** Place the sample in a test tube. Add 3 drops of alcoholic guaicum resin (1%) or alcoholic benzidine (1%) and 3 drops of hydrogen peroxide.	Development of blue colour.	Indicates the presence of Coumarin glycoside.

KEY POINTS

- Glycosides are composed of sugar (glycone, genin) and nonsugar (aglycone, agenin) moieties and have nutritional value.
- Glycosides include, O-glycosides (e.g., salicin), N-glycosides (e.g., adenine), S-glycosides (e.g., sinigrin) and C-glycosides (e.g., barbaloin).

62

Physicochemical Characterization of Natural Products

62.1 Determination of Acid Value

Theory

Acid value (AV) is an important indicator of vegetable oil quality. Acid value expresses the amount of potassium hydroxide (in milligrams) necessary to neutralize the free fatty acids present in 1 g of the fat sample. The amount of free acid present in most of the fixed oils is generally low. The acid value is used to eliminate low-grade and rancid oils, which tend to have higher acid values. A high acid value is indicative of a stale oil or fat stored under improper conditions.

Principle: The acid present in the sample reacts with base and convert into corresponding salt form. The completion of the neutralization can be detected with the help of acid-base indicator. The appearance of faint pink colour by the phenolphthalein indicates the end point.

$$\underset{\text{Acid}}{\text{R-COOH}} + \text{KOH} \longrightarrow \text{R-COOK} + H_2O$$

Procedure

Chemicals required: Fat (or oil), Potassium hydroxide solution (0.1 M), Ethanol-ether mixture, Phenolphthalein solution.

Experimental steps

1. Transfer 10 g of the substance being examined (or the quantity specified in the monograph) into a conical flask.
2. Add 50 mL of ethanol (95%) and ether mixture to dissolve the sample. (equal volumes of ethanol (95%) and ether, previously neutralized with 0.1 M potassium hydroxide to phenolphthalein)
3. Heat to dissolve the sample, if necessary.
4. Cool the mixture and add 2 drops of phenolphthalein solution.

5. Titrate against standard potassium hydroxide until the solution remains faintly pink colour after shaking for 30 sec.
6. Note the volume of potassium hydroxide consumed (titre value, **a**) and calculate the acid value from the following formula.

$$\text{Acid value} = \frac{\text{Titre value, a} \times 0.00561 \times 1000 \times \text{Molarity of potassium hydroxide (actual)}}{\text{Molarity of potassium hydroxide (standard)}}$$

Note:

- If the oil has been saturated with carbon dioxide for the purpose of preservation, gently reflux the solution of the oil in ethanol (95%) and ether for 10 min before titration.
- The oil may be freed from the carbon dioxide by exposing it in a shallow-dish in a vacuum desiccator for 24 hr before weighing the sample.

62.2 Determination of Saponification Value

Theory

Saponification value is the number of milligrams of potassium hydroxide necessary to saponify 1 g of the fat sample. The saponification value is a measure of both free and combined acids. The saponification number is a measure of the size of the fat molecule, or more specifically the size or molecular weight of the fatty acids in the fat. A high saponification number indicates the low molecular weight and vice-versa.

Principle: Saponification value can be determined by refluxing a known amount of the sample with excess of standard alcoholic potassium hydroxide solution, and then titrating the unused alkali against a standard acid solution. Since each molecule of triglyceride (fat), regardless of its size, requires three molecules of potassium hydroxide to saponify it, it is evident that the saponification number really indicates the number of fat molecules per gram of the fat.

$$\begin{array}{l} H_2C{-}O{-}\overset{O}{\overset{\|}{C}}{-}R \\ \;| \\ HC{-}O{-}\overset{O}{\overset{\|}{C}}{-}R \\ \;| \\ H_2C{-}O{-}\overset{O}{\overset{\|}{C}}{-}R \end{array} + 3\,KOH \longrightarrow \begin{array}{l} H_2C{-}OH \\ \;| \\ HC{-}OH \\ \;| \\ H_2C{-}OH \end{array} + 3\,R{-}COOK$$

Fatty acid ester — Potassium hydroxide — Glycerol — Soap

Procedure

Chemicals required: Fat (or oil), Alcoholic potassium hydroxide solution (0.5 M), Hydrochloric acid (0.5 M), Phenolphthalein solution.

Experimental steps

1. Transfer 2 g of the substance being examined (or the quantity specified in the monograph) into a flask fitted with reflux condenser.
2. Add 25 mL of ethanolic potassium hydroxide (0.5 M) and a little pumice powder.
3. Boil under reflux on a water-bath for 30 min.
4. Add 2 drops of phenolphthalein solution and titrate immediately against standard hydrochloric acid.
5. Note the volume of standard hydrochloric acid consumed (titre value, **a**).
6. Repeat the operation omitting the sample; note the volume of acid consumed (**b**).
7. Calculate the saponification value from the following formula.

$$\text{Saponification value} = \frac{\text{Titre value, b-a} \times 0.02805 \times 1000 \times \text{Molarity of hydrochloric acid (actual)}}{\text{Sample weight} \times \text{Molarity of hydrochloric acid (standard)}}$$

Note:

- If the oil has been saturated with carbon dioxide for the purpose of preservation, gently reflux the solution of the oil in ethanol (95%) and ether for 10 min before titration.
- The oil may be freed from the carbon dioxide by exposing it in a shallow-dish in a vacuum desiccators for 24 hrs before weighing the sample.

62.3 Determination of Ester Value

Principle: The ester value is the number of milligrams of potassium hydroxide required to saponify the esters present in 1 g (1000 mg) of the substance. This can be calculated by using the formula

Ester value = Saponification value – Acid value

Procedure

Chemicals required: Fat or oil, Alcoholic potassium hydroxide solution (0.5 M), Hydrochloric acid (0.5 M), Phenolphthalein solution, Potassium hydroxide solution (0.1 M), Ethanol-ether mixture (equal volumes of ethanol (95%) and ether, previously neutralized with KOH to phenolphthalein).

Saponification value

1. Transfer 2 g of the substance being examined (or the quantity specified in the monograph) into a flask fitted with reflux condenser.
2. Add 25 mL of ethanolic potassium hydroxide (0.5 M) and a little pumice powder.
3. Boil under reflux on a water bath for 30 min.
4. Add 2 drops of phenolphthalein solution and titrate immediately against standard hydrochloric acid.
5. Note the volume of standard hydrochloric acid consumed (titre value, **a**).
6. Repeat the operation omitting the sample; note the volume of acid consumed (**b**).
7. Calculate the saponification value from the following formula.

$$\text{Saponification value} = \frac{\text{Titre value, b-a} \times 0.02805 \times 1000 \times \text{Molarity of hydrochloric acid (actual)}}{\text{Sample weight} \times \text{Molarity of hydrochloric acid (standard)}}$$

Acid value

1. Transfer 10 g of the substance being examined (or the quantity specified in the monograph) into a conical flask.
2. Add 50 mL of ethanol (95%) and ether mixture to dissolve the sample. (equal volumes of ethanol (95%) and ether, previously neutralized with 0.1 M potassium hydroxide to phenolphthalein)
3. Heat to dissolve the sample, if necessary.
4. Cool the mixture and add 2 drops of phenolphthalein solution.
5. Titrate against standard potassium hydroxide until the solution remains faintly pink colour after shaking for 30 sec.
6. Note the volume of potassium hydroxide consumed (Titre value, **a**) and calculate the acid value from the following formula.

$$\text{Acid value} = \frac{\text{Titre value, a} \times 0.00561 \times 1000 \times \text{Molarity of potassium hydroxide (actual)}}{\text{Molarity of potassium hydroxide (standard)}}$$

62.4 Determination of Peroxide Value

Theory

The autoxidation of lipids is major cause of their deterioration and hydroperoxides formed by the reaction between oxygen and unsaturated fatty acid is the primary product of this reaction. The peroxide concentration usually expressed as peroxide value, gives early measure of lipid oxidation. Peroxide value is the number of milli equivalents of active oxygen that expresses the amount of peroxide contained in 1000 g of the sample.

Principle: Peroxide value can be determined based on iodometric principles. The peroxide present in the sample oxidizes potassium iodide under acidic condition and liberates iodine. The liberated iodine can be titrated against standard sodium thiosulphate using starch mucilage as an indicator.

Procedure

Chemical Required: Fat or oil, Glacial acetic acid, Chloroform, Saturated potassium iodide solution, Sodium thiosulphate (0.01 M), Starch solution.

Experimental steps

1. Transfer 5 g of the substance being examined (or the quantity specified in the monograph) into a glass stoppered conical flask.
2. Add 30 mL of a mixture of 3 volumes of glacial acetic acid (18 mL) and 2 volumes of chloroform (12 mL).
3. Swirl to dissolve the contents and add 0.5 mL of saturated potassium iodide solution.
4. Allow to stand for 10 min, with occasional shaking and add 30 mL of water.
5. Titrate gradually, with continuous and vigorous shaking with standard sodium thiosulphate until the yellow colour becomes faint.
6. Add 0.5 mL of starch solution and continue the titration, shaking vigorously until the blue colour disappears (**a**).
7. Repeat the operation omitting the sample, note the volume of sodium thiosulphate consumed (**b**).
8. Calculate the peroxide value from the expression.

$$\text{Peroxide value} = \frac{10\,(a-b) \times \text{Molarity of sodium thiosulphate (actual)}}{\text{Sample weight} \times \text{Molarity of sodium thiosulphate (standard)}}$$

62.5 Determination of Iodine Value

Theory

Iodine value of a fat or oil may be regarded as a measure of its degree of unsaturation and gives an idea about its drying character. It also helps in finding the adulteration in a fat or oil and judging its suitability for making soap.

Iodine value of

Non-drying oils (e.g., ground nut oil, mustard oil)	=	85-105
Semi drying oils (e.g., cotton oil, seed oil, sesame oil)	=	105-120
Drying oils (e.g., linseed oil, soyabean oil)	=	$\geq$120

Principle: The iodine value is the number of grams of iodine taken up by 100 g of fat or oil. Iodine reacts very slow, hence iodine monochloride or bromine in pyridine is useful in the determination. The known excess of iodine monochloride reacts with the unsaturated component of oil (or fat) and produces addition product. The unreacted iodine can be determined by titrating against standard sodium thiosulphate using starch mucilage as an indicator. The disappearance of blue colour indicates the endpoint. The difference between the initial volume added and the volume of iodine detected is basis for the calculations.

Procedure

Chemicals Required: Fat or oil, Carbon tetrachloride, Iodine monochloride, Potassium iodide solution, Sodium thiosulphate (0.01 M), Starch solution.

Experimental steps

Iodine monochloride method or Wijs method:

1. Transfer accurately weighed quantity of the substance being examined (the quantity specified in the monograph) into a 500 mL glass stoppered conical flask.
2. Add 10 mL of carbon tetrachloride and 20 mL of iodine monochloride solution, insert the stopper and allow to stand in the dark at a temperature between 15 °C to 25 °C for 30 min.
3. Place 15 mL of potassium iodide solution in the cup top, carefully remove the stopper, rinse the stopper and the sides of the flask with 100 mL water.
4. Shake and titrate with 0.1 M sodium thiosulphate until the yellow colour becomes faint.
5. Add 0.5 mL of starch solution and continue the titration, shaking vigorously until the blue colour disappears (**a**).
6. Repeat the operation omitting the sample, note the volume of sodium thiosulphate consumed (**b**).
7. Calculate the iodine value from the expression.

$$\text{Iodine value} = \frac{\text{Titre value, a-b} \times 0.0127 \times 100 \times \text{Molarity of sodium thiosulphate (actual)}}{\text{Sample weight} \times \text{Molarity of sodium thiosulphate (standard)}}$$

a = Volume of 0.1 M sodium thiosulphate consumed by the sample (in mL)

b = Volume of 0.1 M sodium thiosulphate consumed by blank (in mL)

Preparation of Iodine Monochloride Solution: Dissolve iodine trichloride (8 g) in about 200 mL of glacial acetic acid and dissolve iodine (9 g) in carbon tetrachloride (300 mL). Mix the two solutions and adjust to 1000 ml with glacial acetic acid. This operation should be carried out in fume cup-board. Iodine monobromine in glacial acetic acid, may be used in place of Iodine monochloride.

Preparation of 0.1 M sodium thiosulphate: Dissolve about 25 g of sodium thiosulphate in freshly boiled and cooled water and make the volume up to 1000 ml. Keep the solution aside and filter if necessary (if cloudy).

62.6 Determination of Alcohol Number

Principle: Alcohol number represents the number of milliliters of ethanol at 15 °C obtained from 10 mL of tincture or alcohol containing preparations.

Procedure

Chemicals Required: Sample, Alkaline phenolphthalein, Sodium hydroxide, Potassium carbonate.

Experimental steps

Pretreatment

For the following samples pretreatment is necessary

1. ***Glycerin:*** Add sufficient water to the sample.
2. ***Iodine:*** Decolourize with zinc powder.
3. ***Volatile substances (Chloroform, ether, camphor):***
    - Mix 10 mL of the sample with 10 mL of saturated sodium chloride present in separating funnel.
    - Add 10 mL of petroleum ether, shake and collect the aqueous layer.
    - Extract the organic layer with two 5 mL volumes of saturated sodium chloride.
    - Combine the aqueous layers and distilled.
4. Convert volatile acids slight alkaline by adding sodium hydroxide.
5. ***Others:*** Render them slightly acidic with dilute acid.

Amount of distillate after pre-treatment

Ethanol content (vol %)	Distillate (mL)
> 80%	13
80-70	12
70-60	11
60-50	10
50-40	9
40-30	8
< 30	7

Procedure:

1. Transfer 10 mL of sample to the distillation flask and maintain the temperature at 15 ± 2 °C.
2. Add 5 mL of water and add boiling chips.
3. Distill alcohol carefully into the glass stopper volumetric cylinder.
4. To the distillate add potassium carbonate (5 g), alkaline phenolphthalein solution (2 drops) and shake vigorously.
   - *If the aqueous layer shows no white turbidity agitate the distillate with additional potassium carbonate.*
   - *If there is no clear boundary surface between these two layers add few drops of water and shake vigourously.*
5. Allow it to stand in water bath for 30 min and maintain the temperature at 15 ± 2 °C.
6. Read the volume of upper reddish ethanol layer in mL.
7. The volume measured indicates the alcohol number.

Note: Render the sample acidic with phosphoric acid or sulphuric acid to prevent bumping during distillation.

KEY POINTS

- Acid value (AV), an indicator of vegetable oil quality, which expresses the milligrams of potassium hydroxide necessary to neutralize the free acids present in 1 g of the sample.
- Saponification value is the number of milligrams of potassium hydroxide necessary to neutralize the free acids and to saponify the esters present in 1 g of the substance.
- Peroxide value is the number of milli equivalents of active oxygen that expresses the amount of peroxide contained in 1000 g of the sample.
- Iodine value of a fat or oil may be regarded as a measure of its degree of unsaturation and gives an idea about its drying character.
- Alcohol number represents the number of milliliters of ethanol at 15 °C obtained from 10 ml of tincture or alcohol containing preparations.

63

Quantitative Determination of Natural Products

63.1 Estimation of Quinine Sulphate

Theory

Quinine sulfate is a natural alkaloid present in cinchona bark (*Cinchona officinalis* L) has anti-malarial property. It also has mild antipyretic, analgesic and anti-inflammatory potential. Quinine nucleus results by the fusion of quinoline and the bicyclic quinuclidine rings.

Principle: Quinine sulphate is a weak base. The weakly acidic and weakly basic drugs does not produce sharp endpoint, hence aqueous acid base titration is not suitable. Non-aqueous titration is suitable for the weakly acidic (pKa < 7) and weakly basic (pKa > 7) drugs. Therefore, this base can be titrated against perchloric acid using crystal violet as indicator.

HO, H_3CO, N, N, CH_2, $.H_2SO_4$

Quinine sulphate

$\xrightarrow[-H_2SO_4]{HClO_4}$

HO, H_3CO, N, N, CH_2, $.HClO_4$

Quinine perchlorate

Procedure

Requirements: Quinine sulphate powder, Perchloric acid (0.1 M), Chloroform, Glacial acetic acid, Crystal violet solution.

Experimental steps

1. Accurately weigh about 0.2 g of the substance or the quantity specified in the monograph into a 250 mL flask.
2. Add 10 mL of chloroform and 20 mL of acetic anhydride and shake well.
3. Titrate the contents of the flask with 0.1 M perchloric acid using crystal violet as indicator.
4. Each mL of 0.1 M perchloric acid = 0.0249 g of $C_{40}H_{50}N_4O_8S$.

Preparation of 0.1 M perchloric acid: Slowly add perchloric acid (72%, 85 mL) to glacial acetic acid (900 mL) with continuous stirring. Add acetic anhydride (30 mL) to the above mixer, stir and adjust the volume to 1000 mL with glacial acetic acid. Allow the solution stand for 24 hrs.

Standardization of 0.1 M perchloric acid:

1. Weigh accurately about 0.5 g of the potassium hydrogen phthalate into a flask.
2. Attach reflux condenser (fitted with drying tube) and add glacial acetic acid (25 mL).
3. Warm until the solution is dissolved.
4. Cool and titrate with 0.1 M perchloric acid using crystal violet as indicator till the green colour persists at least for 30 sec.
5. Perform blank titration omitting the sample.
   Each mL of 0.1 M $HClO_4$ = 0.2041 g of potassium hydrogen phthalate

$$\text{Molarity of perchloric acid} = \frac{\text{Weight of potassium hydrogen phthalate}}{\text{Volume of perchloric acid consumed} \times 0.2041}$$

63.2 Estimation of Ascorbic Acid

Theory

Ascorbic acid (vitamin C) is an essential antioxidant plays essential role in the protection of body from infections and diseases. It is not synthesized in the body, hence should be supplied through diet.

Principle: The amount of ascorbic acid can be determined by redox-titration using iodine (iodimetric titration). Ascorbic acid reduces iodine into iodide and gets oxidized to dehydroascorbic acid. Iodine reduction to iodide will continue as long as ascorbic acid is present. The excess of iodine can be detected by the reaction with starch indicator, which gives blue colour with iodine. This method is applicable for ascorbic acid present in fruits, food and pharmaceutical formulations.

Ascorbic acid (Vitamin C) + I_2 (Iodine) ⇌ Dehydroascorbic acid + $2I^-$ (Iodide)

Sample preparation: Ascorbic acid is susceptible to oxidation by atmospheric oxygen, hence should be prepared immediately before the titrations. It can be minimized by the addition of small amount of oxalic acid.

- ***Fruits and vegetables:*** Cut into small pieces and grind in a mortar and pestle (blending fruits and vegetables also can be done). Add distilled water and decant the liquid into flask (repeat this operation for several times). Strain the decanted portion through cheese cloth and dilute it with distilled water.
- ***Fresh fruit juice:*** Strain the juice through cheese cloth to remove seeds and pulp (otherwise blocks the pipette).
- ***Packaged fruit juice:*** Strain through cheese cloth, if it contains pulp and seeds.

Procedure:

Requirements: Citrus fruits, Sulphuric acid (1 M), Iodine (0.05 M), Starch paste.

Experimental steps

1. Pipette 20 mL of sample solution into conical flask.
2. Add distilled water (100 mL) and starch paste (1 mL).
3. Titrate the mixture with 0.005 M iodine solution.
4. The appearance of persistent dark blue-black colour due to the starch iodine complex is the end point.
5. Repeat the titration for correction.

Preparation of 0.005 M iodine: Dissolve 2 g of iodate-free potassium iodide in 30 mL of distilled water in a glass-stoppered flask. Add 1.27 g of resublimed iodine to above flask and shake well until iodine dissolves. Make the volume up to 1000 mL and stored in cool and dark place.

Standardization of iodine:

1. Weigh accurately about 0.15 g of arsenic trioxide and dissolve in 20 mL of 1 N sodium hydroxide (warm if necessary).
2. Add 40 mL of water, 2 drops of methyl orange indicator followed by dil. hydrochloric acid until pink colour is obtained.
3. Add 2 g of sodium bicarbonate, dilute with 50 mL water followed by few drops of starch solution and titrate with iodine solution until a permanent blue colour is produced.

$$\text{Molarity of iodine} = \frac{\text{Weight of arsenic trioxide}}{\text{Volume of iodine consumed} \times 0.04946}$$

Note: Any excess of sodium hydroxide added to dissolve arsenic trioxide is neutralised with hydrocloric acid. Iodine may react with NaOH to form sodium hypoiodide (NaOI). Sodium thiosulphate which is recently standardized can be used as an alternative to arsenic trioxide.

KEY POINTS

- Non-aqueous titration is suitable for the weakly acidic (pKa < 7) and weakly basic (pKa > 7) drugs, since weakly acidic and weakly basic drugs does not produce sharp endpoint in acid-base titrations.
- Quinine sulfate is a natural alkaloid present in cinchona bark (Cinchona officinalis L) has anti-malarial property.
- Ascorbic acid (vitamin C) is an antioxidant plays essential role in the protection of body from infections and diseases.

64

Degradation of Natural Products

64.1 Degradation of Trimyristin

Theory

Trimyristin is a glyceryl ester of myristic acid (triglycerides) obtained from the roots and leaves of Myristica fragrans (Family: Myristicaceae). Saponification of trimyristin with potassium hydroxide produces the potassium salt of myristic acid, which on acidification releases a myristic acid.

Principle: Trimyristin on alkaline hydrolysis (excessive potassium hydroxide) liberates myristic acid (potassium myristate) and glycerol. The sodium myristate salt upon acidification with hydrochloric acid precipitates myristic acid. It occurs as white to yellowish grey solid with a melting range of 56 to 57 °C.

$$\begin{array}{l} H_2C-O-\overset{O}{\overset{\|}{C}}-C_{13}H_{17} \\ \;| \\ HC-O-\overset{O}{\overset{\|}{C}}-C_{13}H_{17} \\ \;| \\ H_2C-O-\overset{O}{\overset{\|}{C}}-C_{13}H_{17} \end{array} + KOH \xrightarrow{C_2H_5OH} \begin{array}{l} H_2C-OH \\ HC-OH \\ H_2C-OH \end{array} + 3\,C_{13}H_{17}COOK$$

Trimyristin; Potassium hydroxide; Glycerol; Potassium salt of Myristic acid

$$C_{13}H_{17}COOK + HCl \longrightarrow C_{13}H_{17}COOH + KCl$$

Potassium salt of Myristic acid; Myristic acid

Procedure

Chemicals Required: Trimyristin, Ethanol (95%), Potassium hydroxide/Sodium hydroxide, Sodium chloride solution (35%), Distilled water.

Experimental steps

1. Add the trimyristin (1 g), along with 20 mL of ethanol (95%) and 0.20 g of solid sodium hydroxide to a 100 mL of round bottom flask.
2. Reflux the mixture on a water bath at 85 to 90 °C for 15 min.

3. Cool to room temperature, and then add 20 mL of water, followed by 20 mL of sodium chloride solution (35%).
4. Sodium myristate forms as white voluminous solid (if not place in an ice bath) which is vacuum filtered and washed with 30 mL of sodium chloride solution (35%).
5. Allow product to dry and recrystallize from ethanol.
6. The melting range of pure myristic acid is 56 to 57 °C.

64.2 Degradation of Atropine

Theory

Atropine is an alkaloid obtained from the roots and leaves of *Atropa belladonna* (Family: Solanaceae). It is a racemic mixture of hyoscyamine.

Principle: Atropine is a tropyl ester of tropic acid. The alkaline hydrolysis of atropine releases tropine and tropic acid.

$$\text{Atropine} \xrightarrow{Ba(OH)_2} \text{Tropine} + \text{Tropic acid}$$

$Ba(OH)_2$

Atropine

Tropine

Tropic acid

Procedure

Chemicals Required: Atropine, Barium hydroxide (10%), Chloroform, Distilled water

Experimental steps

1. Transfer atropine (200 mg) into reaction flask (100 mL).
2. Add barium hydroxide (7.5 mL, 10%) to the flask.
3. Boil the mixture for 45 min, maintaining the temperature at 95 °C.
4. Extract the reaction mixture with chloroform (5 mL) three times.
5. Atropine degradation products (tropine and tropic acid) enters chloroform layer.
6. Combine the chloroform extracts and evaporate to dryness.
7. The degradation products can be detected through chemical identification tests.

KEYPOINTS

- Trimyristin is a glyceryl ester of myristic acid (triglycerides) upon saponification with potassium hydroxide produces the potassium salt of myristic acid.
- Atropine is a tropyl ester of tropic acid upon alkaline hydrolysis releases tropine and tropic acid.

www.ingramcontent.com/pod-product-compliance
Ingram Content Group UK Ltd.
Pitfield, Milton Keynes, MK11 3LW, UK
UKHW061533190726
13845UKWH00005B/85

9 789349 562301